M000219373

CREATION OF THE UNIVERSE

SAVE YOURSELF

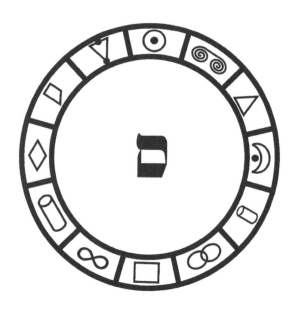

**Arcady
Petrov**

CREATION OF THE UNIVERSE

SAVE YOURSELF

Jelezky publishing, Hamburg 2011

Jelezky publishing, Hamburg
www.jelezky-media.com

Copyright © Original Russian Language Version:
Arcady Petrov, Moscow

**English 1st Edition, july 2011
(1st Edition)**

©2011English Language Version
Dimitri Eletski, Hamburg (Editor)

English Translation: Lingua Communications Translation Services, USA

Whatever we might be doing and wherever we might be going, we were moving toward one goal – to one's inner self, to remembering oneself. People who have lost the memory of their past and their future are akin to children who are ready, day after day, without ever tiring of it, to ride on their favorite carousel.

Something always changes around us – one day the sun is out, the next it rains the leaves appear on the trees and then fall off, first one set of people come along to see how these carefree folks who behave like children whirl on the carousel, and then others come to watch.

We turn around a closed circle, squealing with delight at the speed, forgetting that at some point we were truly able to fly and that our exaggerated excitement is nothing but a vague memory of who we once were.

ISBN: 978-3-943110-08-1

CREATION OF THE UNIVERSE

SAVE YOURSELF

"The most beautiful thing we can experience is the mysterious... He to whom this emotion is a stranger, who can no longer pause to wonder and stand rapt in awe, is as good as dead."

Albert Einstein

All the events depicted in this book didn't happen somewhere on a distant planet. They occurred here, on planet Earth, and involved people who are our contemporaries. Those who will take the time to read this book may perceive it as fiction or as reality, since all the events described here are associated with such an unusual phenomenon as controlled clairvoyance. People who have this ability can soar through their conscience into celestial spheres or dive deep down to the bottom of the ocean. They can travel in time to the distant past and penetrate the secret world of the biological cell...

My story is autobiographical. I have written down what I know and am sharing this knowledge with you in chronological order, presenting it exactly the way I received it, moving from one stage in the Initiation process to the next, leafing through the pages of my life. I was bestowed the right to share with you whatever I find to be essential at this particular point in time.

Humanity has apparently been interconnected with the mysterious world of unfathomable and rationally inexplicable phenomena throughout its entire history. There were always a select few who possessed a rare gift: the ability to foretell the future, control atmospheric events, cure severe diseases, and so on. Even though this type of knowledge and corresponding skills were carefully concealed, there is, nevertheless, sufficiently abundant literature about such phenomena.

Regretfully, most of these books will be of little value to the reader who will definitely learn about many bizarre things and become familiar with a dozen or so new terms but that is probably all. Knowledge of the secret and the hidden continues to be passed on from teacher to student over many years, or through some unknown channel, unexplainable even to the clairvoyants themselves.

Meanwhile, the spiritual processes taking place in the world today are of global, even cosmic proportions. It is not accidental that during the past century our knowledge of man's nature, his world and the purpose of his existence within the Universe has changed dramatically. Everybody is talking about the advent of the Age of Aquarius, about the new era... At the turn of a millennium, people tend to be filled with mystical expectations. Just as Virgil, the great Roman poet, foretold the coming of Jesus Christ ("The age renews itself/ Justice returns, and man's primeval time,/And a new progeny descends from heaven," – "Eclogues." 4.), present-day prophets are now predicting His second coming.

This indicates that it is time for people at large to have access to the secret teachings, which were unattainable to them in the past. Of course, transmitting esoteric knowledge and skills will not take place instantaneously. Just as any other process, it will require some time for humanity to master this new knowledge and set of skills. But it is important to make a note of the fact that many of the Initiated have been granted permission from the higher authority to reveal their sacred knowledge.

I am asking those of you who are atheists to keep an open mind and not perceive everything you find in this book as sheer fantasy. Those of you who are believers, I am asking not to view its contents as heresy. Let me reiterate: my story is autobiographical; the people in this book are real, and many of them are alive and well today, when you are reading these lines. I have tried to write predominantly about my personal experience and the meaning of esotericism, instead of focusing on its methods or technical aspects.

How and for what purpose do a select few receive this sacred knowledge? What level of spirituality is required for a person to be Initiated? How should we live our lives, and what is the meaning of life? If my book causes the reader to ponder these questions, if he decides to work on overcoming his own limitations in order to reach another level of being – I will consider my goal accomplished. Each and every one of us has his own path to God, and each will serve Him in his own way. I am simply trying to help those who aren't afraid of the extreme cold of outer space or the heavenly fire of mysticism to find the right direction. I am doing my best to help those who are prepared to serve in spheres about which they presently have no idea.

"Many are called, but few are chosen" (Matthews, 20:16). Some people are unable to traverse this road. If you aren't prepared for the difficult road ahead, if you are too tired and fainthearted or overwhelmed by worldly concerns it would be better if you didn't even try. There are plenty of schools and teachers in the world that are ready to offer their students elementary training in extrasensory perception for daily use. Perhaps, it would be advisable for most people to limit themselves to such training. Whatever the case may be, it is essential to know already today that a wonderful and magical world of the unknowable exists out there.

This book is written in a somewhat unusual style. That which appears to be unreal is intertwined in it with reality. Paradoxically, many of you will perceive what is fantastic as real and what is real as imaginary. You are given the opportunity to choose, among the two suggested roads, the one which will help you find your own unique path. Please accept my apology for not providing comments to some of the important facts that I present and for the absence of explanations to certain pivotal events – I expect you to hear the voice of truth within you without my help.

I wrote about my own personal experiences and the people around me who have helped me on my life's journey. This book is about events that occurred in the past-present and future-current events. Time coordinates exist in space precisely in this order, because the present always takes place along the continuous interactive flow between the past and future. For the word "Now" to sound, somebody had to utter it in the Past and hear it in the Future.

At the end of the second millennium many people, some with trepidation, others with hope, awaited the first year of the new millennium and the events prophesied in the Holy Scriptures –Armageddon, Apocalypses or the coming of the Golden Age. After they took a good look around them, some gave a sigh of relief: nothing at all happened; others were disappointed: "Is everything going to stay the same?" They must have forgotten that in the beginning was the WORD. Which of you has the sharp vision to see what God has done or whose hearing is so perfect that he can hear the judgments He pronounced?

Yes, of course, later, when the will of the Creator puts the celestial spheres into motion, it will be seen and it will be heard. All the more so, since the motion has already begun. And the End of Times for those who are accustomed to act as irresponsible middlemen between the Creator and His creation, between the Creator and that which He created, has actually come.

After reading this book, you will understand why immortal Man, succumbing to his fate, was banished by his Father. You will know the meaning of original sin, and what awaits Man and the human race in the secret realms, which are opening up before them today. The trilogy I have written – "Save Yourself," "Save the World Within You," and "Save the World Around You" – will be the first in the third millennium to lead you into a new world, to new knowledge. These books will guide you from death to immortality, from fear and passive anticipation to a recollection of yourself and your place in the eternal Cosmos, which has long been

10

waiting, with endless love and patience, for your awakening.

It took me quite a while to decide what the title of my book should be. In the thousands of years of the existence of writing, numerous people have tried, on multiple occasions, to figure out their place and purpose in this world and their connections to other worlds. Many have attempted to write the book of their destiny or at least to be able to read it. That is why no matter what title I chose, I couldn't come up with anything original – someone had already used it before! But I didn't want to give my book a title somebody had thought of before me because I was convinced that so far no one else had described an experience identical to mine. I finally chose the title which those reading my book already know. It makes me extremely happy that through the process of ultimate initiation I had the opportunity to acquire extraordinary knowledge, which is of tremendous significance for all those presently living on Earth, and that I was able to transfer this knowledge onto the fresh page of the new millennium.

Chapter 1

In June of 1996, I was admitted to the hospital. Severe kidney failure brought me to the Moscow Medical and Sanatorium Association located not far from the Circle Highway, near the Mitino district. My morale was at an all time low. This illness was like a steam-roller, its crushing force destroying my life without mercy, breaking my plans and forcing me to go back on my commitments and promises.

Only a few months prior to my hospitalization, I was appointed Director of "Khudozhestvennaya Literatura"* Publishing House. Not that long before, this was one of the largest publishers in the world, but it was in a sorry state for a number of years now, faced with multibillion debts (in rubles, – *Transl. Note*) and relying on a disorganized staff, demoralized by constant layoffs. Equipment and supplies were virtually non-existent. To give you just one example, the former director merged all computer support into a small-size enterprise, which was at some point dissolved, with all the equipment and the director himself vanishing into thin air. A number of distinguished Russian writers wrote to President Yeltsin about this shocking situation at the publishers. They urged the government to intervene and put an end to the plundering of the company, comparing the cultural significance of the "Khudozhestvennaya Literatura" to that of the Bolshoi and the Moscow Tretyakov gallery. Some of them compared its ruin to the sinking of "Titanic."

The generated alarm signal was transmitted to the media and caught up by numerous articles in major newspapers and in collective petitions signed by prominent cultural personalities and public figures. Some of those concerned felt that any local efforts to revive the publishing company were doomed and futile, whereas others requested additional government funding to delay its final demise. As usual, the government could not spare any money, but it responded in its customary fashion by demanding better accountability and performance from top management. Replacing company leadership would not require major investments and had the appearance of effective intervention in the public eye. Actually, the future director was also promised a certain amount of financial assistance alongside moral support.

It was at this point that I was contacted by Boris Andreyevich Mozhayev, a man for whom I had the utmost respect. This famous writer who was at the time in charge of Russia's Federal Publishing Program suggested that I should try out for the top administrative position at the publishing house. This suggestion came as a total surprise. I already had my own publishing company "Kultura"** in Pushkin, a small town not far from Moscow. I was both its founder and general director. Things were going well, and I was quite optimistic about the future. What else could I ask for?

I was aware from reports in the media of the publishers' stifling debt and the array of pending criminal charges against it. "Khudozhestvennaya Literatura" hadn't published a single book for almost an entire year. Experienced editors who were fluent in several languages subsisted on a meager monthly salary of 146 thousand rubles (146 rubles after the reform). Since the publishing house was unable to pay its bills, providers threatened to cut off their electricity, heat and phone services. The prospect of declaring bankruptcy, with plans to auction the company building, became a reality, even a welcome one to some people. The very same

* "Khudozhestvennaya Literatura" – the name of the publishing house means "fiction" in Russian.
** "Kultura" – the name of the publishing house means "culture" in Russian.

individuals who contributed to the publishers' financial ruin were now eager to buy the building on Basmannaya Street, which was occupied by the company, and move in not as guests or tenants but as legitimate owners.

I was also reluctant to accept the position of director because just a month before the offer, in December of the previous year, I was elected Vice-President of the Humanities Department at the International Informatization Academy. I realized how hard it would be to hold these two responsible positions. True, I was tortured by doubts but I was also tempted by the prospect of working for what used to be the most well-known publishing house in Russia... Besides, how could I let down Boris Andreyevich who had such high hopes for me?

Boris Andreyevich and I met a long time ago, and in the years of our friendship I not only grew to admire this man, his character and his perseverance, but I also tried to emulate him, in part consciously, mostly on some unconscious level I couldn't explain. I realized that the stalwart protagonist of his novel "Alive!" Fyodor Kuzkin – the "statistical average" – was the essence of the author himself. His own life was not a bed of roses. Yet though he went through hard times and faced trials of many kinds, he responded with unrelenting resolve. He would shake off his problems: "Alive!" – isn't it a pleasant surprise? And he would proceed with his work.

As any true artist, he understood that his destiny was a path to Golgotha. Perhaps this destiny was not as significant, historically speaking, and not so carefully rehearsed by the powers that be as the path of Solzhenitsyn, whom he courageously defended, but it was no less thorny on a personal level. Unlike Alexander Isayevich Solzhenitsyn, who could never forget about his historical significance, Boris Mozhayev carried his cross with a smile, his eyes squinting merrily at the communist apparatchiks

14

following him. As many of his contemporaries, he was painfully aware of the government's disdain for the individual. He realized that for the Soviet bureaucrat a human being was not the most precious entity in creation, but only a small, insignificant stone to be used in the building of a utopia. The Soviet system, while brazenly and with impunity invading our souls, could not figure out that the main threat to its existence came from those seemingly agreeable men and women who were carefully preserving the core of the Russian character. They were the simple people whom Mozhayev portrayed with such warmth.

He wrote that a new society couldn't be built on blood, through crimes and violence. He called for harmony in spiritual life. He observed with regret how in place of the old system a new one – equally heartless and with the same sovereign indifference to man – was being created over the past few years. But by that time Mozhayev had already published his novels, and his long and short stories, which gave those readers, who had lost direction confronted with the destructive processes of Russian reality, some clues as to the purpose and meaning of their lives.

How could I say "no" to the request of such a person? Besides, his faith in me and his positive comments about the dynamic life of the "Kultura" publishing company were extremely flattering. So I finally accepted the offer.

The State Publishing Committee held a contest to fill the open position of director at the "Khudozhestvennaya Literatura" Publishing House, which I won. So they now had a person in charge, the appropriate procedure was followed – they went through the motions and could now get the real problems of the publishing company off their minds. I believe that these urgent issues would have been addressed if Mozhayev hadn't fallen gravely ill. My appointment as director was approved in January, and on

March 2, Boris Andreyevich passed away.

Maybe it was the ensuing sense of abandonment that escalated my ill-ness. Despite my mature age, there were many things I failed to recognize or comprehend at the time. "What is life and what is death?" I didn't have the answer. During the funeral, over my teacher's grave, I solemnly pro-mised to do everything in my power to rescue the publishing house from total ruin. Just three months later, when we only started to resolve some of the most urgent problems, both my kidneys suddenly stopped working. The situation was so dire that doctors recommended removing the left kidney. Despair and utter hopelessness didn't leave me for a moment: the knowledge that no effort of will could change my plight was unbearable.

During one of those hapless days something clicked deep inside me like a switch. I suddenly began to visualize, with utmost clarity, distant events that took place thousands of years before but were so closely and with such accuracy interconnected in their essence with our times, with my personal situation that this couldn't, most likely, be coincidental.

No, these weren't dreams, they were visions. Besides, the brightness of these images so far surpassed the human capabilities of our regular visi-on that this in itself produced a stunning effect. I instantly forgot about my condition and agitatedly began to jot down the things which the strange screen of my inner vision was presenting to my consciousness.

Two years later these notes were assembled into my novel "Eldibor" (M., "Bibliosfera," 1999). An average reader will see this novel not as sci-ence fiction but as something called fantasy in the West. It doesn't provide an explanation or prediction of some scientific innovation like Jules Vern does, but is more likely perceived as a didactic fairytale, such as those written by Ray Bradbury, for example. However, I saw this "fairytale"

16

with my own eyes! It is impossible for these remarkably vivid visions to have been simply a product of my imagination. After all, imagination is mostly a mental process, not an emotional one. Anyone who finds this intriguing enough might want to read my novel. Consequent events, however, were so closely intertwined with what I uncovered while writing "Eldibor" that I finally realized that my visions were part of my real life. I didn't need to supplement them with figments of my imagination or artificially combine the revelation that emerged from the spiritual world with any kind of fantasy. This revelation was, in fact, part of my real existence, part of my destiny. I simply had no right to give my visions away to some fictional heroes, to phantoms of virtual reality.

It all began during a dream. I felt as though some unknown force suddenly jerked me out of myself and flung me into the darkness. The darkness picked me up, twirling me and carrying me faster and faster along a spiral – was it up or down? – until it finally threw me out onto a hard, rocky surface.

I stood up with difficulty, while my willpower tried to curb the stabbing pain piercing every inch of my body. I looked around me. The place where I was propelled by an unknown force was permeated with flickering light as if coming from a crystal ball. I couldn't see a thing as I was enveloped in dense shreds of swirling fog, floating swiftly beside me, beneath my feet, and anywhere else I tried to look.

All at once I was overcome with impatience and disappointment, and even though these feelings did not have time to become transformed into thought, it seemed as if they were ripped out of me and pointed in the direction of my glance. Growing many times stronger from some incredible power instantly connected to them, they hit the mist with a hard, physically

17

tangible wave, and the fog in front of me swayed, and then began to move and melt away.

I barely had time to spring back, seared by the intense heat of the boundless flames. The entire space around me was aflame, the blaze rising and falling as an orange fog in the scarlet light, ejecting plumage-like shafts of sparks. Twinkling, dissolving, and reviving again inside the curves and splashes of moving plasma, the wavering tongues of fire caused tonic vibrations that combined into a melody of flaming patterns.

Everything ahead of me was a composition of sound and color, raging like the flood of a fiery river during a volcanic eruption, and yet delicate like a cobweb in the autumn forest. Blue, green, yellow, brown, and pink colors interplayed, flowed and fluttered, alternating with blinding flashes of light and shiny black stretches of lava.

It was music of Genesis, which revealed the body of the Universe in this dance of self-revelation. The sounds soared up on the tongues of flame and swooped down, merging in their fall and rise into the quiet murmur of billions of fiery creatures, oblivious to the purpose of their existence, then into the fearsome roar of the frenzied plasma, or the melancholy songs of constellations, overlapping on the intersections of time and space.

The person who was Me and not Me at the same time and who should be referred to as He, made one step back and almost lost his balance an arm's length away from the edge of a giant tornado vortex. Inside its gigantic belly he could hear sounds of sobbing and voices, and get glimpses of vague silhouettes, fragments of dissected reality, blocks of ice and water columns. Intense discharges of lightning pierced the pitch darkness and bolts of thunder momentarily overpowered the roaring of the gaping abyss.

The world had come to an end. It no longer existed. Remaining alone among the obscure and the unknown was the liberated madness known as Chaos.

He made a few cautious steps back, and saw the abyss covering with a blanket of fog. Once again all around him was a hard surface covered with pebbles. This surface extended as far as the physical eye could see, almost into infinity. He intuitively sensed that if he ventured to walk across these stones through the uneven twilight, ignoring the desolate picture before him, he would need more than an eternity to reach the edge of this dull monotony, because the rocky plateau was made out of eternity.

He turned around. The fog behind him did not clear yet but it receded slightly, revealing the same uneven stones and the level surface of the plateau. The horror of being stuck in this monotonous infinity proved stronger than his fear and it compelled him to plunge into the swirling waves of the retreating fog, until they swallowed him completely.

Now he understood that he had to be very cautious: the world around him was extremely responsive to any movement of his soul, to every wish he had, to all the powers hidden deep down inside his being. The fog was dangerous. It could bring the bottomless abyss or the swelling swamp right under his feet at any moment. There was still the possibility of a choice, which would not be possible if he disappeared. The person who absorbed my Ego practically knew this for a fact, because he had been on this plateau many times before, since that place was the starting point of his journey, the end of which was not known to him.

Feeling the ground with his foot, he carefully began to move ahead, even though it made no sense to try and guess the right direction in what was all around him. Space and time in this world took on different dimensions, which could not be evaluated with the help of traditional geometric or physical concepts. In this world moving ahead meant walking along invisible coordinates of time, twisted in tight spiral-shaped cords, into some alternate reality, to which he was unconsciously drawn all the while.

He was not in a hurry and felt the path with his foot before shifting the weight of his body forward, which is why he barely made any progress. But the wanderer was not concerned about the distance he had to cover. He knew, thanks to some deeply buried original knowledge, which in this space between the two worlds could best be described as "intuition" that the determining factor in his journey was not distance but direction. One false step and he would vanish in the endless expanses of the Universe. Therefore, before taking another step, he had to listen attentively to the noises and sounds penetrating his brain, and trust the urging of some of them while rejecting the others.

Suddenly, he felt something moving underneath his foot. That something came alive and started ripping itself out of the stone with a hoarse roaring. He had no idea what it was but could guess that it was huge and threatening. Retreating in fear was as dangerous in this situation as moving rashly forward. The wanderer ordered his brain to release one of the most active regulators of neural excitation – acetylcholine – into his bloodstream to lower his blood pressure and slow down his heart rate. He didn't permit even an ounce of fear to enter his heart, inhibiting the first symptoms of adrenalin rush by taking control of his mind.

The ability to control his body's internal processes by his willpower saved his life. The creature rising from the stone calmed down and grew quiet, once again merging with the motionless stone surface, which extended into the outside world but emerged from the inner world. The wanderer no longer belonged to either of the two worlds.

He had to decide which voice he should trust: the voice of fear or that of intuition. Danger lay ahead of him but it was danger that could be

20

tamed by his willpower, which he had successfully done at least once al-
ready. The unknown was awaiting him in every other direction. There was
no way he could predict whether this unknown was going to be supportive
or hostile.

It was unfortunate that the voices in his head were too unclear and
numerous for him to understand. But one of them suddenly seemed fami-
liar. It was coming from the place that almost swallowed him and which
was now in front of him. The wanderer made his choice. He stepped on the
stone that came to life and dashed into the fog, disregarding his former
caution. The surface under his feet started shifting again but not to such
an extent that this could knock him over – it was more like a minor earth-
quake measuring 3-4 on the Richter scale.

He clearly couldn't delay even for a moment now. Mustering all his
strength, but doing his best to keep his inner calm, he rushed into the unk-
nown across the sporadically quivering stone, which was trying to take
the shape of something different. He ran into the unknown through the
fog of many universes, times and spaces: he ran somewhere ... forward or
backward, up or down, past or future.

After a few more large jumps he finally saw the one who was summo-
ning him. The ghost-like figure of a man wearing a ragged, blood-splatte-
red tunic became somewhat visible through the shreds of fog. His neck was
twisted unnaturally, probably as the result of an injury. His long tangled
hair and disheveled beard were shaking from an uncontrollable tick but
his eyes, ablaze with hatred, stared unblinkingly at the stranger.

– Stay exactly where you are! – The all-consuming hatred in the voice
of the one who stood in the wanderer's way and his halting gesture forced
him to obey the command, even though the stones underneath continued to
tremble as if they were alive. Suddenly the half human-half phantom made

21

a convulsive movement, crossing out the space with some special sign, and everything around began to seethe and churn. The wanderer could hear the powerful flutter of giant wings right near his face.

Automatically, without thinking, as if the knowledge that propelled him into action was stored within him at the level if instinct, he instructed the shadow of his body to move into the light and become transparent. A moment later the claws of the flying monster slit through him without causing any harm.

— How could you manage to do that? — the half ghost asked in a tensely hoarse, rasping voice. — Have you created Yidam within the Bardo spaces?

— Never give what is holy to dogs, so they don't throw it into manure. Don't cast pearls before swine, — the wanderer responded evasively with esoteric symbolism and inquired solemnly, — Who are you, and why did you stand in my way?

— Who am I? — the man in the tattered robe laughed in his hoarse, rasping voice. — That you of all people should be asking me, who I am? You!

His loud cry cleared the fog, and the wanderer was better able to make out the features of his face. It looked somewhat unreal and indistinct as if hastily put together out of the muddy shreds of fog swirling around them. His eyes, however, were real and brimming with life and power.

— What did I do to you? — the wanderer asked again.

— Good Lord, it's always the same thing! — the one who stood in his way answered with a note of bitter sarcasm, and his oddly crooked, ugly neck began to shake back and forth, while his face twitched violently. — You don't remember, you don't know, do you? What joy — to forget everything. But I am denied such happiness…

He raised his hand again and made some kind of sign. A dull, hypnotic pain pierced the wanderer's brain, and his body became heavy as if filled with lead. He felt that some foreign will had entered him, and was trying to tear asunder and rip apart his brain cells. He had to suppress his anger and discover the balance between irritation and action in his soul, to build an impenetrable wall of calm, and attempt to oust the hostile foreign power, which was too dangerous in this world of dreams, from his inner being.

But this time he seemed to be too late. Accelerating their movement, centrifugal forces had drawn the holograms of life, which were strung on protein strings binding brain neurons, into their dangerous vortex. This strengthened the unchangeable uncertainty of reality and turned the potential for a new condition away from the Inner Potential.

Making one last desperate effort, he retained in his disintegrating mind the thought that came from within his own deep essence: "It is necessary to make two as one, internal as external and the other way around; up as down and down as up; man and woman as one so that man is no longer man and woman is no longer woman; to make an eye instead of an eye and an arm instead of an arm; a leg instead of a leg and an image instead of an image, – then the light from within will show Yidam the way."

The wanderer had the time to show his inner agreement with this conviction, the source of which he didn't know, and the appearing reality fell apart. It was as if the powerful force of his will transported him from death into birth, into a world where the thought seeks after the flesh for its embodiment.

He was blinded by the brilliant vitality of colors radiating compassion and love. Everything around him was filled with a desire to help and protect – all the interplay of light and sound, and the goodwill which permeated the entire space were moving toward him, responding to his prayer and ready to quell his fear. In the fraction of a second, he was able to restore the centrifugal forces of his personal Potential and began to create a new Manifest Reality.

The eyebrows of his mysterious enemy, who gloatingly observed the disintegration of the wanderer's physical body, shot up in surprise when he saw how from the chaotic flickering of energies separated by some magical power, strange entities suddenly emerged, which hovered above them in a clearly defined geometric rectangle. Among these entities was a three-headed dragon adorned with bejeweled crowns, two large spheres – a red and an orange one, and the All Seeing Eye. The dragon looked disapprovingly at the man in a tattered tunic and turned away. A straight beam of blue light shot out from the mouth of his middle head and struck the spot where wanderer had been standing just a moment ago. Similar beams were projected by the spheres and the All Seeing Eye. These four beams then formed an inverted pyramid, the tip of which was pressed against the chaotic splashes of dying energy. Suddenly, in the intersection of beams there emerged a strange silhouette of a two-headed creature. One head was that of a woman and the other that of a man. The creature's rock hard muscles radiated strength unknown on Earth.

This was a god called the First in the Clan. He stretched as if to check the reliability of his new body and glared at the one who was the cause behind his sudden transmutations.

The dragon, the spheres and the Eye had shrunk and integrated into this newly materialized body.

– I should've foreseen it! – the man with the crooked neck cried out, addressing his revived adversary. – The Dragon, the Sun, Jupiter and the All Seeing Eye – with such patronage you can afford to be fearless. Maybe I am not as powerful as you are, – he continued bitterly, – but I have hatred which you don't. I can wait thousands and thousands of years for you to make a mistake.

The tone of voice in which these words were uttered and the look on the face of the man in the tattered tunic once again seemed somewhat familiar to the wanderer who was transformed into god. A vague memory stirred in his mind.

– You must've learned a great deal if you were able to pass through this cursed spot alive, – the man's hoarse voice sounded bitter and awed at the same time. – But it would've been far better if you vanished here, – he bellowed with a flash of renewed anger, – because I can devise an even better scheme, and then your soul will experience the same suffering mine does.

Rage and hatred distorted the face of the one who stood in his way to such a degree that one wondered what stopped the man from attacking god. Just in case, god prepared "to rear up" the space in front of him, though he was well aware of the danger it might pose. But just as suddenly his fit of rage subsided, and the strange adversary calmed down – only his eyes were still burning with hate.

– Why did you attack me? – asked god.

– I'll explain, I'll tell you since you're asking. Because of you I've been roaming around in the world of Dreams for nearly two thousand years with one single goal and one single thought – to avenge my suffering. I will await you for eternity and guide you to the most deadly places. The spot where you are now standing has seen much bloodshed. Many conceited magicians have found their graves here. This space knows the taste of blood and it craves for more. If it weren't for your accursed skill, which, I must admit, you have mastered quite admirably, your journey would've been cut short right here, and I would've taken possession of your earthly body, using resonance waves to carry me back. But we still have time – you and I... Wherever you may be going, you won't be able to change

anything out there, and all your suffering will be in vain. Oh, my hatred for you is such an intolerably heavy burden to carry!"

— Still, I can't understand why you hate me so much? — god said with genuine regret. — Don't get in my way anymore. I must find my path.

— Go ahead, go, — said the one who stood in his way, and the creature's lips twitched, baring his teeth in a frightening grimace. — Staying here any longer would be a waste of time. But remember, apart from magical skill and high patronage, there is something called luck, and don't expect luck to always be on your side.

He suddenly made a step forward, and his face, contorted into a fierce scowl, moved closer to god's face.

— Remember, I'll always be waiting for you. I'll never forget this, — and he pointed his finger at the ugly, rugged scar running across the nape of his neck, where it was bent sideways. — I will never forget it, trust me.

And with these words he vanished into thin air, as if he never even was there. This man, who had summoned the wanderer from the darkness, dissolved without a trace among its murky shadows.

God stood, lost in reverie, for a moment, and then he took off again, as if propelled by some outside force. His mind was filled with a vague expectation of imminent changes.

All of a sudden, the fog disappeared, clearing both in front and behind him. The hard endless surface of the plateau, strewn with small fragments of stone, was also gone. The sun was shining bright, and the sky was blue. God was standing on a mountain top, with other mountains dressed in lush vegetation all around. The splashing of sea waves could be heard from far away. Streams and waterfalls were running down the steep slopes toward the sea across a narrow valley. Never on earth had he seen such unbelievable beauty, and yet this place was somehow familiar. It was as

26

though he had been to these mountains before... An indefinite feeling that
everything happening to him now had occurred before, stirred within him
as a clear anticipation of events about to happen. Once again, he relied
on his willpower to subdue these vague memories before they could ac-
quire the form of a wish and set into motion new space transformations.
This would have been dangerous because he wasn't able yet to assume full
control of his memory.

There was a small, winding path running down the side of the moun-
tain. God stepped on it with confidence and started walking down the slo-
pe. With every step he took he became increasingly convinced that the
space around him had acquired stability of form. It seemed as though
these forms had been extracted from the very depths of his being, which
he couldn't entirely remember or fully comprehend and which were hi-
ding within him as a vague perception of some hidden mystery. He strode
ahead at a rhythmic pace, abandoning doubt, and positive that he had
finally found his own way, regardless of what his destination might bring
him: death or immortality. Inspired by his thoughts, god failed to notice
the dramatic changes in his appearance. His two heads once again beca-
me one. His short hair had grown so long that it now almost reached his
shoulders. A stubble beard covered his chin, his nose straightened out and
became more pointed, and his eyes sunk deep in their sockets as though
he had suffered from insomnia for many days. His whole body shrank
and withered, acquiring the kind of unreal lightness he never experienced
before. His clothes were also different. He was now wearing a long robe
out of some coarse fabric, with a dark, dust-coated cloth draped over one
shoulder and belted around the waist. He had sandals on his feet, suppor-
ted by leather laces strapped around the ankles, and his head was covered
with a white linen scarf.

In his new disguise, god walked through groves of olive trees, the chirping of birds, and the fading rays of the setting sun. He could hear rustling noises in the thicket and the trees groaning lightly in the wind. These sounds merged together into a long, sorrowful whisper. His feet finally felt safe and secure on this surface of land, and his skin gratefully accepted the caressing, tender breeze.

He descended further and further, mesmerized by his belief that he had finally found what he was looking for. Everything around him seemed very much like that which he had been seeking for such a long time.

The narrow path suddenly merged with a village road. He passed a sheepfold surrounded with a hedge of buckthorn. There were a few carts nearby, loaded with baskets filled with lentils, beans and onions. Donkeys, calves, sheep and goats crowded together next to the carts, with several men and women around them. None of them noticed him. Half an hour later he saw, far in the distance, the panoramic view of a fortified ancient city, enclosed within thick white walls. Temples and palaces rose in splendor high into the sky. Blocks of dwellings climbed in terraces up the nearby hills. He suddenly recognized this place: he had seen it many times before and just as many times, he forgot it. He recalled his destiny in the land that lay before him.

As if transfixed, he gazed at the vistas unfolding in front of his eyes. His pace became faster and faster until he broke into a run. His uncomfortable sandals hit against the soles of his feet, interfering with the rhythm, but he continued running until he felt the dry, scorching-hot air parch his throat. His strength was waning and his legs buckled under him – they no longer obeyed his command. He now forced himself to move forward to his destination, where death and immortality awaited him, by sheer effort of will. A small pebble spun around beneath his sandal under the weight of his body, and he lost his balance, flailing his arms awkwardly in the air and collapsing on the road.

These were the kind of "pictures" I saw – all this was more like watching a film made by a genius director. At the time I didn't know yet that this retrospective chain of the events from two thousand years before was directly connected not only to my present condition but also my future. The future had not yet arrived, but according to the secret laws of the Universe unknown to us, it had already happened in some other dimension. A "link-up" of my past and future was waiting ahead.

At this point I still continued to perceive all that was happening in traditional notions and parameters. I saw everything occurring in my life as sparks of my creative inspiration. Little did I know that this was a significant sign, a precursor of dramatic changes in my life and destiny! This sign spoke of eternity and infinity in the past and future.

I attempted to analyze this amazing phenomenon with the help of my real-life experience. I played around with any number of traditional theories from the natural sciences and philosophy, trying to "tie up" my visions with something familiar to me, until the name of Carl Gustav Jung confidently emerged from deep down within my memory.

This Swiss psychiatrist, the most famous follower and critic of Sigmund Freud, became the founder of a new school known as analytical or depth psychology. He came closer than anyone else to the understanding that man is not a chance phenomenon in the Universe. Jung asserted that there exists a non-material world – the mental substratum. This space contains ideas, thoughts and knowledge of the past, present and future. It was Plato's idealism in its modern interpretation. I am not making the comparison as a label but a point of reference, indicating the connection between

29

different times and traditions. This world does not obey the laws of time and space: it is beyond time and space, and connects to the material world through the psyche, i.e., something associated with the soul. Perhaps it is even the soul itself, which exists in part in the material body, but also merges with this mental substratum through the unconscious. In this case, the unconscious is a manifestation of the non-material space in the material causal world, and the mental substratum is the design for the development of the Universe.

Jung was concerned about the future of mankind. In 1958, when people just started talking about UFOs, he wrote the book "Flying Saucers: A Modern Myth of Things Seen in the Skies." In its preface he addressed "those few who are willing to listen," and talked about the need to prepare for events, which signify the end of one of the greatest eras in world history. At the risk of undermining his reputation as a serious scholar loyal to traditional science, Jung tried to warn mankind about future great cataclysms. "To be honest, I am deeply worried about the fate of all those who will be caught by surprise with the future course of events and, in the absence of necessary preparation, will find themselves bound hand and foot and incapable of understanding what is going on. As far as I know, nobody has so far tried to answer the question about the psychological consequences of these upcoming changes."

As to the world view expressed by Jung, I could relate to his thoughts. The upcoming events didn't seem to threaten my psyche but perhaps the predicted cataclysm had already affected my own mind?

One evening, at dusk, as I lay in my hospital bed watching TV, I shut my eyes for an instant and, all of a sudden, a white, blindingly bright dot flashed through the darkness and exploded inside me. Once again I was neither in my hospital room nor, in general, in this world. Some force sucked me into a tunnel, where I began to speed at an incredible rate down a winding hallway which resembled a flexible hose. Before I knew it, I was in the mental substratum, in which, by Jung's definition, the design for the development of the Universe is constantly being created and made more complex.

Later I found out that this particular event, which resembled a dream, was extremely important for the evolution of any human being. Even a chance visit to this non-material informational space is a ticket to the world of the most incredible adventures in this life, as well as the life on the other side. In fact, at that particular moment a new world is conceived, which liberates the human spirit.

An unusual space, in which a structured and extremely mobile environment was constantly forming well-defined geometric figures, opened up before me. Endless transformations of the environment produced rhombuses and balls, cones and cubes, trapezoids, half-spheres and many others more complicated structures – tetrahedrons, pyramids, icosahedrons and dodecahedrons. These figures instantly became luminous, now gleaming like delicate, orange-yellow ochre, now shining like stern metallic mercury or vivid ultramarine, and they were then carried away, following a complicated but certain rhythm...

Everything is so beautiful, clear and dynamic in this constantly changing infinite space. Everything is permeated with a powerful, mathematically precise life impulse. I am not trying to say that this world is better than ours. It is just absolutely different: a world of mathematics and precise geometric forms in a sequence of endless geometric transformations, impulses and vibrations.

I stood in this space, where there is no solid land and no sky, leaning on emptiness. And each high-speed interaction of multiple geometric ma-

31

nifestations was carefully circumventing my, evidently random, presence.

Suddenly, I saw three dazzlingly white spheres flying toward me, as if they had escaped from a Salvador Dali painting. Moving out of infinity in uneven, though consciously planned zigzags, they were pulling red elastic hoses behind them, which were lightly vibrating with the powerful swift life of a hidden reason. They came to a halt in front of me, as though to study me and decide if my uninvited presence presented any danger. Once they were sure I was harmless, they took off into the expanses of infinite space, carrying with them their endless hoses. The spheres evidently performed the function of guards, and the fact that they displayed no animosity toward me is something to think about.

Before I knew it, one of the pyramids in front of me opened up. Its outer surfaces simply fell apart leaving behind four even triangles. This transformation revealed a device with different objects constantly appearing and disappearing from within it: various tiny wheels, cylinders, spheres, Möbius strips, odd-looking hammers, levers and counterbalances. All of these objects were silently and purposefully performing their inexplicable job around a semi-transparent prism.

I have entered this space on two occasions. The second time it happened during a lecture at the Academy, which was created at my initiative to implement the new energy-information technology devised by the distinguished expert in extrasensory perception Vyacheslav Lapshin from Ukraine. I was elected vice-president of the Academy. In addition to everything I have already described, during this second incident I saw a very strange, completely flat clock. The multiple web-like luminous threads of different color stretching away from the clock in every direction enmeshed everything around them. There was also an hourglass, which turned to the right on its own and initiated a mysterious process of some

32

kind. During this entire time I was not dreaming. In fact, I was constantly in contact with my instructor. This kind of geometrized space is one of many which a person may enter – there are thousands of existing spaces, all very different, and each of these spaces contains yet another mystery of the Universe. The problem is that the facts described by various people who have visited other dimensions do not conform easily to conventional evaluation and research, all the more so since not everyone is capable of memorizing and presenting their experiences with clarity and precision. Psychologists usually classify such stories as autoscopic hallucinations, which are frequently associated with infectious deceases, brain injuries, alcoholism, drug addiction, or epilepsy.

How then can certain facts of reality be accounted for, which clearly cannot be relegated to the category of subjective delusions or hallucinations?

* * *

I shared my hospital room with a man named Boris Orlov. The two of us hit it off and became friends.

The irony was that Boris actually participated in building this hospital. But maybe it was fated to be, considering his profession. At the time, he was the head of "Bekeron," a large building company, and before that, he was the director of the largest construction materials plant in Uzbekistan. That is why, when he moved to the private sector, he was equally capable of maintaining his top position in business. He was a remarkable and gifted man, well educated, with clear thinking and a sharp mind. His strong personality and direct approach combined with the ability to analyze various scenarios almost instantaneously and move toward his goal through complex multi-step combinations.

Boris believed in dreams, omens and the existence of another reality. He was always seeking out opportunities to travel with somebody into the labyrinths of the unknown, even if just by talking about it.

When I told him about my visions, he was not a bit surprised. He admitted that he had been in intensive care three times because of his acute ulcers, and while he hovered somewhere between life and death he saw similar pictures of geometrized space...

Probably it was his familiarity with these strange dimensions of reality that led Plato to conclude in his day that the world of ideas was as real as the world of objects and, perhaps, even more real. After all, Plato insisted that earthly objects were but imperfect shadows of ideas. According to him, our entire material reality was in some sense no more than a hallucination. But don't try to verify how real it is by hitting your head against a wall. Since nature created this world, it means it has some purpose. The illusion of life is equal to life in this world, and the illusion of death is equal to death. Until some other time it would be hopeless on our part to try and change anything. Nothing would come of it.

– There is no doubt some omnipotent force in our world: it is invisible, unknowable and omnipresent, – Boris said. – People call it God or the Higher Mind, depending on what their view of the world might be. Everyone, however, can feel its presence or at least foresee it because life would have been devoid of meaning without it. Just think, if God doesn't exist, then what is the difference between a human being and a moth, which lives only one day? Anyway, what does it matter how long we live, a thousand years or one minute, if our life experience disappears with us and we aren't able to share it? And if we are simply random animal organisms, a matter of blind mutation and chance, and the result of an accidental merging of molecules, why then don't we live by the laws of the animal kingdom? We'd have our hands full struggling for our survival. But for some reason the human species created such a thing as culture... If God doesn't exist, then it was a waste of the amoeba's precious time on earth. Only brainless dummies and your colleagues from the Academy with their exaggerated sense of self-importance fail to understand this concept.

Boris expressed some ideas which I thought to be quite unique. I pondered about them a lot.

– Why do you think people say that life is like a quilt, alternating light and dark strips? Why do happy and unhappy days alternate with such remarkable certainty? Simply because people don't understand that they are responsible for their own decisions. They see it as simple as that: I want something, so I should get it. But what is your collateral? What do you have to pay for the things given to you?

– It seems like we're both paying back for something here, – I answered meekly, hinting at our current bedridden state.

– Yes, both of us are paying for something, – Boris agreed. – But for some reason only you have the privilege of seeing "pictures." Let's look into this. Why did you agree to become the director of "KhudLit?"

– It must be my life's mission to be a first responder, – I retorted jokingly. – Wherever there's a fire or things fall apart, they summon Petrov to help out. I'm not made for a quiet life. If you offered me a position at your company right now with a salary ten times greater than the one I'm being paid at the publishing house, I would refuse. I know you don't really need my help – you have plenty good people without me. But here it's a different story. I promised Mozhayev that I'd save "KhudLit" and I will.

– Stop talking gibberish, – Boris cut me short. – Just think what your "pictures" are showing you. The path of Jesus! Why do you think this is?

35

Don't you get it? Can't you tell where they're taking you? Somebody is deliberately trying to bankrupt your firm. Some very shrewd geeks are sitting at their computers, trying to figure out how to take over this attractive piece of government property bloodlessly. They were almost ready to go ahead with it, when you emerged out of nowhere – a knight in shining armor! It's surprising they haven't attempted to crack your scull in some dark alley. After all, there's some serious dough to be made.

See for yourself: first, they did their best to make the publishers unprofitable. Next, they moved all its equipment to some suspicious small enterprise, after which both the enterprise itself and the equipment vanished without a trace. And finally, they placed representatives from some fake World Book League on every floor of your building. What's more, this "enterprise" had nothing to do with books – it was simply a front for Moscow's notorious Holsten Restaurant, which received all the rights to the property belonging to the "KhudLit" Publishing House. All that remains is to officially announce its bankruptcy. There's even no need to look for a new owner…

– Maybe they'll concoct a plan to privatize the Kremlin, too? – I looked at Orlov with reproach. He was beginning to rub me the wrong way.

– It has been privatized already and divided up with everyone in it, – he grinned. – They decided against inviting you to be there during the transaction. They feared you might start haranguing them about decency or something of that sort.

– I'll do everything I can to prevent the same from happening to "KhudLit,"– I insisted.

– Why then are you here, at the hospital? – In one fell swoop Boris threw me off the pedestal I was desperately trying to climb.

– What does it have to do with anything? – I tried to strike back, feigning surprise.

– Hey, my friend, remember what I hinted at before: What do you have to pay back for the things given to you? – Boris continued, laughing. – So you'd like to save "KhudLit," is that it? What do you have to actually succeed: big bucks, important government connections? Haven't you told me yourself that you were appointed to this position, but the Finance Ministry gave you no money, not even to pay back the debts of the publishing company? We aren't talking about hundred of rubles, or even thousands. It is massive arrears – the firm owes billions of rubles... Before you know it, they'll cut off your electricity, water, heating and telephone.

– They already have...

– You see, – Boris responded with unexpected glee. – And you're still asking why you are at the hospital. It's because you have nothing except for your own health to pay for your wrong and fateful decision. That's why you're seeing this endless film in your mind about Jesus. You're the victim now. You see, you're atoning for other people's sins. Don't you understand? The Laws of the Universe are very strict – you have to pay for everything. What makes it worse – you agreed to it freely, on your own. You were offered the position, and you agreed to take it... You could've refused. What did you want in exchange: fame, recognition? Now you are welcome to enjoy both with an IV stuck in your arm.

What Boris said was brutal, but the honesty of his words had a sobering effect on me, making me seriously reconsider everything that was happening in my life. I now tried to view my situation not from the standpoint of a romantic hero, but from that of a balanced, reasonable individual, capable of understanding that every decision, whether spiritual or material, should strictly correspond to the person's ability to follow it through.

Parallel with these thoughts, a new plot started to resonate within me

37

with growing clarity, though I couldn't tell yet if it was taken from my own life or someone else's. Now the name of the one who was coming into my present from the past was Joshua.

* * *

This sand, may it be cursed, came from the edges of the stone plateau in the desert, emerging from an infinite number of small volcanoes that were awakened by the power of the sun. Bursts of wind, picking up speed in mountain crevices, lifted handfuls of pebbles and stone fragments, and carried them, like a swarm of wild bees, in their cool palms. If a stranger or animal happened to cross the path of these rulers of the desert, they would sting them without mercy as though they were, indeed, wild bees. The only way to protect oneself from the sand was to cover one's head with a keffiyeh. That was exactly what Joshua did under John's scornful gaze.

John's brown eyes, vigilantly surveying the surrounding area, instantly became lined with deep wrinkles. These uneven creases gave his face a sinister, slightly wild look because their sides were covered with a sickly-looking whitish film. The skin on his eyebrows was inflamed and swollen, which didn't prevent his piercing gaze – its fire burning through the film of fungus – from penetrating Joshua's soul. Joshua shivered as if from the cold, guessing to whom John was addressing his contempt.

John detected the state of mind of this newcomer, surrounded by a small group of pilgrims, and he began to walk toward him in a lunging gait. The face of the prophet, whose skin was covered with purulent craters coated in oily layers of lipid, instantly frowned. His soiled, disheveled beard, threaded with gray, was shaking.

– Are you trying to use this head cover to protect yourself against

God's wrath? – the prophet inquired, his searing gaze fixed upon the small opening for the eyes, which the newcomer left in his keffiyeh.

He found the small, frail body of the preacher from Nazareth pitiful and even laughable.

– On your knees!

John's words sounded like a forceful, aggressive command. Its directness stirred up the crowd of pilgrims surrounding them and made them come close and bunch together in awe.

Joshua tried to say something, but John cried out again with hysterical notes in his voice:

– On your knees!

An expression of hate and overwhelming fear suddenly froze in the prophet's eyes.

Joshua figured out what John was thinking and it was not a very pleasant discovery. He sensed the threat in the ensuing deceptive silence, and was overcome with sudden rage and the knowledge that he had to control it.

He sighed and frowned, his face invisible under the cover. The unbearable stench of rotting teeth struck his nose, which worsened his already poor mood. He didn't expect this man – the famous John the Baptist – to be such a mean-spirited ascetic, who had drained every ounce of humanity from his soul.

– What makes you think that this hot dusty wind is the wrath of God? – Joshua asked in a low voice from under his keffiyeh, accepting the challenge.

John did not expect such a display of disobedience from someone who saw him as a teacher, and for a moment he was at a loss what to do.

He finally turned around to face the motionless group of pilgrims who

39

were eyeing him with fierce attention, and, still unsure how to respond, he sat on a rock opposite Joshua.

– If it isn't God's wrath, then whose is it? The devil's? – John inquired in his former mean and sarcastic voice. He placed his staff across his knees as if he were getting ready to spring up from the rock he was sitting on and depart from his disappointingly boring companion.

– I doubt that either of them would concern themselves with such trifles, – the man from Nazareth responded in a calm, quiet voice.

A tortured, apologetic smile flashed across his lips. Once again, no one noticed it because of the cloth covering most of his face.

– I've been told that you preach in the name of God but don't wash away people's sins during baptism, – John said in a somber voice.

He scratched under his armpit, and the stagnant stench of decay escaped from under his ragged garments made of camel wool.

– We have to preach the gospel, – Joshua retorted.

– May the tongue of the one who preaches thus wither away, and may the guts of those who listen to his words without anger or condemnation become rotten and turn into a festering, foul-smelling wound.

The awe-stricken crowd rumbled quietly, waiting. Joshua ripped the cloth off his face and everyone saw that he was absolutely calm and unperturbed. Only his eyes darkened and a spark of rage smoldered in them.

– The pagans used water to cleanse themselves in the Euphrates and the Nile. They also believed that this ritual was going to save them. They thought it would open the heavenly gates before them, even though they worshipped other gods, – Joshua said.

Once again, the rumble of a whisper passed through the crowd. The pilgrims were clearly trying to figure out the meaning of this verbal exchange and decide which of the two men were closer to the truth.

40

– Heresy comes out of your mouth! – John the Baptist exclaimed in a frenzy.

– Judge not, and you shall not be judged, – replied the man from Nazareth.

– You and your disciples are praying to God in your own words. How dare you do that? – John attacked him with new vigor.

One of the men in the crowd, a Pharisee, who had a small leather box attached to his forehead, containing a piece of parchment with prayers, rolled his eyes and gasped in horror. He raised his left arm, with a similar leather box attached to it, in a gesture of protestation.

– No blasphemy! – he shrieked.

John the Baptist turned his sallow face, furrowed with wrinkles, to the Pharisee. His violently dilated nostrils quivered, inhaling the wind and the dust.

– You, monstrous brood of Echidna! I am baptizing you with water as a token of redemption, but the one who is coming after me will baptize you with the Holy Spirit and fire! – John cried in a threatening voice. The fierce glance that accompanied his cry was even more frightening than his words. – His winnowing fork is in his hand to clean up his threshing floor. He will gather the grain into his barn, but he will burn the chaff with inextinguishable fire...

– Men are not chaff, – said Joshua with sadness in his voice.

Murmurs of approval arose from the crowd. John's disciples looked around in bewilderment upon seeing that the approval of the crowd was leaning toward the man from Nazareth.

– The Lord, the God of Israel, be witness! Those who serve the Almighty and preach His Word cannot show pity. He is the stormy ocean and the lifesaving boat on its menacing waves. He is the volcano erupting lava

41

and the unsinkable island of safety in the fire which devours life. You must have faith and only faith. It is not for you to question. Faith moves mountains. As for you, you are serving man, not your heavenly master.

The accusation, which Joshua was afraid to hear, was cast. And again, the crowd of pilgrims around them swayed and began to rumble, discussing John's words.

– It is not true, – Joshua tried to argue, but his unintelligible words had no effect on those who had gathered. His protest was too meek compared to the charges against him directed toward the sky.

Joshua couldn't fail to notice that John was deliberately fanning his irritation and the sense of righteous indignation seething inside him was finally released in a counter accusation.

– Yes, it is true that faith moves mountains but not yours. Your faith only piles them up! – he exclaimed. And immediately Joshua's face was distorted in a grimace of suffering, because he was forced to raise his voice in his own defense to pronounce these words of accusation.

John grew pale with anger. The dirty piece of cloth that covered his head fell over his face, and only his eyes flashed eerily from behind its shadows.

– If you wish to hate me, go ahead, hate me, – said the man from Nazareth. – But don't avoid the issues I'm raising.

– Every tree that isn't producing good fruit will be cut down and thrown into the fire, – the Baptist shouted with fanatical conviction. Cupping his hand above his eyes John peered intently at the one who had the nerve to argue with him.

– He is our Father and we are His children, – the man from Nazareth continued, undeterred. – How can the Father raise an axe against His own children?

42

– If He so wishes, the Lord can create His children even from stones,
– John commented mockingly.

– Are you trying to expose God as someone who has created something useless that requires alteration? – the man from Nazareth reproached Joshua in the same ironic tone.

It was clear that this time John was at a loss what to say to his unexpected adversary who appeared before him for some unknown reason. His eyes suddenly became lusterless and heavy, too weary to stay open any longer. He stood up from the stone and walked quickly away toward a nearby tent, without responding to Joshua's sarcastic remark. He lay down, and the striped piece of worn, sand torn fabric, stretched over his head and held in place with the help of thin long twigs, bending in the wind, hid him from the assembled crowd.

Joshua sighed, covered his face with his keffiyeh once again, turned around and started to walk away from the man, whom he had wanted to call his teacher not so long ago.

The crowd silently followed the man from Nazareth and the few disciples, trudging along behind him, with their eyes.

* * *

In the beginning, I had grave doubts about the authenticity of the plot in this vision. It was in stark contradiction to the Holy Scriptures and to all that we know about John the Baptist. Even later I could never completely figure out what it meant. Perhaps, in contradiction to the design of the Creator, embodied in Biblical texts in the mysterious hologram code of four-dimensional consciousness, the real John the Baptist did not recognize the Messiah, whose arrival he was supposed to proclaim. After all, it is a known fact that the sects of John the Baptist and Jesus Christ were at cross-purposes with each other after the death of their teachers.

Why couldn't it happen that way? The prophet, after being assigned his mission, suddenly, for some secret reason, perhaps due to the interference of some powerful supernatural forces, or because his intuition failed him at the time of their encounter, proved unable to fulfill it.

It couldn't be that John the Baptist's only mission was to baptize God in the waters of the Jordan River, could it? The inconsistency in the story could have fatal consequences. Just imagine, God was not recognized: the one who had to announce His coming and who was instructed to point Him out to the people, failed to recognize Him. Maybe that was the reason why the first coming of Jesus ended so tragically? Following the Baptist, the rest of the world also denied His Kingdom on earth. The earthly manifestation of God was then delayed for any amount of time...

It seemed that the plot of this story had two levels in reality: one showed things as they ought to have been, as they were described in the sacred words of the Bible; the other showed things the way they really were, as they were described in historical testimonies and eyewitness accounts of contemporaries. According to the latter, St. John the Baptist couldn't have baptized Joshua at the time indicated in the Holy Scriptures because by then the imprisoned Baptist was already beheaded by King Herod.

Then again, there was a third level, the one shown to me in my visions.

So what is the truth? How is the fabric of reality created in general? Maybe what I saw happened at a different time and in an altogether different place? Did it take place in the past, or, perhaps, in the future? When?

Frankly, these thoughts would occur to me much later. In the meantime, I was so busy writing down everything I saw in my visions that I didn't notice the remarkable improvement in my health. The symptoms of my condition were rapidly disappearing: the yellowing of the skin and my back pain were almost gone. My health problems weren't on my mind anymore. I experienced the amazing plot involving the participation of archetypal characters as if these were dramatic events from my own personal life. I was beginning to see that this was only the starting point of some very significant developments. Shortly after, I was released from the hospital. As to my prediction, it came true sooner than I had anticipated.

True, at first the events that took place in my life weren't filled with fanfare as my visions about Jesus. These events were gradually sneaking into my life, apparently trying to be as inconspicuous as possible and presenting themselves as part of my everyday experiences. It seemed as though the one who initiated them wasn't entirely sure that he was doing the right thing. He crept toward me slowly, as if fumbling in the dark, trying to find the person he already knew about. He finally seemed to find that person, the Seeing One…

Our meeting took place at the Palace of Congresses* in the fall of 1996, during the Fifth International Informatization Conference. Berezhnoi was right – it turned out to be an acquaintance of major impact.

There was something demonic about Lapshin's appearance: with his close-cropped beard and habit of moving unusually fast and with dexterity in space, he eyed the world with an ironic twinkle. Most importantly, he was a most unusual and interesting person to talk to. He never had a problem becoming the center of attention and arousing the audience's curiosity. Before I knew it, I agreed to help him find suitable premises in Moscow and register the Lapshin International Academy to accommodate his method. The miracle-maker from Ukraine insisted on "International"

* The Palace of Congresses has been renamed the "State Kremlin Palace".

being added to the title.

– Physicians won't be able to cope with the diseases which will attack the world in the new century! – This was the confident explanation Lapshin gave me to support the need for his new organization.

– What makes you think so?

– They don't take into account the energy information structure, now being referred to as the bio-field. As for me, I know how to work with it. Thanks to the interaction in the universal field, the bio-energetic essence of a human being is capable, in a special, altered state of consciousness, to interconnect not only with matter but also with different fields, which are manifestations of the single quantum radiation of outer space. All information in the Universe is organized as a wave frequency-amplitude structure. The human mind is capable of decoding holograms of the past, present and future of both the material and non-material worlds on the basis of this quantum-wave function. Have you ever heard about the bio-computer?

– Just a little. I know only what Berezhnoi told me.

– I see, – Lapshin looked me in the eye with suspicion, and immediately started delivering a long lecture on the subject.

I listened to what he had to say with great interest, quite curious to know more.

– Our cognition is used to interpret things from a linear perspective. But eternity doesn't have the same pattern of movement for everything within it. It is high time we realize that for the Universe our knowledge could be merely a local event. Paleontology has long established the fact that there have been sudden leaps and inexplicable appearances of entirely new life forms, which cannot be explained from the standpoint of an orderly evolution. Man is the highest but not the last link in the chain of life on Earth. As a biological species, Homo sapiens are presently in crisis, which will end with extinction if nature doesn't put into motion the mechanism of adaptation to the new environment.

– Do you know what this mechanism is? – I asked.

– The bio-computer, which we have spoken about earlier, is the product of a superconscient functional system. People can develop phenomenal abilities with its help, such as different ways of seeing, and not necessarily with the eyes alone. They can use unconventional ways to obtain information – through the scanning of space, telepathy, clairvoyance, etc. All this will allow people to discover the necessary tools for their development, transformation and survival.

The Soviet Union has been the world leader not only in the study of psychic processes, but also in developing the latest bio-information technologies, something the majority of people know nothing about today.

– Are you talking about a conveyer for manufacturing supermen?

– Why not? It is absolutely necessary to educate the masses about the human body's super-conscious functions and about bio-informational technologies. This should include the self-regulation of energy-distribution systems in human beings, as well as education about mechanical regulation of the general exchange of these energies. At every turn of our planetary existence we witness something we call a reactivation of a portion of our genetic code or program, which defines a qualitatively new level in our abilities, elevating us to a higher level of being. If we want to survive, we must change ourselves: our habits and our prejudices. What's more, we should abandon almost all of our past knowledge and acquire new knowledge instead.

– So what is this bio-computer? – I tried to steer Lapshin away from a generalized discussion back to his previous, more specific topic.

47

– It is some entity, – he answered vaguely. – And it functions not only in our material space, and at more levels than one.

– How many of them are there?

– More than enough, – Lapshin said with a smile, and there seemed to be just a hint of mockery in his voice.

As I was listening to Lapshin, I struggled with two opposite emotions. One was the desire to help an enthusiast in pursuit of his dream; the other was a gnawing doubt whether this man had indeed discovered the secret key to human existence. My doubts were not without reason.

True, his discourse, especially when he showered the listener with his radical ideas, sounded scientific on the surface. But after thorough analysis one was apt to notice some flaws in his choice of terms, such as, for instance, when he spoke of the "wave frequency-amplitude structure," which seemed an oxymoron to me. He spoke about quantum radiation, and in response my brain asked with some amusement: "Now what other radiation is there, a non-quantum one?" Then again, when he elaborated on the topic of the mysterious bio-computer, Lapshin based his reasoning on the doubtful method of deriving the cause from the effect. And lastly, he was constantly referring to the human brain as a machine.

On the whole, there was much that I found confusing in his scientific rhetoric. And still, there was, hidden beneath his abundant revelations, some mystical light, or, rather, a kind of terra incognita like the mythical Atlantic in the ocean depths. Hidden behind the turbulence of words and emotions, I felt the presence of a genuine mystery, and I found this enticing.

– The left side of the human brain is energy governed, and its activity is directed toward the material plane. The energy channels, acupuncture points and the overall activity of the left hemisphere of our brain all depend on the energy intake of our body. If there is a breakdown in the delivery of energy, people develop pathologies, – the miracle-maker from Ukraine continued.

– Our brain's right hemisphere is connected to events that contain information and are closely associated with the non-material plane, that is, with the function of our super consciousness.

Artists, musicians, poets and writers are people with an enhanced function of the right hemisphere. They receive information through their super consciousness from the single information field, which we call today, the non-material space. In general, our brain activity molds our consciousness. Therefore, the development of our consciousness and, consequently, our sub-consciousness and our entire body depend on the harmonious function of both hemispheres of the brain.

– Is there any risk that training according to your method might harm the human mind? – I tried to clarify for myself.

He started laughing: "To harm the mind, one must have it. Take a closer look at the life around you. Could you call it sensible? But to answer you on a more serious note, we have accumulated several years of research, and not a single one of the students in our program has developed any kind of psychopathology attributable to my system. On the contrary, our students have consistently exhibited great improvements in their short-term and long-term memory, excellent results in switching their attention and dividing it between different tasks. They also exhibit a measurable decrease in stress level as the result of the rise in the sympathetic tone of their nervous system and a much higher than average level of general wellbeing and psychological stability.

This conversation eventually resulted in the opening of the Lapshin Academy, which soon became known not just in Russia but also elsewhere around the world. Based on our preliminary agreement, Lapshin became the Academy's president, while Berezhnoi and I were appointed as vice-presidents.

A month later, Lapshin completed his affairs in Kiev and moved to Moscow. I took care of all the expenses related to the registration of the Academy, and another sponsor found a nice hotel suite for Lapshin and his family not far Moscow. We all set out to work enthusiastically on this new project.

Without putting it off, I also began to study with Lapshin's instructors whom he brought from Kiev, trying to capture the basics of his system.

At the beginning, I didn't feel any energy flow at all. I even began to irritate my patient teachers with my endless expressions of doubt. But then something unusual happened.

It occurred when I was at home, while my wife and I were trying to master an exercise on the "energy cleansing" of the mind. The goal, according to Lapshin's technique, was to enhance the connections between cerebral hemispheres, develop specific parts of the brain, its cortical and sub-cortical structures, the energy and vascular systems of the right and left hemispheres, the homeostatic mechanism, which controls the dynamic equilibrium within energy information exchange, and the blood circulation system. This exercise required a special kind of breathing – the so-called anode-cathode breathing. During a certain moment, while my wife was doing this exercise and putting her hands on my head according to a prescribed pattern, my vision changed sharply. Colors became considerably brighter in my visual perception, and their range became much wider.

My vision continued to be perfect during the following days and months, and it is perfect to this today.

Incidentally, another student from our group – Professor Anatoli Be-

50

rezhnoi – observed similar changes in his eyesight. He was able to stop using glasses altogether to the surprise of his colleagues and family.

Sometime later, I became aware of changes in my memory as well. The most remarkable thing in this process was that these changes, just like the ones with my vision before them, happened all at once, instantaneously. They took place after four weeks of training.

I came home one evening, had dinner, went to bed, and suddenly a strange projector seemed to turn on in my brain. The things I saw in my sleep through this projector weren't dreams – they were more like a slide film. I saw my own childhood years and my youth up to about of 25 unraveling before me with tremendous speed but in strict chronological order. The various events that took place in our courtyard on Stalin Street, in the small town of Balashikha-3 near Moscow, were presented with great attention to detail.

There we were, my friends and I, sitting on benches around a wooden plank table, listening to Peter Bychkov playing the guitar and singing. I couldn't hear the music or the lyrics – it was just a picture, but both the tune and the lyrics were restored in my memory, and I instantly recalled the names of my friends, whom I hadn't seen in over 40 years.

Next I saw our lake in the grove near the stadium. That day Tolya Malyshev, Kolya Samokhin, Valeri Eliseyev and I cut classes and ran to the lake. We could spend hours swimming, without getting out of the water. The mysterious projector illuminated our puppy faces lit up with infectious enthusiasm. Then, something horrible happened – we saw a man drowning. Everyone at the lake, including the four of us, dived into the water to rescue him. Somebody pulled his body out of the water. The ambulance arrived, and the team of physicians tried to resuscitate the man – nothing worked. They were about to leave but the man's wife – a fragile young woman – continued to give her husband mouth-to-mouth and wouldn't let the ambulance take him away. The doctors and nurse tried to reason with her. She refused to listen to them and continued to perform CPR, spreading and folding his arms on his chest. Giving up, the team of doctors got into the ambulance and it started slowly to drive away. A minute later the man came to life and we rushed after the ambulance, telling the team to come back.

Day after day, hour after hour the slide film returned me into my youth, and everything it showed me was revived in my memory and acquired the features of reality.

These incredible events, certainly unusual as far as my life was concerned – the sudden improvement in my health, the strange transformations in my memory and the fact that I finally started to feel the impact of energy and could produce the same effect on others – all this compelled me treat the idea of collaboration with Lapshin much more seriously. I advanced to the second stage in my training (it was like moving to the second grade) and was given access to the bio-computer –the mechanism of internal and inter-dimensional vision. It was then that true miracles began and the mysterious unknown world reached out to me.

Already in the very first days of my work with the bio-computer the mysterious things hiding behind the threshold of consciousness decided to present me with their potential. They did this with a touch of light, friendly humor and obviously without any intention to intimidate me or bring me under their control. All they wanted was to show me how uncertain and subject to variation was the line between that which we consider to be certain and real, i.e., reality, and that which Carl Gustav Jung called the mental substratum, which contains ideas, thoughts and information about the past, present and future.

This happened in the morning of an otherwise unremarkable day. I was awakened by the bright sun. For some reason I already knew it was time to get up, particularly since I planned to finish reading "The Roots of Consciousness," a book by Jeffrey Mishlove, which I bought the previous week, before leaving for work.

I opened my eyes. The digital clock showed half past six. I put on my slippers and got up. Walked to the bathroom, brushed my teeth, washed and shaved my face. My wife and children were still sleeping, so I slipped quietly into my office, opened the book and began reading. The chapter was titled "The Ecology of Consciousness." I underlined in red the paragraphs I found particularly interesting. After reading several pages, I suddenly noticed everything change around me. I looked away from the text and realized that I must have gotten into serious trouble with the bio-computer. The walls were losing their clear outlines and becoming weirdly distorted. The room was contracting in size. It now looked more like a pantry, and the rough, uneven masonry of its new walls was covered with dark blue oil paint. These walls reminded me of something from long before, from my childhood. In addition, someone was giggling from out there (not maliciously but amicably) and preventing me from getting up from my armchair.

We had been warned that something like that might happen and even told how to shut down the bio-computer, when it turned on voluntarily, without our command. The point is that energy training, by increasing the potential of the brain in its interaction with super consciousness, or the mental substratum, initiates arbitrary transcendental functions that are beyond the limits of our world. Since the work of the bio-computer requires considerable use of energy, it is unacceptable to permit it to act on its own in establishing contacts. That is why I did what was required to close it down: I shut my eyelids, activated an energy surge by mentally transferring energy into the frontal part of my head through the spinal cord, after which I expelled it through the eyes, lifted my eyelids and saw the following: I was still sitting in bed and the clock was showing half past six.

I walked to the bathroom, brushed my teeth and washed my face. Everyone was still asleep, so I slipped quietly into my office and opened Jeffrey Mishlove's book lying on my desk. I found the bookmark exactly where I left it the day before – at the beginning of the next chapter. But when I started reading I realized that I knew the content of the next few pages very well: I read them when the bio-computer switched on without my command. Mind you, none of the paragraphs were underlined in red, which I had done in my "strange dream." The text, however, was not just familiar to me – I actually remembered it by heart line after line.

These visions are perfect illustrations of the ability to create events in our material world through hallucinatory features of a higher creative reason. All that happened was simply a manifestation of the possibilities of the world concealed from us behind the wall of consciousness. It is significant that none of the senses – neither my hearing, nor my vision, or sense of touch, or smell – sounded the alarm or warned me that what I saw was an illusion, a vision so real that it was able to absorb reality, mimic it and even include in the past a future that hadn't yet occurred (unread pages from a book, the content of which I was able to memorize).

When our perception of life undergoes changes so does life itself. The famous British physicist James Jones once remarked: "When one electron vibrates, the entire Universe experiences a shock." The great advantage of this new vision of the world lies in its infinite ability for creative self-development in its interaction with Universal Reason. Every person is an infinite world that can have access to the cosmic super-computer. Those who win the right to interact with it acquire new possibilities for their development.

It is not that difficult to develop contact with the bio-computer once you go through a series of training exercises and study the necessary safety measures. A special command is issued and a white screen instantly appears before you, despite the piece of cloth with which you must cover your eyes to make sure that you are not distracted by the sunlight. This screen usually resembles a TV or computer screen. This, however, is only the beginning. With time, if you make good progress in this direction you will receive a considerably more powerful tool for your interaction with non-material space. For instance, you will be able to see events "on the other side" and "right here" simultaneously and even influence them; all that, of course, while observing the inviolable Laws of the Universe. You will be able to infinitely ascend the steps of evolution until you violate one of these laws … and if you do, you will lose it all. You must be very careful when you climb up those steps. I know what it means to fall down, because this has happened to me.

Chapter 2

It appeared that Boris Orlov took my situation at "KhudLit" very much to heart. He paid me more or less regular visits, advised me on current issues and analyzed all the steps I was taking. The fact that the State Publishing Committee proved incapable of providing regular financial aid to help the publishing house repay its debts, as it had previously promised, made my situation quite dire. By that time I had already made a promise to the staff that I wasn't going to resort to the more traditional approach used during bankruptcy, meaning blanket layoffs to reduce expenses.

–This was a stupid promise, – my new friend said disapprovingly. – You continue to have a suffocating multimillion-ruble debt from the past strangling you. Isn't that enough trouble? Now you decided to allow your own staff to squeeze your throat even harder? Do you expect them to have a lighter touch? Judging from the series of articles about the hell they've raised before, these people are no sacrificial lambs.

Boris was reclining in a relaxed position in the armchair but despite his deceptively laid-back appearance he was like a tightly bound spring – staying focused on the issue. I was so used to it by now that I was no longer surprised by his ability to be in a constant state of alertness.

– Let's air your dirty linen, – he suggested.

– Go ahead, – I agreed, knowing in advance that his analytical reasoning always provided me with much that was useful.

– So you've got this debt now adjusted to account for the newly uncovered accounting errors and taxes unpaid by your predecessor, do you?

– Yes, we're talking four and some billion rubles, – I immediately responded to his questioning tone.

– What are your current assets?

– Zero.

– What's the turnover for your printed books?

– Right now we estimate it to be approximately three years.

Boris stared at me fixedly as if to check whether I was making fun of him.

– Level of profitability?

– Twenty percent.

Boris grew visibly paler.

– Now I see you've been discharged from the hospital too early. You're definitely not well. Do you know of any economic theory which allows you, in your situation, to believe in a better tomorrow and make promises to your employees that they will all keep their jobs?

– No, I don't, – I gave the honest answer.

– So what's your plan of action?

– My deputy, Sergei Kolesnikov, has arranged for us to receive paper on loan, – I reported to him the steps that had been taken.

– What's the amount of credit?

– One billion two hundred rubles.

– What else?

– I am taking a bank loan, using my stocks at the Buddyonovsk Oil and Gas Plant as collateral.

– How big a loan?

– Seven hundred million rubles.

– Is that all?

– There's more. We also have agreements with the printers that they would print out books on credit. The credit amount is one billion rubles, – I added, knowing that he was going to ask for that number anyway.

– So the total is about three billion rubles, – Boris summed up. – What if you lose all your stocks? What then? – he snapped irritably. – Have you been promised "KhudLit" as a gift if you save it?

– No, I simply think that losing such a publishing house as "KhudLit" would be tantamount in its negative impact to losing the Bolshoi or the Tretyakov Gallery, – I shrugged.

– Oh, you think so? – Boris raved. – And what does the government think? Judging from the fact that it denies you even the help it originally promised, the government couldn't care less about you and your castles in the air! Get back to earth, my friend. You're just one step away from Golgotha. It looks like carpenters are building the cross for you and have already picked out some rusty nails, nice and long ones…

– There's something I forgot to tell you. We have also completed the proposal for the "Golden Collection," and we are now looking for a suitable investor, – I wasn't going to give up so easily.

– Alright, – Boris suddenly calmed down. – It's time to do the final calculations. So you have three billion rubles with a three year turnover. Nine years, right?

– Yes, – I agreed unwillingly.

– With a twenty percent profit margin, please multiply nine by five. What we get is approximately half a century, and that only if you haven't erred in your assumptions.

– You are not exactly right, – I stubbornly refused to accept the truth.

– Well, well.

– We have several other projects that are bound to be of interest to investors. Incidentally, these new projects will have over a hundred percent profitability and a turnover of about one year.

– Hopefully your economists haven't goofed up.

– What economists are you talking about? We did the calculations ourselves.

– I see, – Boris sounded more agreeable again. – So you have several fantastic projects in mind but you can't start them because you haven't got the funds. Mind you, if you should decide to start these projects anyway, without sufficient funding, you risk losing not only your anticipated profit but also your actual production expenses because you won't have the money to properly market your products.

– We must, therefore, beat our competitors both in the quality and price of our books.

– Good, – Boris praised me. – One can immediately tell you have at least a college degree. Only remember, you won't be asking your college professor for money – you will have to go to the bank. There you will find a polite but stern-looking gentlemen sitting at his desk, and he will, of course, express his willingness to give you a loan at a ridiculously high interest rate, but even in this fortunate scenario he will not forget to ask: "What assets can you pledge as collateral for such a credit amount?"

– Yes, he will.

– So what do you have as collateral – the building?

– No, the building is owned by the state.

– The stocks then?

– Yes, I have these internal foreign currency bonds but the state refuses to honor them. They have postponed making payments until the next millennium...

– You see, – Boris suddenly perked up again. – The situation becomes even clearer. You are being offered participation in an elimination racing event. The track is a killer and other participants are like wild beasts. And our beloved government has forgotten to pour even a drop of gasoline into

59

its own government-owned car. Why don't you guys push the car ahead all the way to the finishing line for a hundred dollar monthly salary? Isn't it like that?

– Yes, it's true, – I was forced to agree. – There aren't any government investment funds where we could take out a loan for various publishing ventures. And it looks like nobody intends to set up any fund of that sort. I asked some folks at the Publishing Committee about it and was told that this should come under the purview of the Federal program for book publishing. But we can't get any funding from this program either.

– What is the proportion of publishing expenses in your cost estimate? – Boris continued to question me.

– It's 50-60 percent.

– This is outrageous. No commercial enterprise will allow itself to exceed 10 percent. You should bear in mind that every ten percent of operating expenses mean losing at least fifteen percent in profit. After the most basic calculations you will see that unless you resolve this problem – and it brings you directly to the necessity to make drastic cuts in your pool of employees – your publishing house is destined to die a slow and tortuous death.

Boris looked at me expectantly, assessing how well I understood what he had just said.

I didn't say a thing. He really saw the root of the matter. High operating costs were our biggest problem. To be precise, what was killing us was the hidden cost associated with our building. "KhudLit" had long gone past the point when its large premises stopped being an advantage and turned into a liability. Nobody had ever bothered to calculate how much the building cost us. Every single meter of underutilized space was equivalent to losing twenty two thousand rubles a month. The money was mostly spent on communal payments and services. We had huge meeting halls and the entire first floor was taken up by a library and storage facility. Many of the rooms were occupied with storage containing old chairs, closets and all sorts of junk. It was unthinkable to be using valuable space in the heart of the capital for such useless rubbish!

I already had a plan for how we could clean out these rooms and facilities, decrease storage and fit the library in the space it once occupied. In the vacant space we could open a high-end store named "Pegasus." This would give us the floating funds which would make it possible to keep up with payroll. The most important thing was to move slowly but surely toward solvency. Our greatest threat was stagnation.

I told Boris about my plans but he didn't get it.

– It is easier to start everything from scratch than to correct the current mess-up in your affairs, – was his final verdict. – The path toward success lies in fast adaptation to ever-changing external and internal conditions. How are you going to adapt to anything when you have been shackled to the past? How can you break these shackles and who will help you do it? The market has one immutable law: you should never produce anything that entails losses. This is the basic formula for success. If you know of any other one, God speed you on your way – be the trailblazer. Don't delude yourself – the life to which you are condemning yourself will be more like a nightmare. And worst of all, the very moment you, standing at the very edge of the abyss, miraculously grab onto something called luck, someone will come and say: "We'll do it ourselves from now on. Go have a rest, stupid. If we see some other thing falling into the abyss later, we will be sure to ask you for help."

These last words Boris said to me ripped right through the festive shell of my melodramatic side. The shell slipped under the feet of my

61

vanity like the Emperor's new clothes. I suddenly realized that my goal was nothing but a chivalric fantasy of a deluded Don Quixote. If not for any other reason, it was absurd because the original Don Quixote never dreamed of standing solemnly on the high pedestal of history. I must admit: I did anticipate a barrage of applause after I rescued the publishing house. I wasn't in it for the money, or the lucrative position, no. I wasn't looking for such rewards. All I wanted was flowers and applause. But Boris showed what awaited me if the miracle of rescuing the company was accomplished, and he did it pitilessly, with harsh precision. I would be lucky if the winner didn't step on my fingers at the moment of parting. After all, "KhudLit" was truly a gem, for which new publishing giants might come together to fight it out. They weren't interested in it right now because of its sorry state – it was more like a decomposing corpse. But if I helped reanimate the publishing house and it was once again perceived as an actual competitor, the situation would change. An attempt to destroy the competitor would most likely be undertaken when the company's potential became obvious and it was seen as a future threat.

Boris, who was closely watching my face for the barely noticeable signs of self-rebuke, noted significantly:

– I think you now understand how dumb it was to accept this position, this role of a businessman and savior combined in one. Such a role is impossible in the real world around us. A businessman looks for ways to make money. You, on the contrary, have found a place where you can spend what you have. The day will come when those for whose sake you are risking everything you have, will make you into a laughing stock. Did you finally get it?

I got it... he was right... But what do I have left, what can I hold on to now? Only my promise at my friend's grave to save "KhudLit." Save it

…but at what price? We never spoke about the price. All I did was make a promise...

Once again, parallel to the events of the day, my night dreams unveiled visions of events from two thousand years before – and in them I saw the path, the path of Jesus.

* * *

...Leaving the vineyard, Yeshua walked westward with a confident stride, toward Mount Carmel. Behind his back, the first rays of the morning sun were already lighting up the canyon between Sulem and Tabor. The night dissipated softly and quietly, hiding in the distance. The vast space ahead of him was gradually filled with the faint gray of dawn; the trunks of fig trees around him were becoming more distinct and sharply defined, as was the lush foliage of the orchards surrounding Nazareth.

The road now meandered uphill, and the horizon behind the valley, which seemed very narrow before, started to expand. The peak of the Chechem Mountains, a sacred site honoring the memory of the first Patriarchs of Israel, was becoming visible far off ahead of him. Yeshua walked faster now, as if under the spell of the summons of the ages, which resounded in his soul from these petrified witnesses of events of yore, swallowed by the relentless waves of oblivion.

But the world did not wish to know anything about the past. All around him life, carefree and cheerful, was waking up together with the rising sun. Dense forests replaced the orchards on his path. Long, woody lianas entwined the tall and powerful tree trunks. Dove-colored blackbirds bustled about in the grass. Crested larks hopped from branch to branch. Some of the old trees had green clusters of parasitic plants attached to their bodies. Responding to the warmth of the rising sun, their delicate flowers began to spread out their petals, disturbing the solemn stillness of the forest with their barely audible rustling.

Though he was exhausted, Yeshua hurried on. He was walking toward the bend in a small creek, with a steep cliff rising high into the sky next to it. The edges of the cliff were carved out of deposits of shiny white limestone. The cliff's pure white color and its surface, free of any growth in the very midst of such luscious greenery, produced a strange, mysterious and fascinating impression.

Deep inside the caves carved out in the cliff, in almost complete darkness, there were several tombs. The mountain exuded a delicate, sad aura of mysticism arising from this ancient land, and just like subterranean waters that are forced out onto the surface by the weight of layers of clay-rich sediment, its invisible emanation trickles down the rough boulders into the green grass, the underbrush and the trees.

Yeshua was looking for his Father here. He wanted to pour out his doubts to Him and ask whether true religion required priests and rituals.

It was not Yeshua's first visit to that cliff. He liked to indulge in solitude, sitting on a large boulder, at the foot of which a spring flowed from below to the surface of the earth. Here he would slip into reverie, contemplating that which filled his soul day after day. Here, as though growing out of the roots of this mountain range, Yeshua could hear with special clarity the rebukes of the Old Testament prophets. His soul trembled at the Words of the Lord passed on by the Prophet Isaiah, heavy and malleable as a metal bell. "To what purpose is the multitude of your sacrifices to me? I am full of the burnt offerings of rams, and the fat of fed beasts ... incense is an abomination to Me ... your hands are full of blood. Wash yourselves, make yourselves clean. Remove the evil of your deeds from My sight.

Cease to do evil. Learn to do good ... And then come."

This was a spot where Yeshua often had the sensation that time was about to stop, flow backward or, quite the opposite, flow forward, doubling its speed. The cliff was like a small island in the ocean of centuries, with waves from the past, the future and even from the times which had never existed and never will, lapping at its side. This cliff concealed a secret, one that lured the prophets and also the voice of the abyss, which it was unable to restrain.

Yeshua stopped and looked around himself. The golden needles of the sun's rays had awakened the entire area: they shuffled the grass, unfolded the leaves on the trees and disturbed the insects. Yeshua was standing on a stretch of land, where the path ended abruptly. On one side it was cut off by the vertical cliff, and on the other, by the steep slope of loose rock debris. These stone fragments would undoubtedly start to slide down and carry with them anyone who had the audacity to step on the precipitous incline. There was a crevice behind the slope, with a narrow rocky ridge winding snake-like across its bottom.

The boulder lay at the end of the flat stretch of land, the surface of which was polished to a shine by rain and wind.

Yeshua came closer to the boulder. A sad smile flitted across his face, almost instantly disappearing in his thick moustache and copious beard. He sat down on the boulder. The spring was gurgling below, right at his feet. Yeshua parted the grass, creating a tiny pool of water framed in dark green and the many colors of mountain flowers scattered around. In the mirror of the pool Yeshua saw his own reflection. He was short and fragile, like a young shoot of grass pushing its way to the sun through the dry crust of the earth. Death had already disfigured his face with its imprint. But his youthful eyes were shining in contrast to his frail body, ablaze not

65

with the feverishness of sickly impotence but fired by his dream. His were the eyes of a man who never turned his glance away from anything he was looking at, unless this was his own intention.

And yet he was miserable and pitiful, equally miserable and pitiful to those whose pain and suffering he had decided to mold into the faith of brotherly love. His dark hair was parted as was the custom for men from Nazareth. His beard was also divided in the middle. He cast a disapproving look at his reflection in the water. A small river turtle with meek sparkling eyes crawled out of the grass toward the spring and froze in fear upon seeing a human being. Yeshua snickered:

– Now what exactly are you afraid of? You're here because you're thirsty, aren't you? Drink then.

But the turtle didn't listen to him. It turned around and shuffled away in funny, awkward little steps.

The day before, Yeshua had returned from his pilgrimage to Jerusalem. As always, his path lay through Genea and Chechem, past the ancient sanctuaries of the Pool of Siloam. His plan was to meet with the Father at the Temple of Jerusalem but he only found priests inside and their strange establishment, which had usurped the right to act as mediators between man and God.

– Abba, Father, – he called in a quiet voice, and the echo of his whispered words slipped into the ravine. – Tell me, why do Your priests stand between the son and the Father? Can't I turn to You with a pure heart, without the mediation of these men, who defile the faith with false mimicry and with their attire bearing the insignia of false righteousness? Won't You hear the voice of my soul without the intervention of those parading their worthy deeds and selling faith in Your temples?

He spoke with such profound conviction that his body suddenly felt

66

limp and covered with sweat from the strength of his emotion.

– You, Who can see the hidden, know for Yourself that the goal of their service is not the pursuit of truth but power.

Yeshua straightened the kuffiyeh on his head. Tears welled up in his deep dark eyes.

– Tell me, Father, why do I remember my life there? Why haven't You rid me of memory, as you did the others, but forced me to enter this world with knowledge of the past?

Yeshua lowered his face closer to the water. A ray of sun from behind his back caught the water on fire, and multicolored little stars lit up, sparkling, in its cold depth. He looked intently as they moved haphazardly to and fro, trying to stop their odd dance with an effort of will, but they lit up even brighter, then gradually grew darker and disappeared altogether, leaving only an obscure dark spot behind them. It stirred and turned back and forth, as if trying to find a comfortable position at the bottom of the spring, looking for its place in the infinite chain of time, both already past and that which barely indicated the contours of its movement.

Darkness pulled Yeshua's glance down, and it began to pulsate in accord with this darkness in a steady rhythm with the opening chasm of space. The chasm called, beckoning to him, so Yeshua cautiously moved his consciousness into the depths of that open chasm. And the expanse, the chasm took him in.

It seemed to him for a brief instant that someone's image floated up from the dark rippling water and appeared on the surface, only to melt away into the depths, as if it were trying to pull Yeshua's glance in its trace. He didn't even have enough time to get frightened by how unusual the vision was, since the significance of what was happening was barely recorded in his consciousness.

67

When Yeshua inadvertently shut his eyes, exhausted by his previous exertion of will, a blindingly bright little star seem to explode before his inner eye. It lit up and stretched out into a pulsating horizontal line, which a moment later unfolded upward and downward into a white rectangular space, resembling a window into another world. A light, first small and tremulous, then growing increasingly brighter, turned on, its many colors moving to and fro in this window and gradually expanding. It was a beautiful, bright and luminous light, but the outlines of the dark mouth of the Corridor of Imaginary Time were visible as a barely perceptible turbulence in its very center. Its unconquerable force already captured the emanation of torturous anticipation, which Yeshua's consciousness was engaged in. As it tuned in to the emitted vibrations, this unstoppable force fragmented into a handful of shimmering light reflections and pulled into its endless black gut what only a moment before was a human being.

Yeshua felt this due to that imperceptible shift of consciousness from the external to the inner, which makes the body absent. Now he himself had to become light, so that he could become transferred, through the funereal summons of death, from the dusk of material space into the brilliant world beyond. And he entered Death, who silently allowed him to enter inside her.

He and Death became one. And for an instant Yeshua became aware of the weight of his incorporeity. However, this unpleasant sensation lasted only briefly, until the waves of fire awakened within Yeshua, and the mysterious external gravitation once again pulled him into the dark and narrow space of the Corridor.

Yeshua turned into something similar to a balloon filled with hot gas. His consciousness became painfully tense, and a kaleidoscope of images began to swirl within it with ever increasing clarity and distinctness. This procession of images grabbed him, pulling him into a chain of infinite transformations. Now he rose upward as a tree, trying to squeeze its roots deeper into the ground, and he felt the juices he was sucking in trickle down the tree's trunk and branches. Suddenly everything was transformed, and he became a lizard, lying motionless on a rock under the warm caressing sun. He then turned into a beast, following his pray through the heavy underbrush. All the nine states of the first minor circle of development were presented, successively alternating in his memory: man-plant, man-animal, man-beast; then sacrifice, provider and master; and, finally, man-knowledge, magician and saint. It was the entire cycle of transformation of energies at the transition to the all-encompassing universal level.

Once the transformations ended, he became clearly aware that a potential for a new state had grown out of their subtle interaction. He was enveloped by a brilliant transparent sphere and pushed out of the Corridor into the intermediate Bardo channel – an intersection of worlds where everything began and everything ended, from which came needs and desires, and toward which satisfaction was directed. The brilliant world accepted his body, which had become separated from the black flow of darkness, and it wrapped him in an enveloping wave of shimmering reflections of light.

Yeshua could feel that he was like a weightless, intricately moving snake, curling its body into pliable and mobile rings. He was keenly aware of his powerful energy essence and its saturation with unsteady, shifting vibrations of life and death, light and darkness, non-existence and immortality. He now possessed everything – wisdom and blind passion, the cure and the poison, God and the Devil. Knowledge, strength, deceit, sophistication, and cunning penetrated within each other, blending into a feeling that he was capable of every possible spiritual interpretation.

The vibrations grew stronger and became structured within the intersection of complicated interactions between the material and non-material space, information and energy, and the soul and consciousness, until they called forth a reciprocal reaction from the Bardo channel. Across from them, the clear image of a six-headed dragon appeared amidst the prominences of flares.

The guard of the Border was at the same time beautiful and awe-inspiring. His heads, resembling those of a huge alligator, were topped with bejeweled crowns. Each crown had an enormous diamond in its center, right above the Dragon's eyes – the stone of perfection, satisfying all wishes and allowing one to see the soul of things.

The precious stones on the crowns sparkled, and there were also shiny diamonds and rubies on the creature's glittering silvery gold scales and elongated crest. His powerful paws, with its nails ending in odd triple spikes, were trembling slightly. His muzzles spat out tongues of fire. The eyes, sunk deep in their sockets, were of indefinite color: his expression seemed to change all the time, depending on how low the creases of his massive leathery brows hung over his eyes.

A lightning speed revelation brought back all of Yeshua's former incarnations. He recalled that years ago, in the Golden Age of the ancient times, the Dragons of Light lived among humans, revealing knowledge to them and helping them to comprehend the purpose of man's evolution. These Dragons were called Masters of Wisdom. They taught people how to control their own energy, become masters of the elements, and work together with the gods and spirits. All this ended after the old continents and oceans were swallowed up in the chasm of the Earth, and new mountain chains appeared, where they had never been before.

No one could now ascend higher than the sixth Sefira of Tefiret – the

House of Jesus. The universe, divided between Light and Darkness, guarded its borders with the help of powerful and ferocious entities that obeyed only Cosmic Laws.

The six-headed Dragon was their master, and he was emblematic of the perfect balance between the two great forces of the Universe – the male and female. He was the embryo of two opposite sources contained in the circle of cyclic movement. He was also the ferocious Sentinel of the Border.

The Master of Dragons, whose name should not be pronounced, blocked the path, and no one had the right to continue on their way without special permission.

The pulsations of alarm, which were brought on by the appearance of the Master of Dragons, began to expand and spread around concern about all that was happening. The Dragon heard this. One of his middle heads bent over toward Yeshua. The black irises, surrounded by yellow sparks like those of a wolf, were hidden for an instant behind a whitish mucous film which dropped from under the creases above the dragon's eyebrows. When it lifted, the eyes of the Dragon emitted tiny, delicate blue rays which pierced through the stranger, and he felt secure inside his energy.

– Did that which was asleep, awaken? – Yeshua heard his inner voice.

– Yes, master, – it confirmed, also without words.

– I know that you were summoned, but I can't let you through.

– Why not?

– You have already merged with the egregore* of Jesus – the live God, but the Yidams within the Bardo channel and material space have not yet

*Egregor is a concept representing a thought-form or collective group mind, an autonomous psychic entity made up of the thoughts of a group of people and able to influence them.

71

recovered fully within you. The inter-dimensional transitions in the physical body could disrupt the program.

– Who has requested the program? – Yeshua asked.

– The system has, – the Dragon answered tersely.

– What is its ultimate goal?

– To conceive a child who has memory not only of the past but also of the future, in order to implement what has been predicted. Then the number six hundred sixty six will turn upside down and the double-headed Androgyne will arrive once again to separate Good from Evil.

– How am I to do that?

– Your spiritual vision will soon become activated. This will help you, – the Dragon responded, nodding his fire-spewing heads, which symbolized the twelve forces interacting between the two worlds, and determined the mutual impact between static and dynamic laws.

– What next?

– Hidden information, – the Dragon stated calmly, without any signs of irritation. – You will find out about your future after the complete merging with the egregore of the program.

– Cold you at least show me this future until the inter-dimensional transition?

– Here, look at it, – the Dragon agreed, and a large oval mirror materialized out of empty space.

Yeshua peered into the mirror, as its surface parted and fused with the frame, revealing new space, from which twelve glowing spheres emerged and surrounded.

Yeshua on different orbits. They then began to circle around him as though he was the center of their small dynamic system. Together with their movement, a melodious sound appeared and started growing in volume. Its vibrations pierced the stranger and brought about a synchronic sequence of pulsations, which blended into luminous circles of different color. These bright lights intertwined into complex patterns of secret symbols – voices of harmony. They appeared and disappeared, until the image of an ancient city spreading out across several hills emerged out of the delicate shades of the sounding colors.

Yeshua recognized this city; he saw its people and heard their voices. Desperation pierced his heart.

– The Church will consider the miracles I am about to perform to be the doing of the devil, – he lamented sadly. – Many clerics think that not only God the Father but the devil, too, has that kind of power to revive the dead.

– Then prove to them that you come from the Father, – the Dragon suggested.

– How?

– Through self sacrifice. The devil would never sacrifice himself – he only accepts sacrifices.

– You have snatched me out of nothingness, Abba, You may also take me back! – God-man shouted, raising his head.

A light breeze freed itself out of the ravine and brushed against Yeshua's sun-scorched face. Large white bubbles of gas swelled up at the bottom of the stream and burst loudly, splashing around tiny fountains of boiling water. Yeshua looked down and saw that all the grass and flowers around the water spring had darkened, and the petals had fallen to the ground.

Chapter 3

A year went by. Strange enough, despite the fact that the government did not give us any financial support, the situation at "KhudLit" began to improve. After a number of successful publishing ventures, the rational re-structuring of the company's internal economics and realization services, accounting and storage facilities, combined with the changes we introdu-ced in our relations with authors and literary agents, and our conservative estimation of our possibilities in the production of new books, our over-head expenses began to decrease continuously, whereas our profitability started to show tangible signs of growth.

The executive staff, which we were fortunate enough to assemble, played an important role in our successes. Sergei Genadiyevich Kolesni-kov came to us from "Prosvesheniye"* Publishing House and he was now my first deputy. I developed very good friendly relations with the editor-in-chief, Valeri Sergeyevich Modestov, and soon afterwards, Inara Bori-sovna Stepanova, who used to work for "KhudLit" before as accounting deputy head, returned to us from "Sovetsky Pisatel"** Publishing House, now in the capacity of head of accounting. Incidentally, many of the pu-blishing house's former employees who decided to quit during its former management, were now coming back. Almost all of them were losing mo-ney in the transition, but the strength of their desire to put the publishing house, in which they had invested so much hard work, back on its feet and their belief that it was now possible, were serious considerations in favor of their comeback.

* "Prosvesheniye" – the name of the publishers can be translated into English as "education."
** "Sovetsky Pisatel" – the name of this publishing house means "Soviet writer" in Russian.

"KhudLit" was no longer a "Titanic" being drawn into the vortex of nothingness. On the contrary, everyone who worked there was keenly aware of its good prospects. We were able to raise the salary for many of them, and people now had a positive feeling about the future. Mind you, they were, for the most part, the same people who were employed a year before when the publishing house was confidently approaching its inevitable demise.

"KhudLit" was no longer tumbling rapidly down. It floated, light as a feather, in the air, halting in one place occasionally, thanks to the almost invisible but already quite tangible upward streams of inner transformations, and, once in a while, it even soared up.

The media started to take notice – positively, I must say – of these welcome tendencies. Here is one such publication:

– Previous management left it a legacy of the most adverse circumstances. During the years of political and social stagnation "KhudLit" produced hundreds of titles of books annually; in the downcast 90s, they nevertheless produced 20 to 30 book titles, but in the second half of 1995 not a single book was published. The outstanding balance of the publishing house contains two billion rubles of debt and monthly fines.

The new management intends to continue the main directions of its publishing work, which was initiated by writer Maxim Gorky and implemented in different ways during different periods. "KhudLit" was envisaged as the guardian of world and classical Russian literature, everything that is the pride of our own and other nations' cultures.

We will never forget the unique collected works by a wide range of authors published by "KhudLit" and its series of poetry collections in one or two volumes. The publishing house is convinced that books of the highest quality are needed today; there are few such books on the market and there is a demand for them. The plan is to fulfill its obligations to subscribers and complete the much delayed publication of collected works by Heinrich Böll, Hoffmann, Fallada, Kuprin, Ehrenburg, Leonid Andreyev, Alexander Grin, George Sand, Graham Greene and others, all together about twenty multi-volume collections of belles-lettres ("Vitrina" magazine, 1996, issue 10).

Here is another quotation:

– A year ago, "Khudozhestvennaya Literatura" Publishing House was compared to the drowning "Titanic." The body of this giant of Soviet book publishing, managed by a strong but incompetent executive, received such damage in the tumultuous sea of the current Russian economy that it seemed to be doomed. Books with the logo of the famous publishers did not appear on the market for all of eight months. Nevertheless, a year later new books by the publishing house come our regularly, among them new volumes of collected works. The classics continue to be held in high esteem here. So how did such a miracle occur? ("Kuranty," 1997, issue 29).

I must admit that it gave me great pleasure to read such commentary, all the more so since similar materials came out pretty much regularly.

Could I ever imagine that one day I would head the famous "KhudLit" – and, even more, that I would join it during its most critical times in the role of a rescuer, or that I would become a well-known writer? No, I never had this kind of foresight. And yet, if I were to strain my memory…

There is a "legend" in my family, really more of an anecdotal memory, in which I am the main participant.

It happened in 1951. I was four years old at the time. The place where it all took place was quite a prosaic one: it was the communal kitchen.*

---

* Because of the shortage of residential space, most Soviet people lived in communal apartment in those years, housing several families, where they had a shared kitchen and bathroom facilities.

I remember walking into the kitchen when a few of our relatives and neighbors were there, but no one paid any attention to me. The adults were fully occupied with their daily chores. For some reason I very much wanted to be noticed at that moment. Yet no matter how loudly I sighed and puffed, no matter how much of a nuisance I made myself, getting in their way, they continued to ignore my presence. Then, grabbing the leg of a stool standing nearby, I dragged it to the center of the kitchen, which appeared huge to me at the time, climbed on top of this improvised "podium" and, bringing my little fist to my mouth and cupping it, I announced in a loud voice, though still failing to properly pronounce some of the letters: – *Attention! Attention! I, joulnalist Alkady Petlov, will now lead my poems...*

Of course, at that time I hadn't written any poems and couldn't have, but already then I felt a certain inner rhythm within me which sought expression, and that is why, imitating what I saw grownups do, I made a clip-clop sound with my tongue right into my clenched fist, the "microphone," straightened my shirt solemnly, bowed to the "esteemed public," and then dropped to my knees and cautiously climbed down from the stool onto the floor.

Where, from what future, did this child get the strange urge to play the role of a man of letters, or, to be more precise, the strange hybrid role of a "poet-joulnalist?" The odd thing is that this was exactly what happened years later...

Not everyone has a sense of rhythm, a good ear for music or a proclivity for art, toward seeing the world as a pictorial and coloristic vision. As they say, this is a gift from God. A gift such as that is like money – you either have it or you don't! Everything here is as clear as day. But climbing on top of a stool ... you need to have guts for something like that; after all, you could easily fall down and hurt yourself, and what's worse, eve-

77

ryone would see you falling… However, going back to this naïve "family legend," I can assert with confidence that already as a young child I knew my calling in life. And any new endeavor, any new beginning, always entails risk, to some extent.

I was always carried forward on the waves of fate. Whether I wanted to or not, I somehow always seemed to be turned in the direction Providence had in mind for me, where the vocation chosen for me by someone from above awaited me. Say, my mother, ignoring the fateful prompting she heard in the kitchen, arrived at the decision to enroll me at a chemical-technological college. What next? Strength of materials – it entered in one ear and straight out the other – my hand was jotting down poems instead of taking down notes at the lecture… I dropped out of college during the third year.

After my military service, where I grew quite proficient at weaving rhymes, I decided that this was the right time to pursue a career at a newspaper. For some reason, I thought that all poets were employed either at newspapers or at magazines. I will never forget the mute amazement of Oleg Alekseyevich Vavilkin, the editor at the Balashikha city newspaper "Znamya Kommunisma,"* when in response to his question: "What skills do you have?" I responded by saying quite innocently, "I write poetry!"

Oleg Alexeyevich literally roared: "I am ready to exchange four poets for one journalist without a moment's delay!" That is how I learned that a poet and a journalist were not one and the same thing.

Still, in the end I did become a journalist.

It actually happened the very next day. Oleg Alexeyevich gave me an assignment to write an article immediately, which was a pedagogical move on his part, I now assume. And he gave me a topic to write about.

* "Znamya Kommunisma" – the name of the newspaper means "banner of communism" in Russian.

I spent the evening urgently gathering relevant information, and the following morning I handed in the article. As he read it, Oleg Alexeyevich occasionally crossed out words and wrote his own suggestions on top. I instantly lost all confidence in myself and grew very sad. By the time he was through making the corrections, I had become quite ashamed of myself. So I stood up, apologized and walked to the door, completely dispirited. The sound of Vavilkin's voice stopped me. "And here's how my co-workers write, graduates of the Moscow University!" he cried out, showing me pages of text that were entirely crossed out and then totally rewritten by the editor. Oleg Alexeyevich was my first mentor in journalism. It was he who later gave me a recommendation when I applied for membership at the Journalists' Union.

Nevertheless, "You can lead a horse to water, but you can't make it drink," as the shrewd Yankees say...

Our country has entered new times, as for me, I have taken on a new burden. Is that it?

What's with those strange reminiscences about events that took place two thousand years ago and were allegorically so closely intertwined with my concerns about the present? Then again, this strange man, Lapin, indeed, so very strange... What does it mean? Why? What was the moral behind these recollections?

* * *

When the screen of our inner vision is opened, it reveals another world, which is always near us but we fail to see or notice it. We are no different from Geppetto, Pinocchio's father, who had no idea that there was a secret door into a wondrous land hidden behind the cloth with the painted

79

(unreal!) fireplace on the wall of his little house. It is not surprising that being just as curious as Pinocchio, I began to actively search for conventional scientific proof of those phenomena, which so unexpectedly and forcefully burst into my life – the life of a common person. I discovered, not without amazement, that hundreds of labs, university departments, academic institutions and special services of different countries were actively engaged in developing theories that would explain the accumulated factual instances of clairvoyance, telepathy, levitation, teleportation and extra-sensory perception. Some written material about such phenomena was also available in print, and I, too, had some knowledge of these facts. But in my specific case, that is, during contact with the bio-computer, the phenomena that shock the imagination of an average man were displayed merely as facets of possibilities of some amazing instrument of the unknowable noumenal world. The bio-computer was capable of performing miracles, in retail or wholesale, as they say, and that was not all. It turned out that all famous psychics, clairvoyants and prophets fully relied on how wide this remarkable masterpiece of subtle technologies opened up its unlimited possibilities before them.

I wasn't aware at the time that the degree to which the bio-computer is connected to this or that program is directly linked to the accomplishments of each individual along the path of evolution within the chain of successive incarnations at the earthly plane of being. Nor did I know that the finishing line for this race was already quite near: it was indicated by a number, or, rather, a date in a regular calendar. The last day of year zero, the millennium year, i.e., the year of change – that was the visible boundary line, which cut off the departing world from the newly emerging one – the cosmic age of mankind.

Truthfully speaking, not everyone will be able to cross that boundary line. Many will have to continue their path along the spiral in the old conditions, where cause and effect is rigidly regulated by the law of karma: if you wished trouble upon your neighbor, expect trouble to pay you a visit; if you dug a hole for somebody else, you yourself will fall into it. If you did something bad or nurtured evil thoughts in your head, it shouldn't surprise you if your health suddenly deteriorates and you develop chest pains or liver problems.

It does happen that bad karma strikes with its wand of destiny not the guilty person but a member of his or her family: a son, daughter, mother or father. People have long been complaining about the unfairness of destiny. For instance, the Belarusan writer Vasili Bykov, perhaps the best author of books about a people at war, ends his novel "The Quarry" with the following bitter complaint: "One has to pay for everything – for the good and for the bad, which are so closely interwoven in this life, but the issue remains: who must pay? In the end, the person who pays is, of course, the one who is least to blame, who never expects to be the winner, who is destined from birth to give, unlike those who have learned only to take from others and to demand as by virtue of a right."

What can I say, that is also true. But this is our human truth here on earth. We don't know what our Lord, our Father, thinks about it and what His plan is in this regard. That is why each of us should carry his cross with dignity. After all, when Jesus was a man He, too, complained that He was forsaken by the Father and deprived of His grace.

So what does science say on this score, how does it explain the miracles that take place right next to us – miracles, which we ignore for the most part, considering them to be insufficiently reliable or unconfirmed by scientific and technical means of registration. The latter, incidentally, though it is the most widespread demand in determining the veracity of a

81

phenomenon, is also the most absurd. Just imagine what would happen if some Daedalus tried to convince the citizens of ancient Rome that it was possible to create a flying machine out of iron and soar into the sky in it. No doubt someone like the Soviet era Academician Kruglyakov would have immediately accused him of displaying pseudoscientific mentality and would have urged establishing a committee, demanding the death sentence to the culprit. And he would be right in a way, because the laws of physics that said this was possible hadn't been discovered yet. Someone like Kruglyakov is incapable of discovering these laws and, consequently, he demands that whoever dares to cross the threshold of his personal ignorance be put to death.

In order to explain these phenomena, which have recently been witnessed more frequently, new laws of physics must be discovered and an interpretation must be found for the new forms of the transfer of energy and information.

No doubt, these discoveries will strike yet another blow to the half-ruined building of the classical vision of the universe. No doubt, they will undermine the prestige of a number of highly respected scientists. What's new? The mechanistic picture of the world has over the past hundred years been gradually reduced until it became merely a fact of history, dragging behind it vulgar materialism, Darwinism and other "isms." We must admit that primitive idealism is also becoming a fact of history. The central question of philosophy: what is primary, matter or consciousness, has lost all meaning. Let me, once again, quote the selfsame Carl Jung.

"Both these opposing concepts – the materialistic and spiritualistic ones – are no more than metaphysical prejudices. The hypothesis according to which any living matter possesses a psychic aspect, whereas psychic substances possess a physical aspect corresponds to obtained experimental data much better. If, however, we pay para-psychological data the attention it deserves, we will be forced to develop a hypothesis asserting that the psychic aspect reaches beyond biophysical processes in living nature and to expand it to all matter, including non-living matter. From the standpoint of this hypothesis, being is based on a certain substrate, which has of now not been identified, that possesses both material and psychic qualities."

As for science gurus, it's impossible to carry the torch of truth without setting someone's beard on fire, as they say. It's the same in science as everywhere else: "For every one with a plow, there are seven with a spoon." Don't you remember that some twenty years ago, every fourth scientist in the world came from the Soviet Union? Everybody knows exactly what these scientists were working on and what kinds of fruit they were giving to the people who gave them their bread and butter.

Yes, of course, facts are the oxygen of science. A scientist's honesty lies in his dedication to finding rational explanations to phenomena. But once a phenomenon manifests itself, one shouldn't hide from it – one should study and try to comprehend such a phenomenon.

I must admit that despite all this denial, some things were being done.

Lapshin told me the truth in our first conversation: the Soviet Union was, indeed, a world leader not only in the research of extra-sensory processes but in its achievements in the field of bio-informational technologies, with which most people weren't even familiar.

The sensational discoveries made by the Russian Chinese Dr. Tszyan Kanchzhen, outlined in his work "Theory of Field Control" attracted the attention of the science section of the Communist Party Central Committee years ago and were classified as top secret. Dr. Kanchzhen determined that "DNA is not simply a 'cassette' with recorded data; its material carri-

83

ers are bioelectric signals." In other words, the electromagnetic field and DNA comprise a combined genetic material, which exists in two forms: the passive one – the DNA and the active one – the electromagnetic field. The first stores the genetic code, which ensures the stability of the body. The second, however, is capable of altering it. This can be accomplished through the impact of bio-electromagnetic signals, which contain energy and information simultaneously.

Dr. Tszyan Kanchzhen brilliantly confirmed his theory in practice, creating a device, which could read the information from the DNA of one living object and direct it toward another. This resulted in changes that could be pre-planned. For instance, following the distance effect of the bio-field of the green mass of wheat upon the germinated seeds of corn, peculiar ears with grains similar to both corn and wheat developed in place of panicle formation. These new characteristics were preserved in several generations, in other words, they were genetically transmitted. The bio-field of a melon influenced the germinated seeds of a cucumber, as a result of which the cucumbers tasted like a melon and their DNA, the foundation of the genotype, underwent a change. The influence of a duck's bio-field on chicken eggs led to chicks developing membranes on their feet. Their heads became flat and their eyes changed their shape. The impact of the bio-field of young green shoots of various herbs on a person resulted in changes in hair color (grey hair disappeared) and hair structure. Subjects participating in the experiment began to look more youthful. Their health, specifically their immune system, showed signs of improvement.

Thus, for the first time it was experimentally proved that extrasensory influence is an extremely powerful and effective tool in an area where world science had until now achieved only minor results.

Dr. Tszyan Kanchzhen's works have been patented and are essentially the first to have made a serious dent in the credibility of numerous orthodox deniers of the psychophysical makeup of reality. Until then traditional science considered the hypothesis about the active participation of the mind and consciousness in the processes under research to be an absurdity. The thought process was viewed merely as a sequence of neurophysiological reactions that could not have any original, primary energy, i.e., any energy acting in advance of such neuro-physiological reactions.

If that were true, how could we explain the abilities of the famous Israeli psychic Uri Geller? Through willpower and the strength of his mind he was able to erase the data recorded on computer diskettes. During a television interview, he demonstrated his ability to bend spoons and forks in the homes of TV viewers located hundreds or even thousands of miles away from the studio. Viewers in Britain, France and the USA were able to watch the program where he demonstrated his abilities.

I was engaged in a polemic regarding this phenomenon with the Vice President of the Russian Academy of Sciences, Yevgeny Pavlovich Velikhov. During the TV show "Good Day" he listened to my comments about the abilities demonstrated by Uri Geller. In response, he smirked and stated that the famous American magician James Randi had exposed Geller, proving his so-called psychic powers to be nothing but trickery. This denouncement, however, failed to elaborate on how Geller was able to learn his magic tricks.

It is true that such accusations actually took place, but this story also had a continuation. Top American scientists, who participated in Geller's experiments, publicly censured Randi, pointing out the difference between magic techniques on the stage and the research conducted by physicists in scientific studies. There was a trial and Uri Geller won the case. Yevgeny Pavlovich was either unfamiliar with these developments or preferred to ignore the facts.

Similar half-truths, concealment or outright falsification are used against the most celebrated healers. The European Health Association – quite a traditional institution! – initiated a study of certain psychics from the Philippines who performed extremely complex operations, including cancer surgery, without the knife. The authenticity of the phenomenon and the effectiveness of this unusual treatment method were reported in voluminous documents. There was also a chapter in the published conclusions of the commission, which exposed charlatans who are invariably attracted to any sensational and lucrative business. It was precisely this chapter, which was immediately picked up on the pages of the Russian media, with "helpful" prompting from a number of officials from the Russian Academy of Sciences. What can I say, "à la guerre comme à la guerre" – all is fair in love and war. God forbid that before long we may not need any surgeons, therapists or drugs!

Let us, however, return to Russian psychics.

In the meantime, Professor Yuri Petrovich Pytyev, who has a PhD in physics and mathematics, was conducting research involving experts who had undergone training at our Academy and were able to "see" with their eyes closed.

Professor Pytyev proved that a mysterious radiation was being emitted during extrasensory perception of an object, which is a process operating at the millimeter wave scale. While this happens, the sources of the radiation are located outside the psychic's head (similar to virtual "eyes").

As for perception itself, in his experiments with a diffraction grid the scientist determined the following: perception resembles a holographic process. Incidentally, the wave nature of this phenomenon was tested with the help of the Fresnel zone plate, which acted as a collecting lens in this range of wavelengths.

The closest analogy would be echolocation (acoustic location, acoustic sight) in bats and dolphins. They emit ultrasonic sounds that are scattered among surrounding objects and then listen to the echoes of those sounds with the help of acoustic receptors.

Pytyev rightly concluded that consciousness is responsible for the interpretation of both extrasensory and visual perception: "We have to assume that it (consciousness – Trans. note) is simply not sufficiently trained in most psychics to interpret extrasensory information as visual. For instance, when they bring their hand close to a magnet with their eyes shut, psychics can feel the 'heat' or the 'cold' but they aren't able to 'see' them.

As a physicist I can only believe in phenomena that can be registered with a device. So the fact that we were able to establish the close link between extrasensory perception and electro-dynamic processes is extremely vital."

Pytyev was not the only scientist who conducted serious research of the mysterious phenomenon. Publications about the activities of our Academy, which regularly appeared in the press, prompted the head of the Laboratory for Brain Research at the research institute for traditional treatment methods at Russia's Health Ministry, Olga Ivanovna Koyokina, to engage in a series of experiments on the remote bio-energetic interaction between the brain of the operator (healer) and recipient (patient). This interaction was expressed every time in the synchronization of the bio-potentials which characterize a specific part of the operator's and recipient's brain. It was suggested to view this new reality as the virtual brain, which functions due to the activity of various parts of the operators' and recipients' brain.

Similar results were also obtained in other countries. In Sweden, one of the most eminent experts on cancer, Bjorn Nordenstrom, used the subtle energy of the body in the treatment of malignant tumors. Nordenstrom directed resonant frequencies of subtle energy at cancer cells, which resulted in their transformation into healthy cells.

The virtual eyes registered by Professor Pityev and the virtual brain discovered by Master of Medicine Olga Koyokina are anything but routine events commonly discovered in science research. They can be likened to Archimedes' Lever, with which it is possible to quite literally "move the world!" The scope of knowledge that people will obtain by developing these discoveries will become a power of global significance.

Many TV programs have already demonstrated people who can see with their eyes closed and can read books with the help of alternative vision or the screen of inner vision. Experts are often invited to participate in such shows – well-known scientists or prominent specialists in their respective fields. There is only one drawback to an otherwise good idea: these individuals encounter the phenomenon, which they have been invited to comment on, for the first time during the show. Not surprisingly, their observations always lead them to the banal conclusion: "I bet they're peeping through a tiny hole..."

In general, I firmly believe that a genuine scientist shouldn't express his opinion publicly, to show off on the TV screen, unless he has studied the issue in depth and conducted all the necessary research. I see as a model of scientific integrity the position taken on this particular issue by Academician Natalya Petrovna Bekhtereva, a world renowned expert in the field of neurophysiology, USSR State Prize Winner and director of the Institute of the Human Brain. In one of her interviews about a TV program, which showed that children who were blind could instead receive another, alternative vision, she stated the following: "The demonstration was convincing. These children read texts from randomly selected books, rode bicycles, carefully avoiding obstacles in their way, and performed other acts, which usually presupposed the presence of normal vision.

When I spoke to an expert who is well known in circles associated with extrasensory perception, he told me: 'I saw it myself – they were peeking.'

But I was also watching closely. No, they weren't peeking. (Information Bulletin 'The Beginning,' issue 2)."

After that Natalya Petrovna did what others should have done before her: she started a research program to study the strange phenomenon. For this purpose, she invited a number of well-respected experts with promising results in the discovery of alternative vision, and suggested that they continue their work together with a group of her specialists within the premises of the Institute of the Human Brain, to be followed by the registration of results with the help of special research equipment.

Larisa Pavlova, the daughter of one of the Institute employees, was chosen as a candidate. She had lost her sight at the age of six when attacked by a maniac, who pierced her eyes with a sharp-pointed awl, and she was now to demonstrate the discovery of alternative vision. Twenty years had passed since the horrible attack. Here is what Natalya Petrovna Bekhtereva wrote in the same information bulletin about the results of the research:

"The study uncovered a number of interesting facts (mechanisms), the most significant of which is the ease of using, during high visual load conditions, instead of one's usual vision, specially developed alternative vision, both with one's eyes open and closed. The brain can easily switch to this method of receiving information, perhaps a more effective one. The

results obtained emphasize the physiological foundation of the training in progress and of direct (alternative) vision."

This is an example of how a true scientist acts when in doubt. A scientist of such caliber undertakes an exploratory research study, and, as a result, with further help from intuition, makes a new discovery of world importance.

After all, it turns out that traces of extrasensory influences are recorded by research devices. Truth be told, I am personally very skeptical about the possibility of discovering the essence of such phenomena through traditional scientific research methods. The point is that the people who are engaged in such studies have an overdeveloped left hemisphere of the brain, which "speaks" for the brain as a whole. Such an overdeveloped left hemisphere has no interest in becoming equal with the right hemisphere, and it will not give up its privileged position without a fight. That is why it blocks the information arriving through the channel of intuition, and even if it allows it to enter the person's consciousness, it tries to cut off any knowledge about the theory of the phenomenon and its original source.

Even the famous Edgar Cayce, one of the most outstanding healers of the 20th century, knew nothing about the mechanism he used in his treatment. Entering into a self-induced trance, he diagnosed health problems of patients he had never seen and determined the course of treatment for thousands of people. Cayce had no medical degree and was frequently attacked by people representing the so-called medical circles, despite the fact that the commission of the American Society for Clinical Research, which had subjected to scrutiny 100 of his diagnoses, admitted that they were all correct.

Moreover, in six instances Cayce disproved the diagnoses reached by

90

medical professionals, who insisted on surgical intervention, and he actually protected these patients from undergoing unnecessary surgery.

The archives of medical institutions in the state of Virginia currently hold more than 9,000 medical case histories of Edgar Cayce's patients. They have all been reviewed, and the help which the healer provided was deemed to have been life-saving. Cayce did more than diagnose medical problems. He predicted the exact dates of the beginning and end of two world wars, the outcome of the battle at the Kursk Bulge and the collapse of fascism. Several months before his death he was able to "see" the disintegration of the Soviet Union.

People who acquire access to the bio-computer undergo a change in the nature of their thinking: they frequently begin to think in images, which is extremely efficient. This is associated, first and foremost, with changes in the right hemisphere of their brain. It is interesting that famous people who suffered a trauma to the right hemisphere couldn't find any original solutions in their field of work, even though they fully retained their ability to think logically. With the bio-computer, reality is reflected in artistic images, in all its multiple links and contradictions simultaneously. In this case, information doesn't have to be streamlined – in non-material space it remains close to its natural condition. The Universe thinks in images. By developing this ability in ourselves, we come closer to mutual understanding with the Universe...

Among the ruins of the cities of Sumer, the most ancient on earth, archeologists have discovered clay tablets with images of the solar system. The sequence of the planets, their position and the distance between them has been indicated absolutely correctly. No less than two thousand years of astronomic observations would be required to obtain such precise results. But archeologists insist that there was no developed civilization

91

capable of such observations two thousand years prior to the appearance of the Sumer people.

I find it necessary to specify that they are talking only about a developed technical civilization. The traditions of western science only allow for a strict linear interpretation of causality of events. Democritus could have never developed his atomic theory of the structure of matter either, in the absence of the complex equipment of physical labs, proceeding merely from the cause and effect historical suppositions. No doubt he had no electronic microscope at his disposal, and he therefore used some other method in his research. I am positive that the instrument used by Democritus and many other world geniuses was none other than the bio-computer.

The American physicist Heinz Pagels gave a clear description of the science community's conflicted attitudes on this subject: "The view of the new physics suggests: 'The vacuum is all of physics.' Everything that ever existed or can exist is already there in the nothingness of space ... that nothingness contains all being."

Once again we are being told that information is ahead of matter in its manifestation!

There is a well-known instance of prediction, which occurred on June 5, 1968, two months prior to the assassination of Robert Kennedy. Alan Wogan, who was studying synchronia at the Institute for Frontier Areas of Psychology at Freiburg University, had a sudden premonition that Robert Kennedy was going to be assassinated and that this event was part of a complex plot, which also involved the assassination of Martin Luther King. Alan Wogan sent a letter in the hopes that Kennedy would be warned. Probably the warning was not taken seriously, and it didn't save the lives of either the Attorney General or Martin Luther King. But shortly afterwards, the Central Premonitions Registry was established in the United States.

This is a perfect example of how an event that hasn't yet occurred displays itself in our reality long before it actually happens. And we are not talking about a single episode.

In 1981 the American neurophysiologist Roger Sperry received the Nobel Prize, among other things, for the discovery of how thought-forms within the mind develop "causal potency," a force, which initiates everything that takes place in a person's life. Sperry's research indicates that causal potency is created in the mind as a built-in bioelectrical system, similar to a high-volume capacitor battery. The more actively one charges such a "battery," the greater the amount of energy it produces, giving people the opportunity to personally influence events of the so-called objective reality. It may appear strange at first, but physicists know very well that a device with two 4.5 volt batteries may generate an energy impulse of 20 kilowatts of power. This shows that under certain conditions energy can become transformed from a latent to an apparent form.

It seems that man is himself involved in the anomalies of this world, and it is impossible to study these anomalies without taking into account the mind's influence on events.

Each thought activates molecule-carriers in the brain. This means that any thought impulse automatically turns into biological information. What if we deal not with the brain of a usual person, included in the average 3-4 percent, but with the brain which is capable of working at full capacity? The mind of such a person would be capable of contact with the mind of the planet, with cosmic consciousness. That is the ultimate goal: to bring the human brain to the level of the possibilities with which nature has endowed man.

The bio-computer is not a usual phenomenon. Unlike various technologies, which man uses to compensate for the difference between his desires and abilities, the bio-computer unquestionably has a mind and intellect of its own, and interaction with it is only possible with compromises being made by both sides. What is hidden behind this? Research is absolutely essential and very serious research. The only thing that we cannot afford is inaction.

Any household devices, from a TV set to an iron, are sources of electromagnetic radiation. In these circumstances bio-computers may frequently open spontaneously. When this happens, people become horrified and run to psychiatrists for help. However, shrinks, who don't have any, even elementary, knowledge in the area of super-conscious functions, prescribe them powerful drugs. This increases the numbers of mentally ill people and those suffering from drug addictions.

It would be impossible to stop the process which has begun. I actually suspect that computers and other "intelligent machines" are merely simulators given to people so that they can prepare themselves for work with material and non-material space through the bio-computer. In very much the same way, the magic flying carpet preceded the appearance of present-day flying machines, while seven-league boots presaged the appearance of land motor vehicles.

It is not so easy to study this phenomenon. For certain reasons associated with their age, adults can only rarely attain the maximum level of proficiency in their access to the bio-computer, which makes possible inter-dimensional communication with other planes of the Universe.

It is easier for children – they are open to contact with populated spaces of other worlds, and to do that they have absolutely no need for gigantic radio telescopes. Contact occurs spontaneously. Why does this happen? Children don't want to know. It would be the same as asking them how

94

they are able to see or hear.

They see with their eyes, hear with their ears and establish contact with the bio-computer – this is probably how children would explain people's make-up.

However, let's recall Kornei Chukovsky's wonderful book "From Two to Five." Why does this totally amazing advance in comprehending reality occur within a child at a particular age? Show me an adult who would be able to give me a convincing and well-substantiated explanation for this mass phenomenon. It is much easier to study a foreign language, learn how to swim and acquire numerous other skills at an age strictly determined by nature. The same is true of the bio-computer.

Jesus said, "Let the little children come to me…"

Sooner or later millions of people will learn how to use the bio-computer. And once again, we are faced with the age-old dilemma of the ethical aspect of these new abilities, of creating a culture which is oriented toward acquiring esoteric knowledge.

The world experience of the last centuries allows us to formulate the following thesis: higher energies require a higher level of morality. Regretfully, so far humanity has nothing to its credit in this respect. We see over and over again how new discoveries lead to their abuse. From gun powder to Chernobyl, from the homunculus in vitro to genetic engineering – there is no end of examples. Everyone agrees that computers are a great achievement, but they have already given birth to computer viruses, hackers obtaining illegal information for a profit, and new health problems.

Occult energies pose the same issues. From the pages of newspapers masters of white and black magic, healers and clairvoyants promise to "remove damage," "cast a love/lust spell on someone" and other such amazing results. How can we expect an ordinary reader to cut through pure hype and figure out where the light is and where the darkness? Even pop music has become psychedelic. Many performers use magic musical formulas discovered in pagan cults and insert satanic spells in their compositions.

About ten years ago Anatoly Kashpirovsky gained popularity through his TV lectures. He preached emphatically: "I set the guideline toward good! I give you only good!" The issue is what he understood as good? Did he feel the dialectics of good and evil; did he know that their polarity could change instantaneously; did he realize how relative these concepts were? The healer brings the patient's body organs to a normal state ... but what is the norm? And can the norm be the same for millions of viewers sitting in front of their TV screens, considering how different and unique each of them is? A psychic directly addresses the person's field structure, the source of the harmony of body and soul – he influences him through the person's subconscious self, which is why he should be aware of his special responsibility for his actions.

Psycho analytics have proved long ago that many neurotic responses are associated with deep, profound personal issues. To treat neuroses head-on would mean only exacerbating the original disease. This happens in medicine all the time, when physicians fight negative symptoms instead of the original cause of the problem. Moreover, health is connected not so much with a "healthy lifestyle" as with the overall cultural level of the person's view of the world. Physical diseases have an ethical meaning – every true person of faith understands this. So what is it that requires treatment: the disease of the flesh or moral depravity? At the same time, each of us can come up with examples of how a grave illness or congenital physical defect raised a person to a higher moral plane. In general, life can't be limited to middle-class obsession with physical comforts.

So what kind of "good" can psychics such as Kashpirovsky offer us? Unfortunately, all too often they can offer only a flawed perception, one conceived by them personally at the "level of their own depravity," and corresponding to their individual level of intellect. And this vision of "good" is fraught with such unexpected bouts of evil that it would have been better if they just left the person alone, with all his health issues.

Man's haughty arrogance is both dangerous and boundless. Knowing nothing at all about the psychophysical characteristics of our space and the Universe, about the impact of any thought, even the most insignificant one, on the dynamics and potential of events taking place in the world, man over and over again plunges himself and his fellow beings into a series of horrible, endless disasters.

Man fights injustice by increasing use of force, which ends in greater injustice. He tries to conquer nature, as the result of which there is no clean water, land and air left on earth. He is poisoned by the waste from the latest scientific technologies that are a source of pride for scientists. He fights against everyone who, like Jesus Christ, tries to bring humanity back into the Realm of Reason! This is accompanied by more hurricanes and more diseases. Man cringes helplessly, powerless in the face of the elemental forces of nature. Then – the heart-rending cry: "O Lord, why are You punishing us?"

It would be hopeless to expect that the secrets of nature will reveal themselves to cruel and aggressive people. Only secrets that increase violence and cruelty, which like a boomerang will come back to us sooner or later, reveal themselves to such people.

Chapter 4

The visions from biblical history and from an unusual life that I couldn't understand were apparently linked directly to what was going on in my usual day-today reality. Concerned and embarrassed, I was trying to put two and two together. I constantly recalled Orlov's ominous question: "What can you offer as security?" Perhaps my visions were actually "recollections of the future," a warning that fate was about to present me with a serious choice?

By then I was already convinced that we were, indeed, an inseparable part of some higher power, which people are accustomed to call the Creator for lack of reliable information or on a whim from this power. So we are a part of God, but which part? I recalled the ancient myths and legends I knew. Maybe we are His dream or His breath? Or, perhaps, a toy, with which He entertains Himself? A myriad of prophets living in different lands and centuries elucidated the complex relationship between Man and God each in their own way.

Until now I, personally, was a spontaneous materialist and atheist; in other words, I stood on the tested ground of the accomplishments of natural sciences. Of course, I found the Christian doctrine more to my liking and closer to my understanding of things: God is not just the Creator, but our Father. He is the Lord in the sense that He treats us as a father treats his son, and not as a slave-owner treats his slave. Hence, Love is equal to Truth, and there is Freedom of Choice and Grace, which is above the law. Clearly, the visions I am being "shown" are purely biblical, relating directly to the Passion of Christ. But who shows them to me? Could it be that God Himself has so little to do that he is willing to spend hours with me

98

personally? And if it isn't Him, who is it? What is the hierarchy up there?

At this point one issue was clear to me: every person has his calling, his own individual goal and his own role to play. And we are all being carried into the unknown by a stream of cause-and-effect interrelationships within an incomprehensible reality, which we are somehow able to perceive (individually and collectively).

Incidentally, this is not a novel idea. "As if goaded by the invisible spirits of time, the sun-steeds bear the light chariot of our destiny onward, and there is nothing we can do but grasp the reins with firm resolve, occasionally turning to the right or to the left, now steering the wheels away from the cliff, now away from the precipice. Where are we in such a hurry to arrive, who knows? Actually, only a few of us know even where they come from." These are the images Goethe used in his "Egmont" on the topic we are discussing. Other authors used different images.

So we hold the reins of our chariot, and we are, therefore, partially free to do whatever we please in this stream of life: we can completely lose our mind or do all we can to develop it; we can grieve or celebrate life, love or hate. Until a certain point, before the counter-positions of the subconscious become expressed, the world will remain the way we have created it. Only you shouldn't forget that, unlike us, God has many days… He can afford to make things, break them and then make them over again, seeking the kind of perfection only He knows. We, people, only get one chance to become co-creators of the Universe, instead of living the life of weak-willed, anemic "extras" – for this they need to know themselves. The sages said in ancient times: know yourself, and you will know the world. True, they also warned us that this was the most difficult thing of all.

But which of us ever took the trouble to engage in such a quest? As for the sages, those recognized bearers of truth, how many of them have really found it?

"Actually, only a few of us know where they come from." To speculate about the future, we must understand the past. Perhaps then the goal of the human race as a whole and the personal calling of each individual will become clearer to us. Hence, one of the most important tasks is to understand the origin of life, to discover the criteria for its appearance. All opinions on this issue are basically reduced to debates between evolutionists and advocates of creationism. The evolution theory is accepted by the majority of scientists, because they consider it to be the only plausible explanation for observed natural and social phenomena. Creationists, to the contrary, adhere to the concept that the entire world around us was created by a supernatural power, that is, God, and not over any lengthy period of development, but all at once, as a single design, over six biblical days of Creation.

I have two books in front of me. One belongs to the great science fiction writer Isaac Asimov and is called "In the Beginning." It is a comprehensive and multifaceted scientific exegesis of the biblical portrayal of how the world and man were created. Asimov (1920 - 1992), who was a biochemistry professor, called himself an atheist, but his work is not at all a hymn to absence of faith or the evolution theory. He was honest in his efforts to figure out the truth, and there must have been a reason why one of the editions of his book was published with the subtitle: "Science Faces God."

The second book I am referring to is "The Evidence for Creation." It was penned by three authors, two Canadians and an American. Both Canadians – G. S. McLean and his son Larry McLean – are pastors, while the American, Roger Oakland, is a biologist and former evolutionist, who had become an advocate of creationism as the result of research and reflection.

Both these books, written by people from such diverse backgrounds, share a similar respect for different viewpoints, and present an attempt to provide an in-depth analysis of all the existing evidence and proof. All four authors conscientiously seek the truth: it shouldn't be surprising that in many ways they arrive at the same arguments and conclusions.

Do all those who display an interest in these matters act that way? Unfortunately not... So many of them end up serving those they idolize, or overestimate themselves and refuse to recognize their limitations. So many don't seek the truth, but only victory in a dispute... They will never admit their limited knowledge, saying, "I don't know and don't understand it," and they only trust their own experience, which is why they will deny any reality outside their narrowly understood categories of space and time.

How much effort went into gathering, one by one, the grains of knowledge accumulated over the centuries, then compressing them into blocks of research trends and erecting the magnificent edifice of materialism! Well, "everyone steals from eternity, but eternity is there, like sand by the sea "(O. Mandelstam). And eternity has deceived these enthusiasts: it turned back into sand that which they created out of sand. In very much the same fashion, centuries ago, Orphic and Pythagorean doctrines were scattered into disparate phenomena, losing the cohesion of a millennium-long synthesis. Just as then, now, too, the features of the ancient Temple have become vaguely visible behind the ruins of collapsed structures.

The cycles of creation and destruction, birth and death consistently turn the giant spiral of cosmic genesis. And once again, human consciousness is being tormented by the selfsame agonizing questions: where does, what has happened, go to? Where does, what has come, appear from?

Where are the roots of what we call the future?

The future hasn't come to us yet but it already exists somewhere else. The super solid link between the consistent cause-and-effect transformations leads the incorporeal idea to its unavoidable materialization, not allowing it to deviate arbitrarily from Providence and Destiny. There were more than a few people in the history of man, who were capable of seeing what hasn't happened yet, – new beginning, events and destinies.

Perhaps there truly is a world where that which hasn't happened yet is already a reality, a world separated from us by an invisible boundary line, a well-guarded and inaccessible world? In it gods, magicians and dragons play around with the past, which hasn't disappeared, and they control the future, which hasn't yet arrived. The planets are toys for the entertainment of Superior Creatures. The destinies of nations are their self-delusion, their passions and dreams. And all of this taken together is the theater of immortal film directors, masters of virtual illusion, of indescribable Maya. Could it be that the One, Who acted out the mystery of His earthly existence under the name of Jesus, was trying to warn us about it?

He knew the past, predicted the future and saw what was distant across various obstacles and distances; he could treat the sick by the laying on of hands and return people back to life by the secret word. He could encourage the wretched by humility and strengthen the faint-hearted by hope; and He could show the blind a path toward transformation. What have we understood of the things, which He was trying to explain to us? Have any of us seen the light, to which we should strive? Perhaps these weren't miracles at all, but fundamental abilities inherent in each of us?

Twenty centuries have gone by, two millennia, yet we are still unable to comprehend that the greatest illusion of the Universe is the correspondence of conventional truths to the essence of occurring events. So let us try, one more time, to determine Being through Consciousness...

* * *

In the meantime, the affairs at the Academy were not bad at all. Producer Igor Shadkhan made a film about Lapshin (I was one of the screen writers). My book on the same subject came out simultaneously with the film, as well as a publication on the training methods used. The Academy was attracting an ever growing number of people. There they really acquired what they were looking for – health, optimism and faith in the future. Many were able to open access to their bio-computers. They unexpectedly found themselves in the position of people who had lived their lives without even realizing that they were born with tinted contact lenses on their eyes.

But now these lenses were removed, and they understood that without the tinted filter they were able to see the world in a totally different light. They realized that a person was capable of seeing much more than he ever thought possible. He is able to see even internal organs, cell processes and the aura, as well as the information damage that the aggressive environment inflicts upon it. What is more, a person can diagnose his own health problems and find treatment for them without the help of doctors.

During all this time I was seriously studying everything that might provide me with a clue toward understanding the Lapshin phenomenon in a scientific way. It puzzled me that the author of the method did not produce the impression of a well-educated man. At the same time any, even the most distinguished scientist, could only dream about the kind of results he was able to achieve.

Well, similar anomalies existed in history before. And the people, whose names have been inscribed in the annals of science, sometimes produced the impression of completely illiterate upstarts. On the other hand, everyone knows how many brilliantly educated people are capable only of speaking about things they have read or studied – they can really do little else. During a conversation with such a person you may marvel at his encyclopedic knowledge. But was he able to move even an inch beyond what he had learned from others? Have his life and his destiny added a page or even a phrase to the chronicle of Being?

Why am I bringing this up? The point I am trying to make is that there are different realities, including unidentified spiritual ones, which penetrate our consciousness mainly through the pineal gland and the right hemisphere of our brain, and which affect our lives. That is why some people "know," while others – "discern." But knowledge fluctuates: it is volatile and constantly needs verification; it can also be rejected and replaced by other knowledge... Whereas discernment is an irrational path, which leads us to the source of things, even to what existed before our time. Along this path one doesn't need to know anatomy to cure a person. It is enough to place oneself in the position of the Creator, and success will be yours. The question remains whether certain higher forces will allow us to take that position.

In reality, the vacuum, which means "emptiness" when translated from Latin, turns out to be not empty space at all but a certain informational environment that contains over 99 percent of the total information within the Universe. There is reason to assume that new knowledge appears as the product of the interaction between consciousness and what Vladimir Vernadsky called the noosphere (the sphere of reason) – the information field. One gets the impression that man is a psycho-physical object; he exists in the stream of form definitions between the micro-and macrocosm, and is both the object and subject of the transformation process.

Science, especially in areas of direct interaction between different fields, such as physics-chemistry, biology-genetics and computer science-psychology, is now beginning to accept a paradoxical paradigm, which would have been considered blasphemous heresy just yesterday: there is no impassable barrier between the material and the ideal; one can quite easily become transformed into the other. After the discovery of the bio-computer one can even assert that reason and thought, under certain conditions, become tangibly objectified in their direct impact on the environment. Mental and physical processes don't possess any real distinctions – they are merely different states of a whole. Mental impact on material objects is gradually acquiring the status of a scientific fact.

Here is what follows from the above: the world has psychophysical nature, and there is no physical world isolated from consciousness, nor can there be one. It is true that in the beginning was the Word. It is possible for nothing to create something. And virtual processes can create physical force. That is why I insist: man's mental and semiotic space presents not only a structured unity of personal, spiritual, emotional, social and historical experiences, imprinted in his mind and the environment with the help of a special holographic projection of objects, but also a subtle re-transformer of distant properties of any structure in the Cosmos and the physical vacuum. That is why the evolution of man must be viewed as a realization of the potentials that exist in nature as a given.

The issue of a scientific view of the world after the discovery of the bio-computer is no longer merely a philosophical question. It is a matter of humanity's survival and reflects the quest for an alternative path for its development.

These are the kinds of worldview issues we were trying to tackle at the Academy. We had assembled a fairly large group of experts in various fields, including a number of acclaimed scientists. We also organized conferences and symposiums. Nationally renowned academicians paid us casual visits to take a look at the "miracles" we were performing and improve their health along the way. The media regularly and consistently informed people about the Academy through newspaper and magazine articles and radio reviews. Igor Shadkhan's film, which I mentioned before, was shown on TV several times.

As it happens, there were occasional embarrassing incidents, rather comical from the standpoint of eternity. Here is one of them.

A close friend of mine found himself in a fix on account of the virtual world. He brought his young son for training at the Academy, and three weeks later the boy was able to open access to the bio-computer. He could now see what nobody else in the family could. He saw how and where his dad was spending his time, so he knew where to find him. Even if his father made a point of not telling anyone at home about his whereabouts, it didn't exclude the possibility that the phone would suddenly ring with alarming persistence at an apartment no one was supposed to know about, and his son would reproach him in an apprehensive voice: "It's getting very late. You've got to come home right now. Mom is crying and I'm waiting for you."

Now I understood the wisdom of another friend of mine, the well-known writer Yuri Polyakov, who said: "Of course, I would like my daughter Alina to have a bio-computer like that. But it would be so hard to bring her up if she can see right through me." In the end, he didn't overcome his reservations and decided not to sign up his daughter for training at the Academy. No, it wasn't the hesitation of a philistine – it was, indeed, a serious moral issue.

The situation in my friend's household was going from bad to worse. His family now knew every single step he took. This was a source of tension both to those who knew and the one they knew about. This wasn't the outcome he wanted. He thought originally that his son would help him to watch the others. But the child wasn't concerned about the "others," all he cared about was his dad. The boy was spying on him literally from morning till night, and he upbraided his father with childish straightforwardness every time he revealed any wrongdoing.

– What are we going to do now? – asked my friend. – It's killing me, what the little guy is doing! I don't know how to protect myself from him.

–You should open your own bio-computer and install a protection program, – I advised.

– Where am I going to find the time? I have fourteen plants to supervise. The lives of thousands of employees depend on whether I find new work projects or not. I've never had enough time left for myself my whole life.

My friend was feeling nervous and insecure. I was in a quandary. I didn't know how to help him. His son obviously had the upper hand in this battle of personalities, because he believed with the uncompromising position of a child that there is only one truth – the one he understands. The boy placed a taboo on anything that took his father away from the family, which, of course, turned the man's life into a nightmare. These goings-on made me recall the popular song about the wizard: "I tried to make a thunderstorm, but I made a goat instead…" The "goat" was bad news and threatened to gore my friend's married life to death. And I couldn't do anything about it because the bio-computer is more than new human capabilities. It gives one an entry ticket to another world, the dawn of which was already peeking through the fog of the upcoming year of the millennium. In that year, 1997, no one knew yet what the sun of the millennium was going to look like. Will it be the Sun of Light or the Sun of Darkness? No one could tell, not even the gods...

Slowly but surely, the Academy was receiving the reputation of some mysterious institution with wizards and sorcerers on its staff. This happened thanks to the hundreds of people who, after their training, became free of their diseases deemed incurable by physicians. Lapshin was not intimidated by this doubtful recognition. More than that, he promoted it with his regular lectures about making contact with otherworldly forms of existence. I listened to Vyacheslav Mikhailovich and tried to memorize what he was saying. At the same time I couldn't get rid of a deep-seated resentment against the portrait of the Universe, which he was trying to impose on his students and followers. God, the devil, the underworld and working with it – all this was both fascinatingly exotic and not particularly desirable as an orientation, which he was thrusting upon me. All the more so since I considered myself an atheist and regarded all these things as pure mythology. I didn't see how any of it could relate to the daily realities of our life.

True, Lapshin and I never got into an open confrontation. One of the reasons was that, contrary to his rash, rather tactless and boorish conduct with other people, with me he was quite considerate and cautious in his choice of words. And besides, the results spoke for themselves... I had to admit that the cures were real and not imaginary. I witnessed on numerous occasions how blind people, even those quite advanced in age, would suddenly cry out: "I can see! I can see!" Then they would navigate themselves accurately in a room where a moment before they stumbled helplessly, knocking down chairs.

Seeing such amazing results, I could tolerate my inner disagreement with Lapshin's view of the world and accept it as a kind of odd deviation of an otherwise highly honored master.

By that time Lapshin's methods were actually approaching world recognition. Films about him were shot in the Ukraine, Greece, Germany and France. Some time before, then First Lady Hillary Clinton found the time to visit Lapshin's center in Kiev during President Clinton's visit to the Ukraine.

A little boy with a huge bouquet of flowers came out to greet the important visitor. He walked across the large reception hall with tremendous difficulty. The medical establishment's recent verdict for this seven-year-old child, who suffered from cerebral palsy, had been life in a wheelchair. He was now able to walk, albeit with difficulty, across the hall, muttering something under his breath, and smiling happily. He reached Mrs. Clinton and presented her with the flowers. At this point, most of the people assembled in the hall had trouble holding back their tears.

The film shown a number of times on TV brought Lapshin even greater recognition. Those who watched it were amazed that a series of simple exercises helped blind people to develop alternative radar vision during the first stage in the training and to reacquire their ability to see with their own eyes during the second stage. This became a genuine sensation.

It was a true discovery for many that there are cells that can emit and receive electromagnetic waves in the bulb-shaped masses located in the back of the brain, called the thalamus, and that the use of this method of vision has a far better prospect in nature than the traditional use of eyes.

Thus, it didn't come as a surprise when Lapshin was invited to take part in a TV show. He was promised a slot of time for a brief presentation and was asked to bring over one of the children trained at the Academy, so that the child could demonstrate his ability to read when blindfolded.

109

I can't explain why but something alerted me in this upcoming TV demonstration. I had a vague feeling of something threatening or fake. I insistently advised Lapshin to use extreme caution and take along with him one of the blind children, instead of an ordinary, healthy kid, so that there remains no shadow of doubt regarding the reliability of the outcomes.

It turned out that my premonitions weren't wrong.

The TV show in which Lapshin was to participate was organized by a TV company named "Image." The show was called "On Trial," and it represented a dramatized tribunal of practicing healers, psychics, shamans and sorcerers. The organizers did their best to ensure that the staging of the show was consistent with their plan: there was a panel of jurors, lawyers, prosecutors and witnesses. There was even a judge wearing a mantle, though he needed occasional prompting as to what to say and when to pound his gavel.

Anyway, it was a trial like any other. There were those on trial and those who were charging them. And let's be honest – most normal people were apt to experience discomfort, watching plump girls with candles perform ballet steps around self-proclaimed magicians, who were trying to "remove their crown of celibacy," or who were advertising their homemade potions.

I was never a fan of exotic visionary artists who were willing to show their magic and tell fortunes about anything or claim they could treat every disease under the sun. That is why I perceived what was happening on stage as a person unrelated to the "action" taking place at the "trial."

At first, everything appeared to be pretty decent. Lapshin made his presentation trying, as was typical of him, in a manner not entirely intelligible for people who know nothing about the esoteric field, to explain something about the essence of his method. As always, very few people understood what he was saying. Everyone was waiting for a practical demonstration of his results.

Finally, a fourteen-year-old blind boy by the name of Alex came on stage. He had been legally blind since early childhood. Diagnosis: malformation of the optic nerve, retinal detachment and strabismus. In addition, he had developed a cataract in his right eye following a trauma during a bad fall. This was an essentially blind teenager, with his sad life story, which unfolded mainly at a special boarding school for the blind and visually impaired.

Alex walked to the witness stand. They brought him some pages with text from the judge's desk. And the boy tied a dark bandage over his eyes and started reading pretty fast. Then he was given another text to read – the result was the same. There was the kind of silence in the hall, which one only witnesses when people had just gained first-hand access to a miracle. It seemed one could hear the beating of hearts in this silence, and could even feel quite tangible waves of shock and amazement. I triumphed inwardly in anticipation of applause.

But then something strange happened. One of the organizers of the mock trial stood up and invited Mr. Nikonov, a correspondent from "Ogonyok" magazine, for a rebuttal.

A self-assured young man walked rapidly along the aisle, nearly pushing the perplexed child away from the witness stand, and loudly declared: "I'll now expose these charlatans."

Then he explained, unabashedly and clearly, how one could see fairly well, and read texts through the tiny holes in the fabric of the bandage without difficulty, after some training, of course.

– Wherever I appear, – Nikonov declaimed across the hall as a genuine showman, – miracles come to an end.

It was not news that one could read that way after some amount of training. Yuri Gorny was known to have shown similar tricks. But what did any of this have to do with Lapshin? His patients needed to apply a fabric bandage, when they used Radar vision, as a defense against external stimuli. It is used at the initial stage for attention and concentration during treatment for cerebral palsy in children, for diabetes and other pathologies.

Also, Alex was blind. The thought rushed through my mind: perhaps Nikonov would like to first poke the child's eyes out to demonstrate "purity" of the experiment, and only then give the boy texts to read?

Of course, I didn't say anything like that out loud. These were just my thoughts… In the meantime, there was a commotion in the hall, and everyone was stressed out.

Nikonov asked Alex to hand him the bandage and placed it over his eyes… Then he took a page with text and began to read it in a confident voice. Everyone in the hall jumped to their feet and started yelling. Pandemonium broke out. Those who were watching him didn't notice that Nikonov shifted the text to the right side before reading it. Even if they did, they wouldn't know what it signified. It meant that Nikonov was using the same technique of radar vision that Alex used before him. This is how virtually everyone, who succeeded in opening the screen of their inner vision, is able to see for at least the initial two or three years.

The young showman who was yearning for TV fame was not disconcerted either by the teenager's perplexed look, or the desperation of his father, who was trying to voice his objections amidst the wild disorder in the hall. During the intermission I spoke with Nikonov and tried to explain to him how unethical his conduct had been, but the young man openly stated that all he was interested in was the impression he made on the screen during the show. He didn't look at me during the conversation, and his eyes were roaming the hall in search of signs that would confirm his increased popularity. "This is just a show, nothing but a show." He tried to diminish the significance of his pre-planned actions.

No, it wasn't just a show! It was a serious effort to discredit a method, which could help thousands of hopelessly ill people get their health back. The cynicism of the accuser and his immorality clearly surpassed acceptable limits. There were, in addition, several children who recognized the young journalist as one of people they saw taking a training course based on Lapshin's method at the Moscow Institute of Steel and Alloys. This explained why Nikonov was able to freely read a text, which was held not in front of him but to the right side, close to his right ear. I have already mentioned that this is how people read at the beginning, after they've learned to use radar vision, where images are displaced by 60-90 degrees. If this assumption is true, what happened at the TV show was not just a stupid stunt demonstrating the journalist's spiritual callousness, but rather an act of utter depravity and, even worse, a premeditated one.

It was strange that the show organizers chose not to use an expert for their so-called "rebuttal" but a journalist, though there were more than a few professional physicians in the hall – people with an impeccable reputation – and also a number of distinguished scientists, who were personally acquainted with Lapshin himself and the children he had cured. They implored the company administrators in vain to give them the floor. They were told that this was impossible because the organizers had run out of film; besides, the Jupiter lamps had overheated dangerously and there was no more studio time left. Well, everything was going haywire! You know how often this happens...

I also tried to impress it upon the show director that such sensation seeking was quite unethical. It was all in vain. I didn't even recall that the operator who was filming this sham trial, said: "There's something wrong going on here. I had worked on a film script about Lapshin at the Tver Medical Academy. The people presented there were definitely blind, and they were really able to read."

The show was later aired on TV without Nikonov's fraudulent "rebuttal." What rescued the situation was that Alex was, in fact, blind. The organizers of the show didn't expect us to bring a genuinely blind child to participate in their "trial." They miscalculated, probably thinking that everybody around them were frauds just like them.

This episode brought Lapshin and me closer together. He began to show much greater warmth in his attitude to me. He also started to share more and became more trusting toward my ideas and projects.

I must say I was completely shocked by what I gradually learned. The world as portrayed by Lapshin, turned out to be quite a consistent and dynamic system. Apart from well-known esoteric structures, it contained certain details, which a stranger to this world could not know if he was studying it from available literary sources. As a professional in information systems, I was particularly intrigued by Lapshin's thoughts about the informational foundation of the Universe.

When we were alone in the evenings, he would offer me his perspective:

– Information is the designation of the form of space. Every person sees a book as a collection of some gathered information, which has been written down by the author; for me a book represents an inter-dimensional hole, which contains an assemblage of certain entities, and I am a shepherd for these entities, somehow or other. I know how to work with them. The books you currently have on your shelf can destroy whatever health you have left or, conversely, they can cure you. This is no joking matter. I'll explain the direction of it all: why this information is transported through us, why we are writing books, what in general is happening to this information, and how we are supposed to handle it. I will tell you my point of view, and how I work with this and I live with it.

He often referred to the Bible:

– The beginning lines of the Bible tell us that first there were Light and Darkness. God separated Light from Darkness. Few people pay attention to the appearance of the third component: there is Light, Darkness and something in between, a straight line separating the one from the other. Have you heard of the prophetic Yi Jing, the Chinese "Book of Changes"? Based on the "Book of Changes," hexagrams can have two types of lines: one solid and one broken. The broken line represents the interaction between two spaces: Light and Darkness. According to the symbols of numbers, the solid lines are being called "nines," whereas the broken lines are known as "sixes." In the first scenario, we are dealing with closed spaces that do not interact among themselves, while in the second scenario there is interaction between spaces, which eventually leads to a distortion of space in both realms. People have designated as information these forms of distortion and deformation of space.

You see, all the attention in the "Book of Changes" is focused on explaining the qualities and properties incorporated within the in-between state, the dividing line. If we were to examine this issue from a slightly different angle, we would find that it is nothing else than the technology of book magic. If you unfold this line, it will become transformed into a plane. This plane is being simulated in a variety of materials, which people use to write something down on, computer diskettes among them.

In other words, the first appearance of information is directly associated with the appearance of Light and Darkness. There are certain forms of distortion within the spaces of Light and Darkness. And there is a certain kind of information that has emerged as a product of the interaction between Light and Darkness, specifically within the in-between state. This in-between area is also known as Bardo, a Tibetan word denoting the intermediate space, where, according to information provided in the "Apocrypha of Ancient Christians," there are "the five trees of Paradise, which remain unchanged in the summer and winter, and do not shed their leaves. Anyone who knows them will be immune to death."

Lapshin usually accompanied his explanation with drawings.

– I am referring here to different structures, – he said, – specifically, the first, second and so on, although six lines are used to designate the structures of the in-between space. But one's focus should not be on the lines themselves but on the spaces between them. Manifestations of different information depend on how the split occurs between the spaces in this in-between area.

Let us review this in a simplified scenario. The space of Light, where we now are, is astrological space, in other words, the space of God the Son. The intangible, angelic space which is not astrological is the world of God the Father. The intermediate space is the world of the Holy Spirit. Information can either be presented in the form of space distorted in the direction of Light, i.e., the material world, or in the direction of Darkness, i.e., the intangible, non-material world.

– There are, therefore, three types of information, – he concluded, – that of the material, non-material (intangible) and intermediate Bardo world.

Lapshin then proceeded with technical details, which, as it turned out later, were quite close to what I myself experienced.

– The intermediate Bardo information (idea) is incorporated initially

116

on the left as a kind of virtual reality, a design (non-material, intangible space), and then it is transported to the right, to material space, for performance. It is similar to the way a drawing, after it is delivered to the factory shop, acquires the shape and functional properties of the finished product.

This is what the Universe looks like in Lapshin's interpretation. It has the one who places the order (who is he?), a design institute where his ideas are implemented into projects and drawings (the form), and there is also a plant where anything can be produced according to these drawings, including revolution, civil war, etc (when we talk about the human community). Or, quite the opposite, the result can be stability and prosperity.

Actually, if we were to thoroughly analyze history, we would see that at least two competing structures have the right to place the order, that is, select the idea. (Unless we admit their existence we won't get a truthful and coherent picture.) Thus, there are two universal corporations named "Light" and "Darkness." They are in constant competition to sell their respective products in the material space of the Universe. We, human beings, are the consumers at the first stage of the process. At the second stage, depending on whose products or services we chose to use, we ourselves are going to be consumed. Who will do that? It will be one of the two oldest and most highly respected corporations – "Light" or "Darkness." And all of it, taken together, is called basic informational interaction. Only very few of us are able to escape the sequence of repetitive spiral interrelationships between the material and non-material spaces.

Lapshin's words always produced a somewhat odd impression on me. I had the feeling that when he became focused in a certain way, some transmission device became activated within him and began to broadcast, through him, very complicated and sometimes even obscure presentations. At the same time, he clearly wasn't familiar even with basic physics

117

or basic medicine, areas where he attained spectacular results, making the achievements of venerable academics pale in comparison. As soon as this "broadcasting device" was switched off, he immediately reverted to being not just an ordinary, even a mediocre person, I would say. But he knew how to manipulate these "on" and "off" states, and very few people were aware of these strange qualities of his mind.

As a rule, I verified everything I heard from Lapshin, and occasionally discovered curious parallels in the world of "official" sciences, particularly physics.

At the Russian-American seminar "Vision of the Future" (St. Petersburg, 1993) physicists A.V. Moskovsly and I.V. Mirzalis presented a report, titled "Consciousness and the Physical World." In it they wrote: "If we literally follow the structure of quantum formalism, the whole world appears as if split into two. The first plane is a kind of quantum looking-glass land, where all the potentially possible conditions of the Universe exist simultaneously and interact among themselves, observing some unusual laws. The evolution of this world is described, for example, by the Schrodinger equation. So we can speak of a continuous stream of mutually interfering potential possibilities, 'virtual paths,' 'shadows,' 'clouds of probability' and so on – this series of metaphors could be continued, but the important point here lies in the paradoxical interaction, inconceivable in the classical world, of that which, sort of … doesn't exist. The second plane is the real, macroscopic world, the space of actual events, in which there is no room for uncertainty and ambiguity, and when this occasionally does occur, we explain it by our ignorance of what is actually happening in reality."

The position of American Eugene Wigner, winner of the Nobel Prize in Physics, seems even more radical. He thought that the final collapse of the quantum wave packet happened directly in the consciousness of the observer. Only human consciousness possesses the unique characteristic of being conscious of itself. It is like the screen in a movie theater, which makes it possible for the photons in the luminous flux of light to obtain a definite location in space, which they did not have prior to their interaction with it.

From this perspective, "the principle of reality" is contained in the plane of consciousness, not in the physical world. In the plane of Consciousness really, I should add. In other words, everything is exactly opposite to what we know from conventional cosmological theories: the physical is ephemeral, whereas mental processes are real.

A similarly radical approach is developed by Everett, who arrived at the conclusion that our world was not unique, but that there existed a myriad of equal copies. According to the scientist, our mind merely selects one of the many scenarios of the make-up of the world. In other words, it is not Matter that shapes Mind, but the other way around, Mind shapes Matter.

We will not divert into the analysis of assertions that the major factor in shaping the Universe is not its self-development, but the effect upon it of the intangible, non-material field of information. These kinds of broad philosophical concepts should clearly be actively and comprehensively discussed before any conclusions are made. But let us at least maintain for a starter that there are grounds for such a major change of emphasis, and substantial ones, too. As it turned out, the mysterious "emptiness" of vacuum in some inexplicable way captures information before it is expressed. Moreover, at the material level of Being, whatever the original source may have been, it is information that has become the determining force which creates new reality.

It's possible the whisper was born before the lips
And leaves were spiraling in treelessness,
And those to whom we dedicate our trials,
Their features acquired before we were tried.

(Osip Mandelstam)

The world is replete with intelligent devices and machines. The new information space is rapidly organizing and perfecting itself. It also acquires new intelligence that is free of its former excessive emotionality. Everywhere, man is becoming not so much the manager and administrator as the operator and user of global computer networks, which are beginning to have a more or less independent existence. People's spiritual aspirations, their moral quests, increasingly have diminished value in this anthropogenic world, and they are less able to influence society's vital decisions. The standardization of mass culture destroys individuality in the full sense of the word, and it stimulates mediocrity, everything commonplace and conventional.

The developed countries of the world have long since embarked on the path of building an information society, where development of new information technologies takes priority over creating energy or material goods. But the further they moved along this path, the more dependent they became upon their own creation.

The entire life of a modern society relies on the smooth operation of its infrastructures, the intensity of information exchange, and the completeness, timeliness and reliability of the data circulated via the computer and telecommunications systems. The point is that no one, not even the most highly qualified professional can evaluate a project proposed by an information super-system objectively without assistance from the super-system itself.

Due to the principle of distributed processing of information discovered by Academician E.V. Yevreinov, computer technology now operates at a combined rate surpassing the speed of light. And though computer speed for us, users, is different, this fact alone still means that it is basically impossible for Man (in the current situation, at the present stage of his development) to compete with the world of "intelligent machines" which he himself has created. The problem is that while we are engaged in learning, the knowledge we have acquired becomes hopelessly outdated.

Reading, repetition, and learning by heart at school ruins the most efficient type of memory in children – eidetic memory (more commonly known as photographic memory, – Transl. Note). The fact that intuitive thinking is far more efficient than logical thinking is being totally ignored.

Moreover, the illusory standards of what we consider to demonstrate a high level of education create an obstacle rather than developing people's intellect. Regretfully, these standards mainly teach one other people's thoughts, instead of teaching one how to think.

It appears that philosophers may be justified in their concerns, when they warned that the successes of technical sciences have created a situation where only that which is amenable to mathematical and technical modeling is being qualified as man's essence. This opens a new page in history: it is no longer man who creates technology after his own image, but, quite the other way around, modern technologies with their speed, high noise immunity and other functional advantages have begun to make their demands on the structure and functioning not just in reference to the individual, but even to society as a whole. Do we need such a page in history, I wonder? How can we, spiritual beings, respond to it?

Lapshin, however, did not ponder such subtle issues. And more and more often I felt that he and I were on different sides of the dividing line between Light and Darkness. Actually, at the time, I was mostly tormented by the metamorphosis of my consciousness.

It seemed as though my brain that had absorbed the new power lines of space and time coordinates, had decoded them and responded with these strange images of a re-created world. It remained only to muster the courage to find out what kind of world this was, and when exactly all this was happening?

* * *

Yeshua stopped by the threshold and directed a long, probing glance at the gathering of people awaiting him. Upon seeing the Rabbi, the owner of the house, Simon the Pharisee, rose from the bench, on which he had been reclining in the Roman tradition, and an amicable smile lit up his face. Simon considered himself to be a man of broad views and he liked everything that allowed others to see the genuineness and simplicity of his heart. Now, too, having invited this strange preacher from Nazareth into his home, he reserved for him a place of honor on the bench among the elite, next to the table, where the stranger could feel that he was an equal among equals.

— We were waiting for you, teacher, — thus he confirmed his invitation to the preacher, which he originally made through his servant. — Please take this seat by the table and partake of our meal with us.

When he spoke, his black beard sprinkled with grey hair was swinging up and down, as if he were at a sermon in the temple.

Taking off his sandals and leaving them beside the other shoes at the entrance, Yeshua crossed the threshold and halted on the thick, roughly made rug. When he saw that Simon was not going to step forward for a respectful greeting kiss, Yeshua said:

– Peace be with you, peace to your home and everything that is yours.

Simon bowed in response and answered with the conventional:

– God bless you. Come in, Rabbi.

There were several low painted tables in the spacious room, surrounded by low lounge benches. Each table had on it a large dish with rice and meat, lubban soup, and various fruit. Only one seat next to the bench of the owner of the house was vacant, and Yeshua walked to the designated table with his eyes cast down, realizing that his disciples were not going to be invited to partake of the food.

Despite the heat outdoors, the house made of hewn stone stayed fresh and cool. The room's open windows and doors overlooked a large terrace upholstered in wood that afforded a good view of the western shore of Lake Genisaret. The terrace, with its colonnades and cornices which were entwined with ivy, exuded the promise of rest and peace. Relaxing blissfully on their benches, the guests of Simon the Pharisee nodded their heads in greeting, accepting the man who was rumored to work miracles into their circle.

The new guest reclined on the seat set aside for him and looked around. None of the servants approached him with a basin and pitcher, so that he could wash his hands before the meal, no one made any effort to comply with the canon. Yeshua chuckled and sank his nimble fingers into the food, satisfying his hunger with considerable agility. All his movements spoke of his habit not to restrain himself with rules and rituals, and those gathered uttered a sigh of relief – this couldn't the Messiah, as the simple folk said, this was clearly a man.

The house gradually filled with more people. Simon's neighbors came rushing to his place after they heard that a preacher had arrived in Magdala. This rare opportunity to listen and argue was a real treat for them. They crowded by the walls, surrounding the benches of elite guests and pushing back the disciples who came together with the preacher.

There was nothing mysterious about the visitor, and, puzzled, they turned around to look at each other as though silently wondering: "Could this be the one spoken about?"

Sensing the thickening aura of doubt, the master of the house threw a respectful question at his guest, as sweet bait to his famous, highly reputed eloquence:

– There is testimony suggesting that you are an articulate speaker. Where have you learned this skill and acquired the gift to persuade people? It is a known fact that there is no Beth Midrash, or Beit Rabban in Nazareth, where you come from. Yet you can even write, though no one taught you that.

The preacher's head, with its hair divided by a clear parting, was bent over his platter with food. He now raised it slightly and turned his calm eyes to the one who was asking the question.

– My teacher is inside me. I know everything from him.

Glancing around himself in bewilderment, as if he were seeking witnesses, who would confirm that his guest was acting irrationally, Simon commented:

– What could speak within us, except for the voice of divine nature, from which all of us learn, and to whose call we all respond, when she summons us?

Yeshua turned a deaf ear to the banal flattery and looked closely at Simon.

– You aren't learning but stealing, – he said bluntly, without turning

his eyes away from his host's face that reddened with resentment at the insult. – You are stealing her form, without comprehending her essence. And the path of the man-beast, which you follow, illuminates for you only the light of the beast's circle. Soon it will be reflected in the heavenly mirror of God, and in it you will see what you are really like.

– You accuse us of not knowing the path of the Lord? – Simon said with astonishment, in the disgusted manner of a spiritually unblemished man, and he half-rose from his seat. – But we all know each other here, and every day we praise the Lord in our prayers and go to the temple to offer sacrifices and observe sacred laws. What, then, can you hold against us? – he asked in the tone of a man as spotless, as the Lord Himself.

But the wandering preacher was not embarrassed by his passionate rebuke. The shadow of harsh ridicule slipped across his face.

– Prayer doesn't need a temple, – he retorted sullenly. –Prayer needs a pure heart. And you are bringing your sacrifices to the priests rather than God. It is you who create these sacred laws to make it easier to propel people toward sin. Beware that you don't fall into this pit yourselves. "For out of the abundance of the heart his mouth speaks." Isn't this proverb justified for you?

– The mouth is created to speak, – a friend of Simon's remarked sarcastically. He was sitting to his left, almost opposite the preacher from Nazareth.

– Nothing that goes into a man's stomach can make him unclean. Rather, it is the evil that comes out of a man's heart that makes him unclean, – the strange guest rebuffed instantly, unmoved by the mockery. It was hard to deny that he was a skillful orator, and people's hearts were discomfited by the message of his words. – You worship God in the temple, – he continued, – and I worship the Father in spirit and in truth. For this

125

you don't need altars and ministers of the altar.

– Are you implying that we are blind and don't know the way? – Simon tried to clarify.

– Everything you see comes out of Darkness. Everything you hear comes out of Silence. If you are told to go east and you will go there, you will arrive in the west. If you are told that this is God's son, your response will be laughter. The one who understands that the crown grows out of the root – let him get to the root of things. God gives guidance, He doesn't command. He left man to the freedom of his own will.

– But who is the chosen one who can see God's guidance? – Simon shouted out in desperation, realizing that the eloquence of the traveling preacher overshadowed his own oratorical gift.

– Be like a child who runs into his mother's wide-spread arms, – Yeshua answered quietly, – and you will find the way.

A woman who was trying to make her way behind the backs of the men surrounding the tables suddenly attracted his attention. He could see not only her eyes focused on his face, her graceful movements, her thick curly hair and her lean, supple body inviting male gazes, but also the iridescent multi-colored glow around her that was invisible to ordinary people. Tremulous blue and orange rays escaped from the woman's head, radiant like precious stones, and slipped away through the beams in the ceiling. A small plaque made of a silvery metal with a name inscribed on it in gold shone on her forehead, but no one could see it but Yeshua. "Maria," – he read and recalled what was destined for him.

The woman was getting closer and closer. Upon noticing her, Simon's face contorted into a wry grimace. He frowned.

– Don't let her come near, – he suggested to his guest. – She will defile you.

126

His wicked hint didn't produce the slightest effect on the preacher. For a fleeting moment he turned his eyes way from the woman to take note of the sullen faces of the gathered men, and he then addressed her directly.

– Sit at my feet, woman, – Yeshua said calmly.

The woman's face lit up for an instant with a smile of happiness. She slipped past the people surrounding the tables with nimble grace, and lowered herself to the floor, staring askance at the features of the one who summoned her.

– Perhaps you are not aware of it, Rabbi, – Simon intervened again, – but this fallen woman is unworthy to be in our congregation. Her presence will defile us. What do you want with the likes of her?

– It isn't the healthy but those who are ill who need a doctor. And who but the Father knows who is worthy, and who isn't. – Yeshua turned to face Simon. – Don't begrudge yourself anything – neither good nor bad. In the earth – be earth, in the air – be air, in the water – be water, in the fire – be fire, but not a special part of them. Only in this way can purity be connected with purity.

He didn't speak loudly but everyone could hear him, particularly, the woman who was at his feet. Her face now grew red, now suddenly turned pale with excitement.

– Don't be afraid of anything, Mary, – Yeshua encouraged her. Murmurs of amazement rose from all around.

– How did he know her name?

– Do they perhaps know each other?

– He can really see the invisible!

Motionless, as if spellbound, Mary gazed at the preacher from Nazareth, until her strength abandoned her and she suddenly dropped her head upon his feet, wiping them with her hair as if he were a saint. At her

127

waist she had a small alabaster receptacle with holy ointment. She ripped it frantically off her belt, poured out the expensive ointment on her palm, and started rubbing it into the feet and legs of this strange man, who knew her name, though it was never mentioned to him.

From above he could only see the outlines of her cheeks and chin, and her lovely lips swollen from crying. With an uncertain smile, he began to unclasp her hands with such force that they turned white in those places where he squeezed them with his fingers.

Maria quieted down, without raising her head, and several hot tears fell on the preacher's feet. He was startled, and the trembling of his body was immediately conveyed to her. She looked up at him with such large suffering eyes that he couldn't restrain himself and patted her encouragingly on the cheek.

– This isn't a person, it's a weed. You shouldn't feel sorry for her, – Simon practically commanded, watching what was unfolding.

His eyes – two black, unyielding holes – projected contempt for the woman kneeling at the guest's feet.

– Our Heavenly Father is the Gardener, – the Nazarene responded, quietly again. – He wished nothing but beautiful flowers to grow in His garden. He took care of them and watered them. But the buds of many noble plants never opened anyway, because the flower, too, must want to be perfect and beautiful. It should soar on the wings of its dreams. If it doesn't want to, who is there to blame? It is necessary to pick out that which wants to be better, because everything in this world is accomplished not for the sake of the past, but for the sake of the future. God is the Gardener... But who knows what kind of plants may grow and branch out in that garden of His?

–You speak as if you know, – Simon admitted thoughtfully. – But what

do you know? Who is your teacher? Where is your path and the star ligh-
ting it up? Who can witness that you have not veered off the true road
to Our Father? Who can assure me that you are not walking toward the
abyss, blind man, pulling the others after you?

Yeshua's disciples exchanged concerned glances when they heard the-
se dangerous accusations.

– The Father Himself finds those who are looking for Him, – his guest
replied. – I came as a guest to your house, and you didn't give me any
water with which to wash my feet. But she washed my feet with her tears,
– Yeshua nodded toward Maria, – and she wiped them with her hair. You
gave me no welcome kiss, but she has never ceased kissing my feet ever
since she came here. You haven't anointed my head with oil, but this wo-
man has anointed my feet with the precious sacred ointment. I forgive her
many sins, because she has shown much love. Verily I say unto you – only
he will turn into Darkness, who doesn't become Light. Look for a way into
the Kingdom of God inside yourself and not outside. If you don't die here,
you won't die in heaven either.

The confidence in the Nazarene's voice undoubtedly produced a strong
impression. Simon, who never considered himself a devout orthodox belie-
ver, found special poetry and logic in his words, yet something within him
vehemently refused to recognize this shabbily dressed traveling preacher
as the great prophet, or Messiah, as many claimed. There was nothing
mysterious about him, though his speech was captivating. But there were
many others in Judea who could speak quite eloquently!

– If this world reflects a step toward the Kingdom of God, why then
is there so much suffering and injustice in it? – Maria, who continued to
kneel by Yeshua's feet, asked suddenly.

He turned his head toward her and asked:

– Doesn't a woman come to the joy of motherhood through suffering, and doesn't a child enter life through pain? How would it be possible to rejoice in the Kingdom of God without knowing agony on earth? How would one know then what is joy and what is suffering? How would one know the price of the gift? To receive – one must ask for it, to find – one must seek it, for the door to be opened – one must knock.

– We have heard that you raised someone from the dead at Nain. How can this be? – someone from the crowd asked.

– No one is dead for God until He Himself has destroyed the balance between the visible and the invisible. God is within each of us – and so is the Kingdom of God, as I have told you. And those who will not enter the Kingdom of God will be in the Kingdom of the Dead.

– But where is it? – Simon asked mistrustfully. By that time he was almost entirely convinced that the wandering preacher, who was so good at manipulating people, would become a good acquisition for the party of the Pharisees.

Yeshua looked closely into the eyes of his host, as if reading in them his secret thoughts, and replied:

– You asked: where is the Kingdom of the Dead? Don't you know it yourself, dead man?

– How can you tell that I'm dead? – Simon snickered.

– I can see it, – the preacher replied tersely.

– How can you see things that the light doesn't show us? With what eyes do you see them? – Simon continued sarcastically.

– One who is blessed can see without eyes. Look now...

The Nazarene reached down and pulled the shawl off Mary's shoulder.

He covered his eyes with the shawl and tied it at the back of his head. As soon as the darkness became pitch black, he ordered a bright white dot to arise from another space and made it open up in all directions. He could now see everything as though he wasn't blindfolded. Moreover, he could see not only in front of him but also to each side of him and behind him. He could now see what was taking place next to him, and that which was far away, that which was in the past and that which would happen in the future.

Yeshua rose from his seat and walked with a confident stride between the tables. When he approached the servant, who was standing by the door, holding a large dish with a tall pile of fruit, he pointed his finger at a big apple, and asked, turning to Simon:

– Would you like an apple? This is a beautiful one, look at how the sun browned its side? Or perhaps you would like me to give you this wonderful date?

With a confident movement of his hand, he raised the oblong fruit from the dish. The dazed expression on the faces of all those present betrayed complete astonishment. The servant who was holding the fruit began to shake. His lips drooped, and saliva slid to the floor from under them.

– Wipe the drool, – the Nazarene ordered him. – And stop shaking or you'll drop the dish. Perhaps I'll give Simon a grape instead of a date.

Without the slightest hesitation, his hand reached for a large cluster of grapes and tore off a single berry. He then returned to Simon's table in the same confident manner and handed him the yellow grape.

– Here, take it.

– You probably got a sneak peek, admit it? Or perhaps you have a good sense of touch? – Simon said, perplexed, taking the grape into his hand.

– Tell me, isn't the door invisible from where I am standing? – asked the Nazarene.

131

– Yes, it is, – confirmed Simon.

– Go out onto the terrace now. Look, your sister just picked up a sho-vel and is carrying it to the wall. She left it there by the chestnut tree.

Simon did as he was told and looked down into the yard. Terror show-ed on his face.

– You are truly an extraordinary person, – he moaned, acknowledging what he could no longer deny. – How did you do it?

– There is light within a person of light, and its rays illuminate the entire world. If it doesn't, then there is darkness...

The rest of the gathering also ran out onto the terrace, jumping out of their seats. Maria, who had once again kneeled at Yeshua's feet, embraced his knees, nestling her cheek up against them. At that moment, her face seemed almost childlike.

– Will you come with me? – Yeshua asked, and Maria nodded her head silently.

– I will also come with you, Rabbi, – Simon suddenly decided, turning toward the table.

– No, you can't, – the preacher from Nazareth retorted. – It is hard for someone who has lost his sight to find his way.

* * *

Is this a legend, a prophecy, or something else? But our students at the Academy could see the same things, governed by the same laws that were predicted two thousand years ago or maybe more than that.

In both the history of philosophy and the history of mankind there have always been two trends in interpreting the world and its organization that are constantly locked in struggle. One of them is idealistic: God created the world, and this is the only certainty we know. This trend is primarily defined by religion. The other says: No, the world appeared by accident (it "drifted off course" in space or what?). Then it began to develop on its own, to somehow acquire structure, and, therefore, matter is the only thing that exists. Well, what can I say? The first viewpoint is right, and so is the second. When we simultaneously have two correct assertions, it means the time is ripe to look for a third one – the Truth.

It would appear that both approaches form a cohesive whole. Neither can exist without the other. The creator and the creation appeared simultaneously.

When religion attempts to explain the idea of God's spontaneous generation, then it should examine the processes of the world's development as well, since one cannot exist without the other. They are, quite simply, different stages in the existence of a single living organism. After all, no one doubts that a head and a body make a whole. But they have different functions and entirely distinct features characterizing their existence.

Many scientists believe that in the living Cosmos the concept of non-life simply doesn't exist. Life and intellect are inherent in both material structures at the atomic and molecular levels and in subatomic particles lying beyond the space within our reach.

When Einstein destroyed the illusion of space and time, he did this not only in his imagination. Something very real happened – one of the "laws" of nature, considered absolute, was now gone. By eliminating linear time, Einstein also eliminated three-dimensional space. He pointed out that "at the very heart of reality, the concept of linear time fades away."

Thus, there is a reality where linear time does not exist. Some even maintain that this reality is timeless, meaning ETERNAL. That is how the concept of SUPERSPACE was introduced to modern physics, because linear dimensions lost their boundaries in ETERNITY.

How can this new world outlook influence our lives and specific life situations?

"Nature's omnipotence isn't oppressive to us because it gives the living a tangible sense of freedom," wrote Samuil Marshak.* In mechanics, the body's mobility is measured by degrees of freedom. "This sweet word – freedom" stirs up the masses in various corners of our planet. But to what extent does man really need freedom? As I reflected on this, I again ran into Lapshin.

---

* Samuil Marshak (1887 - 1964) was a Russian and Soviet writer, translator and children's poet. Among his Russian translations are William Shakespeare's sonnets, poems by William Blake and Robert Burns, and Rudyard Kipling's stories.

Chapter 5

As a rule Lapshin appeared in my office at the publishing house later in the day. He would sit down at a low end table, while I would take a seat opposite him. My receptionist Tamara Viktorovna Filatova, who was not particularly fond of my strange friend for some reason, nevertheless, placed a white tablecloth on the table at once, following the traditions of hospitality. She also brought a dish with cookies, and served tea or coffee.

He would drink the tea, rarely eating any cookies, and would at some point "switch on" his mysterious internal transmitter.

– Lesson number one: if you want to become god – do it.

– What is lesson number two?

– The soul of a man is a dyad. It consists of tangible and intangible radiation of the vacuum, which is its Organizing Force. But these forces are like ice and fire. Their interaction often ends in cataclysms. Biological life is a mechanism, which makes cooperation between two opposing forces possible; it is also a battlefield where primary forces try to overcome each other. This is why you must learn to control your emotions. The human mind is the intersecting point, or the point of assembly of subconscious and super-conscious processes. This point is our consciousness. If centripetal forces prevail – it will collapse. If centrifugal forces take the upper hand – it will dissolve into the infinite. Both extremes are dangerous if the mind doesn't become a kind of homeostasis of the two opposites. Most importantly, remember: there is nothing that cannot be produced by thought. For instance, we can look in all directions at once without turning our heads; we can pass through walls, and leave this world for the world beyond or the Bardo world.

– Why the Bardo?

– The Bardo world is an intermediate space tunnel. It is like an elevator between the floors, where every floor is a new world. If you are able to create Yidam in the Bardo, the program of immortality will begin to operate within you and you will become indestructible.

–Who is Yidam?

– Yidam is like a double into whom you can move when necessary.

– Will I be able to fly between the different worlds?

– Even on a broom, if you wish to.

– Why do we need to have such strange advantages?

– We need it to conquer the world.

– Wow, so your goal is to control the planet, – I laughed.

He quickly turned his head and looked directly at me with a piercing gaze.

– If we stick together, it will be easy to take over the world. I have all the necessary knowledge to do so. You have no idea what mighty forces support me. I have control over billions of dollars. I can influence events and turn them in the direction we need.

– Why do you need me for all that? You are a magician but I am an ordinary man. What is the purpose of such a union? It's like an elephant in partnership with an ant.

– You know nothing about yourself, – he continued in a serious voice. – You possess the most powerful magic of all – the magic of the Word. Don't you remember: God laid His hands on a book? Not on the globe of the Earth and not on a sword – He laid His hands on a book.

– Look here, at this sheet of paper. – He picked up a sheet of paper from my table to the side of him, pulled out a pen and made a hole in it. – You saw me making a hole. I simulated space that is being pulled apart.

136

What happens when this occurs? The field structure of the sheet of paper changes. Now, streams move up and down through this hole. It seems so insignificant – all I did was pierce a sheet of paper and make a hole. In fact, we now have a most powerful generator. Small things can a make tremendous difference. As the saying goes, "The pen is mightier than the sword."

I could write some symbol or spell here, creating a thought form – and the object would take on entirely different characteristics. A powerful tunnel junction will appear; there will be contacts with outer space and interactions that are even impossible to imagine. This technology is used by demons to trick people into wars or any other desired action.

– So we pierce a hole in a piece of paper, and what then? – I asked ironically.

– To begin with, we'll gain control. It's not as hard to capture power as one might think. We'll give the orders around here in any way we see fit.

– Why don't you do it alone then?

– I need you, – he replied seriously or in jest.

– I have other things on my mind right now. – I politely declined the honor of capturing power in the country. – I'm being shown such things through the bio-computer that I'm ready to run to church.

– But you aren't a believer.

– I've actually become somewhat of a believer lately. The pictures I'm being shown are far too convincing...

He picked up his cup, lazily drank its contents and asked, as if it didn't much matter to him:

– So what are they showing you?

– The story of Christ.

Lapshin grew visibly tense.

137

– Could you elaborate?

I described to him the latest images of the mystery and saw a look of growing alienation in his eyes.

– When nothing changes, it's the same old, same old. The gods created humans and humans created gods, and now they don't know what to do with each other. Why did you get involved in all this stuff?

– It wasn't really me …

I could tell that something wrong was going on with Lapin.

– How long have they been showing you this movie?

– Something like two years.

– Why didn't you say anything to me?

– I didn't think you'd find it interesting.

– You and that Christ of yours! That's when things hit the fan, – Vyacheslav frowned. – Not even a good shower will get us clean now.

I didn't understand what he was talking about. I thought it was just a joke, so I smiled.

* * *

I have a new gift now – the gift of a visionary. Several months before the August 1998 default in Russia, I saw a dream about all the upcoming events associated with the imminent crisis and the overall economic situation arising from it. Moreover, the specific measures that had to be undertaken by "KhudLit" to prevent its basically unavoidable demise, also suddenly became clear to me.

I immediately summoned the entire staff to a general meeting. Of course, I didn't do it to tell them about my dreams. I simply presented a literally month by month analysis of how the events were going to unfold all the way to September and told them the plan of how we could, in my view, counteract the increasingly negative factors in the country's economy.

The things I told them left the staff dumbfounded. On the surface, everything seemed to be the other way round. The new administration headed by Kiriyenko produced the impression of being a team of qualified experts, confident in themselves and the economic strategy they had proposed. The media, including comments by TV gurus, were overflowing with rosy expectations, whereas I was suggesting that we should cut our foreign programs, immediately implement the tightest regime of foreign currency savings, create a dollar reserve and have our assets transferred to Sberbank, even at a low interest rate.

People looked at me with puzzled expressions on their faces, to put it mildly. Mind you, only six months before, I was trying to convince the staff to the contrary. I was telling them that our projects in Germany and France were quite profitable. My deputy Sergei Georgiyevich Kolesnikov and I made a number of trips to Munich and the French city of Dreux, where we urged our partners to agree to months of delays on their "Khud-Lit" orders. We signed a lucrative contract with a Hungarian publishing concern. Essentially due to these accepted delays, we were able to get credit for our projects at the rate charged by Western banks, which was at the time more than ten times lower than the domestic rate. Moreover, these western loans became for us a reservoir of working capital, which we could not obtain in Russia because of the government's apparent strategy to stifle its state-owned enterprises through the mechanism of tax pressure and non-lending policies.

This credit amount allowed the publishing house to defer tax payments until a more opportune moment. It resolved the second problem as well.

And now, after everything seemed to be going so well, I was proposing that we immediately give it up and shift once again to the Russian printing industry, even though the quality of its work was incomparably lower than overseas, and it didn't offer any credit.

There was a murmur of disapproval in the hall. The staff refused to understand my motives. And I had to admit that they had every reason for it. Even my deputies were perplexed. The only person who seemed to grasp that what I was saying made sense was the head of accounting Inara Borisovna Stepanova who was a also a highly qualified economist. She started asking me more specific questions for an analysis that she had already begun in her mind.

I was even more impressed with the position taken by chief editor Valeri Sergeyevich Modestov – one of the veterans of the publishing house, whose hair had turned gray in these walls, and whose authority among the staff was very high. Modestov rose to his feet, and I dreaded to hear what he was going to say about my unpredictability and lack of consistency. Instead, he said:

– I know nothing at all about economics, particularly its present fluctuations. But I do know that if it weren't for Arkady Naumovich, "Khud-Lit" would have long been dead. And our Pegasus would have grazed somewhere else, but definitely not on the slopes of the literary Olympus. What he has just said is very different from how I myself see the current situation. But how can I see it properly when, as I have just admitted, I know nothing about economics? I think that the rest of you present here are no experts in economics either, with the exception, maybe, of two-three people. This is why I will simply say that I trust our director. I know the most important thing of all: he has our best interests and those of the publishing house at heart. So I urge you to trust in him too. Believe him

140

with your heart, if not with your mind. Just trust in him, and that's all. We have to understand that whatever we might say now or recommend will most likely not be of any use. Nothing will be, except for our trust.

After this impressive statement by Valeri Sergeyevich everybody somehow calmed down –the agitation and murmur subsided, and a warm wave of unity and understanding swept across the room. The people gathered were able to suppress their initial outburst of emotion and adopt a more constructive approach.

As the result, the staff accepted all the necessary decisions, though not without an element of doubt. We moved toward reorienting our projects from foreign printing services to domestic ones and began to work on building a foreign currency reserve, which later protected us from the August crisis, when thousands of more successful businesses than ours were destroyed in a matter of days. Thanks to the preliminary defense measures we had taken, we emerged from the default of 1998 without losing a single ruble, and even, to the contrary, due to the increased difference in the rate of American and Russian currencies we secured life-saving stability in the debt crisis that accompanied the collapse of the economy.

After our conversation about Christ, Lapshin didn't come to see me for a while, and he even avoided me. Then he suddenly stopped by. He was planning to go to his home town, Theodosia, for about a month or so. He told me that he will be meeting with people who would help us in our work. Then, looking me straight in the eye, he offered:

– Let's go together.

I thought it over very fast: the affairs at the publishing house had stabilized, the weather was beautiful and if I could also take Nadezhda and one of the children along it would make a wonderful vacation.

Vyacheslav seemed to read my thoughts and he added a few incentives:

– You needn't worry about a hotel. We'll get you great accommodations close to the beach. Theodosia is a very beautiful city and it is also one of the centers of powerful energy flows. I intend to hold some magic rituals there. You will have a chance to see everything firsthand. As a writer, you absolutely must take part in this.

My family was offered a place not far from the seashore in Theodosia, just as Lapshin promised. The hot summer weather enticed the kids to the beach and the water, whereas Anatoli Ivanovich and I tried to spend as much time as we could with Lapshin.

Lapshin was staying in the city center, not far from the Armenian Church. Actually, he was only planning to live there eventually, because his old house wasn't really fit for living. It was in ruins after a fire that took place for an unknown reason several years before.

Whatever was left of the limestone lined structure, stood on a hillside in a large plot of land, surrounded by stone walls and thorny green shrubs. It was rumored that the house was hit by ball lightning and flared up instantly. But neither Vyacheslav Mikhailovich himself, nor any of the neighbors, were inclined to perceive the fact that lightning hit Lapshin's house and not somebody else's as accidental. The local people were alarmed by the suspicious crowd that gathered regularly in Lapshin's back yard at night, and concerned about the shamanic rites with tambourines and loud shrieks. Something was going on that was different from the usual, and this discrepancy couldn't help affecting the atmosphere surrounding Lapshin's life in Theodosia – the locals treated him with suspicion and vigilance.

Several days later, Vyacheslav informed us that everything was ready for a very important ritual of interaction with the elements.

–There used to be a cemetery next to the church. It is now closed but the inter space tunnel into the Kingdom of the Dead remains intact. We are going to use this opportunity. – He introduced us to his plan in a serious voice. A slight smile touched his lips only when he was uttering the last sentence.

Anatoly Ivanovich and I paid little attention to his words about the Kingdom of the Dead and the possibility of interaction with it. Of late, we perceived much of what Vyacheslav was saying as an effort to provoke people.

During our next day's visit, however, we found Lapshin busy with serious preparations. There was a ping-pong table in the middle of the yard with benches around it. On the table we saw a figurine of a woman sitting on her haunches.

– This is an Occult object, – explained Vyacheslav looking us in the eye. – It represents Mother Earth. She was discovered in a Scythian burial mound. In addition to her, it is possible for me to get the scepter of power. What remains is to find the third component of the egregore – the Golden Horse. It was once hid here by Mamai, after the defeat at the Kulikovo Field. If I succeed in finding it – power on earth will belong to me.

Anatoli Ivanovich and I exchanged ironic glances. They clearly expressed what flashed through our minds: "Any bauble of folly will keep the baby jolly. It's fine so long as we find it interesting."

A dozen or so of Lapshin's students were clearing the place designated for the future sacral action from debris.

– That's where the tunnel is, – Lapshin explained. – We'll start at twelve."

– So we're in for a bit of shamanic chanting?" I asked sarcastically.

Lapshin measured me with his eyes. It seemed that he still wasn't sure where I stood in respect to him: whether I was an ally or an adversary. My mocking comments and unwillingness to adopt a clear-cut approach to his strange enterprise definitely threw Vyacheslav off his balance. He tried to beat some sense into me and to make me give up my playful mood.

– A man must take a stance of homeostasis between Light and Darkness. Then he will make them dependent on him. We need to trick both sides. This would be the middle path.

We sat down around the table and listened.

– Preparations for the appearance of a new kind of Man are underway right now. People with entirely new qualities will soon emerge. They will have perfect knowledge of information processes and be able to use them to increase their power. The rest of mankind is doomed. They will start to demonstrate psychic mutations and will eventually vanish.

– Are you trying to tell me that everyone will die out, except for us? – I tried, once again, to shake his confidence of a triumphant leader.

– Well, why not? – Vyacheslav accepted the challenge. – A man dies simply because he didn't know why he was needed here at all. He leaves this system and it isn't clear where he goes. But the center of his assembly remains here, on this planet. So he is passing away here, and dying there – over and over again, forever.

– What do you mean by there? – I stuck to him like a burr to a dog's tail.

– In the Kingdom of the Dead.

– Are you sure we need to go there?

– There's no way to get around it anyway. We'll all end up there! – Vyacheslav tried to turn my counter offensive into a joke.

–You can't make me and I won't go, – I persisted, not ready to capitulate.

– And what about your dragon? He's growing new heads, isn't he? – Vyacheslav pulled out his trump card.

I stopped resisting and shrugged my shoulders. He was right. Something odd was indeed happening to the dragon, some strange development directly connected to my destiny.

While he originally appeared as a character in the land of my inner visions, where he helped me and supported me, the dragon suddenly leaned out half ways, if one can say so, into our reality. The point is that through the screen of internal vision, at the energy information level, it is relatively easy to see not only a person's aura but also a whole sequence of information control structures. By influencing them one can achieve a variety of goals, mainly associated with a person's health and wellbeing. One such structure is the protective quadrant. It envelops a person as an information geometric figure. And in it, archetypal images manifest themselves as the result of various space impacts, with which this or that zodiacal influence is directly connected. Anyway, for some time now a dragon has appeared or, rather, manifested itself, at the top of my square. He grew up and matured, and, before I knew it, he had three heads instead of one. Clairvoyants noticed him and were amazed. There were crowns on top of the dragon's heads, and his body was sprinkled with emeralds. During the treatment of people who came to us with various health problems I often turned to him for help. And in some way unknown to me he actually brought about an effective and almost instantaneous healing.

When I spoke to Vyacheslav about the dragon he would immediately cheer up and begin poking fun at me:

– Just go on growing that little dragon. Only don't forget that you'll have a face-off with him some day. And nobody knows who is going to get the upper hand, whether you'll pierce him with a spear or he'll gobble

145

you up whole.

I didn't understand what he was hinting at, though I suspected that his caustic remarks had a hidden meaning. The thing is that he often mentioned in passing: "Before becoming human, one must first conquer the dragon within himself. But how can he be conquered when he is immortal? It is impossible to kill him or escape from him."

Indeed, something secret and mystical was associated with the dragon. There had to be a reason why he appeared on my protective quadrant and was so actively expanding into "different heads." Will he always remain the kind of amicable assistant he is pretending to be now? Could it be that on some unknown day he might decide to open his toothy mouth and get a taste of his master, who had made him so nice and fat with his passion for esoteric? Then, perhaps, he is the master and not I…

As if he could guess the turmoil inside me, Vyacheslav added fuel to the flames.

– So how many heads does he already have? – He smiled, baring his teeth.

– Three.

– Wow, you must be feeding him well! You've grown a snake ogre here, – he exclaimed with feigned admiration. – Make sure he doesn't grow any additional heads. Even St. George the Dragon Slayer* only fought with a one-headed monster. Are you sure you're growing an opponent you can handle?

– You know, we don't seem to have any intention to quarrel, – I carelessly pushed aside the thought that I might ever get into a fight with the

* St. George the Dragon Slayer – also called St. George the Victorious and
St. George the Conqueror is a Christian Orthodox saint, the patron saint of Moscow
and Russia who, according to legend, had slain a dragon.

harmless and useful little hologram at the top of my protective quadrant.

– Sure, sure, – Vyacheslav suddenly grew serious. – I wouldn't recommend that you quarrel with him either. It's better to strike an agreement on cooperation. He is helping you, isn't he?

–Yes, he is, – I agreed without much enthusiasm.

The people whom Vyacheslav invited to attend the shamanic ritual began to gather at the site toward evening. It was a very diverse crowd, mostly from Moscow – among them was a former advisor to Mikhail Gorbachev, a number of scientists, and even some intelligence staff. There were also a lot of children who were trained in Lapshin's technique and possessed clairvoyant perception.

A circle was formed out of small pebbles in the area cleared of the remnants of the fire, right among the ashes. The figurine of Mother Earth was placed in the center. A storm lamp with a candle inside sent an unusual, convoluted reflection of a secret sign unknown to me toward the figurine. Vyacheslav moved back and forth right next to it, adjusting the position of the lamp with respect to the figurine. The benches and chairs for the guests, who were to witness the magical rite, were placed nearby. One of them approached me.

– Good evening. Vyacheslav told me about you. My name is Dmitri and I work for the Gorbachev Fund. I tell fortunes on the runes.

Dmitri was tall and had good manners.

– Master of the Order of the Dragons, – I introduced myself, as if incited by the sarcastic tone of my previous conversation with Lapshin.

– You know, I already got used to finding the most unusual things and people here, – my new acquaintance agreed with a disarming smile. – Even if a witch were to arrive here today sitting on broom, it wouldn't really surprise me. With Vyacheslav one has to be ready for

147

anything. I realized this during my first visit to this place three years ago.

In the course of the subsequent conversation Dmitri told me many interesting things about the life of the country's former president, who, according to him, had fallen victim to his own kindness and humanity. I agreed with him on this score – I always had a good feeling about Gorbachev. If he were a little tougher, the country wouldn't have been caught in the whirlwind of radical transformations, in the control of people more capable of destruction than creation.

A short while before the beginning of the mystical performance (at least that was how I perceived it at the time), a strange and brief but very furious scandal took place. One of the girls suddenly refused outright to participate in the event organized by Lapshin. She was supposed to play the role of a sign of the zodiac, for which Vyacheslav prepared her thoroughly and for a long time. All his efforts to convince her now were fruitless. He was gentle at the beginning but then started using explicit threats. The young rebel simply turned away from him and walked off.

I had never seen Vyacheslav fly off the handle that way. Threats, curses and desperation were all mixed up in his insulted shrieks about the ungrateful girl for whom he had done so much and who was now letting him down at such a critical moment. Anatoli Ivanovich and I tried to calm him down but all our attempts were to no avail. The refusal of this child seemed to be actually destructive to the deep inner meaning of what was supposed to happen. It also destroyed Vyacheslav's long and tedious efforts.

– A day such as this happens once in a lifetime! – he complained in anguish. – She ruined everything. I have no one to replace her with.

– Try someone else instead, – I suggested lightheartedly. – What difference does it make to you, who of the kids is going to stand around and pretend to be a tiny star or a butterfly?

– The point is that it does make a difference, and a very substantial one, – Lapshin barked out. A phosphorescent flame flashed momentarily in his eyes.

After another failed effort to quell this unexpected revolt, Vyacheslav chose someone among his new students and hastily began to prepare him for the upcoming role in the mystical show.

Closer to midnight Vyacheslav lit the storm lamp and placed twelve clairvoyant children around the figurine in a special arrangement. Then he summoned me and Anatoli Ivanovich into the circle. We took off our shoes, as we were supposed to, and walked barefoot into the center of the action, the scene of esoteric happenings.

A professional shaman who was invited to participate in the special event warned us:

– What is now going to take place is very serious. Please treat it without your usual irony. Make a wish and it will most likely come true.

I made a wish at once to write very many good books. I have no idea what Anatoli Ivanovich's wish was; he didn't want to share it with me since he perceived what was going on somewhat more seriously.

Soon after that, I had to change my attitude too. When the shaman passed by us beating his tambourine, howling and chanting his appeals to the elements of air, land, water and fire, quite perceptible gusts of wind suddenly emerged out of nowhere in the utter silence of this summer night in Theodosia, when you could, it seemed, hear even the whispering of stars. The wind not only hit our faces, but also made a sound similar to roaring that slowly died down. It was replaced by a delicate beam of light shimmering in the moon that fell directly on top of the figurine of the earth goddess. It was barely noticeable and fleeting but still all of us, participants and spectators alike, could see it.

It was then Vyacheslav's turn to act. He appealed to each of the elements in turn, asking if they were willing to cooperate with him. Then he ordered them to open the channel in the center of the circle to the planetary core. I was standing in the center of the circle, right next to Anatoli Ivanovich, and I didn't see anything special happening. Neither my usual sight, nor my screen of inner vision could detect any abnormal phenomena, except for the transient events that occurred earlier and for which my mind had by then found a simple and materialistic explanation: it must have been a random gust of wind and the unusual angle of our vision.

Vyacheslav was shouting something. If what he said could be trusted, an abyss had by now really opened before him. And he was promised from down there the authority and the scepter of power which he could use to establish his rule on Earth. But it seemed to me at that point that he was the only one to hear all this. Since I couldn't see or hear any of it, I continued to perceive everything that was happening as a game, as material I could use for my literary work.

It appeared that Vyacheslav had achieved his goal. The show clearly made a strong impression on everyone present. Perhaps, unlike me, they really saw what Vyacheslav was chanting about. This was indirectly confirmed by another negative incident during the performance: the child, who was unexpectedly asked to replace the rebellious girl, suddenly became ill and had to be hastily taken out of the circle.

In spite of all these successive failures in the design of the script, the performance continued. After he was promised superior power, Vyacheslav announced that the channel was closed. He thanked the elements for their cooperation and completed the ceremony.

The children left, the candle in the storm lamp was blown out and the figurine carried away.

– If I understand right, you've just become the Dark Lord of the Universe, – I said to Vyacheslav caustically. – So what are you going to do? What do you have to run the show?

He looked back at me mockingly. He was in such good spirits that he could afford to be condescending.

– It is now time to take control, – he explained affectionately. – I don't mean right now – it will, of course, be a gradual process, but we shouldn't delay it too much either. I am looking forward to your assistance and cooperation, colleagues.

– The Academy of the Globe or the Milky Way Galaxy! – I exclaimed with ironic admiration. – You sure think big, my friend. And most importantly, you're not humble about it! Modesty is clearly not one of your virtues. Do you believe you have enough knowledge to manage such a colossus? You recently worked at the cemetery hand-chiseling tombstones – and now you suddenly intend to be in charge of the entire planet.

– Yes, with your help, only with your help, – Vyacheslav answered, not taking offense. – After all, you, unlike me, are real academics. So you'll serve as my royal advisors.

Definitely, nothing could spoil his good mood today. Apparently, he truly believed that this night he was given a mandate to govern the Earth. In this case, I would like to know who issued and who approved this mandate. Maybe it wasn't issued or approved but only promised. Between promising and performing, a man may marry his daughter. Stuff happens, you can't plan for it.

***

151

During all the days that followed Vyacheslav was burning with excitement and enthusiasm. And while my son and daughter were basking in the sun at the beach, he dragged Anatoli Ivanovich and me into the mountains, entertaining us with stories about Theodosia and Aivazovsky, whom he called one of the Initiated and insisted that the great Russian artist painted with the help of the bio-computer.

– In general, everything on Earth that is great and significant was created with the help of the bio-computer. – His speech was a triumphant hymn to the mysterious forces of being. – Though the bio-computer is actually nothing more than an instrument, with the help of which information needed for mankind's development is being entered into someone's empty head for an instant or slightly more. This nerd may be sitting in his office, furrowing his brow, empty-headed, when someone from up above shoves a new idea to this numskull. Eureka! We have a discovery!

– Are books written in the same way? – I asked out of curiosity.

– How else do you think? – Lapshin responded with an ironic question.

– Are you saying that everything I've written was actually done for me by some guy from above? – I pressed Vyacheslav for an answer even though I could guess what it was going to be.

Lapshin's face lit up with a cheerful sun-like smile.

– Even you finally got it, Arkady. That which you call an individual, a human being, is really just the outer surface, protective gear. True individuality hides beneath this gear and craftily manipulates its legs, arms and tongue. If you want to free yourself from these manipulations, you must become a kind of homeostasis between cosmic and earthly influences. Remember how quoted the apocrypha of Early Christians to you: "The one who has discovered himself – the world does not deserve to have him."

We must do something for the Earth and the Cosmos to become dependent on us. Not us dependent on them, but the other way round.

I couldn't be quite sure whether Vyacheslav was joking or speaking seriously. Even if I were to consider his position rational and conditionally accept what he was saying as the truth, even then the equation didn't work. So I expressed my doubts, applying for support to Anatoli Ivanovich. After all, he was a mathematics professor and equations were his thing, not mine.

– Just imagine the following identical equation, – I asked him, barely containing my laughter, – Vyacheslav Lapshin equals the Cosmos plus Earth?

Anatoli Ivanovich scratched his head nervously with all five fingers.

– I don't do this kind of equations.

– You shouldn't be laughing, – Vyacheslav grumbled, noticeably irritated. – Look, opportunity only knocks once. Your ambivalent attitude to serious matters is going to cost you...

– You and your opportunities! I'm not looking to get on the bandwagon with you! – I also started to get angry. – It's the moral aspect of this outlandish theory of yours that worries me. The Cosmos has created all life – the Earth and humans. So whatever way we look at it, he is our father, right?

– Yes.

– But you're saying to me: Let's cheat our father and take everything here under our control. What's more, we should also make our parent dance to our tune. That's your plan of action, isn't it?

– What about you? Don't you want to rule the Earth? – Vyacheslav asked incredulously. – All power, all finances will be in our hands. Don't you understand what happened that night? I was promised the scepter of power. And I need you two to help me.

– Who promised it to you? – I tried to find out.

Vyacheslav hid his eyes. It seemed he didn't want any certainty in this issue.

– There are powerful forces that are going to help us, – he replied evasively.

I looked at him attentively and couldn't figure out where his unique, outstanding abilities ended and schizophrenia began? Why couldn't he understand how much one had to know and what remarkable skills the person needed to have in order to become the global president? What did he have to run the show?

It seemed that our conversation and disagreements left Anatoli Ivanovich tired rather than amused. In the evenings when we sat down to eat some watermelon in the gazebo and the children ran to get shish kebab, he would chastise me:

– Why do you grapple with him like that? The man doesn't even have a college degree. His erudition barely covers what he learned in elementary school, why would you talk to him about the Cosmos and the Universe?

– But if he is just that, – I tried again to get to the truth, – then what are we doing here, what are we trying to learn?

– We are trying to satisfy our curiosity, getting a suntan on the beach and swimming. – Berezhnoi listed what we were doing. – There is no need to see such a profound meaning in everything. All we should do is separate the rational from the irrational.

– So what is rational here, the scepter of power or Vyacheslav Lapshin being the Global President?

– Once again, you focus on the extremes, – Berezhnoi cut me short. – All this is silly, of course. But he does return vision to the blind and cures diabetes! What do you say? This means that our conventional science misses something important, doesn't understand something and refuses to admit its helplessness. That is why we must understand these phenomena, comprehend them and attract the public's attention to these matters. Let him deal with his delirium about universal control. Nobody could care less about this craziness. The main thing is to understand the mechanism of the things that bring people back to health.

***

In Theodosia I once again had a vision, but now after the shamanic ritual its content had changed. It was a totally different film, and totally different masters of universal illusions were showing it to me.

Just as in the past, the vision differed from a dream in its unusually bright images and the fact that everything occurring in it was perceived by all the senses. It was a kind of second reality. Perhaps, it was even the first reality because everything in it was better defined than what we are used to seeing in our ordinary lives.

...I saw the Cosmos somewhere not too far from the Earth. Everything in it was so quiet as if all sounds had died. A strange design, consisting of spheres joined together to form pyramids was suspended, motionless, in infinity. One of these spheres lured me and pulled me in. It was the lower one in the lower triangle. But there was also another sphere underneath it, which, although included in the single pyramidal structure, is located apart from the rest. I moved around in this sphere without the slightest effort, as though the elements in the vacuum of space did not create any problems for my existence. It grew and became increasingly larger. The Blue

155

Planet with the outlines of continents... This was Earth, and it was getting closer. I entered the atmosphere, flying over the surface, and the Earth's maternal energies enveloped, caressed and soothed me. I felt like an infant in its cradle. I was content, comfortable and safe in these energy waves from the Earth. I shut my eyes and dozed off on the palms of my native planet. A chain of associations emerged in my consciousness; a sequence of symbols, letters, signs of the zodiac and sacred names floated before my inner vision. I had the feeling as if I knew and understood what they expressed. But how did I acquire this knowledge of the strange cosmic computer, where it was easy to find any bit of information, or make your own wish and command, introducing them into the countless programs of intersecting interactions through a combination of symbols created by the will and the mind?

I opened my eyes and realized that I was asleep – because what was happening couldn't be anything but a dream. I was lying on a cold square-shaped stone slab in a cramped and stuffy dungeon. Its walls of loose gray sandstone had crumbled and decayed from the elements, and there was a cleft high above in one of them. A ray of light, flat as a board, fell through the crack. There weren't any doors or windows in the dungeon, which looked more like a vault.

A wave of foul-smelling, putrid air wafted in from somewhere. I looked down and noticed the floor swaying under my feet, like filthy, oily swamp water. Chilling fear grabbed my throat in a deadly spasm: it really was a vault. I was confined in this vault through a bizarre combination of circumstances, random forces, or hallucinations.

As if pushed up by a spring, I got up from the stone, on which I had been lying, and stood on its edge. Long slimy creatures slid to the floor from under my feet and vanished somewhere down there. I lowered one

156

of my legs cautiously, as if testing the wobbly surface of the grassy cover of the swamp that was hiding an abyss underneath. My leg sank into something disgusting and dangerous.

"So what, – I thought to myself with an unexpected sense of relief, – there is only one honorable way to respond to death, and that is to spit in her face."

Then I suddenly felt that the darkness around me was imperceptibly changing. A cold breeze hit my legs, and icy needles pierced the skin. Their frequent stabs were rising higher and higher up, and everywhere they reached, the body became paralyzed and practically dead. Climbing all the way to my chest, the cold stabs stopped right next to my heart. The very moment when I decided that it was over, a sharp pain shot through my spine. It was as though an icy spear ran through me, and it entered inside my body, like an entomologist's pin goes through the body of a butterfly. My feet were separated from the flat stone, and I found myself hanging in the air on a rod of unbearable pain. A light sigh reached me from behind, and I was turned abruptly to face a spot on the black oily surface under my feet, in the depth of which an obscure play of shadows became discernable. With great effort I could see below me a strange cubic structure of rectangular mirrors, whose surface shimmered with a vivid interplay of energies and colors. A second later, a radiant light appeared on the barely revealed, shimmering mirror surface, to which I felt a strange emotional attraction, the kind one feels to the light of a fire in an ominously dark forest. The light was cold, pure and extremely volatile. A deep, melodic voice emerged from this radiance. It was impossible to tell who it belonged to – a male or female.

– A decision has to be made. Otherwise there won't be any more life or thinking. At this point we can still negotiate an agreement.

157

– Who are you? – I asked, overpowering the severe pain.

– The mediator, – was the terse answer.

– Between whom and whom?

– Between what and whom, – I was corrected.

I humbly accepted it.

– Between what and whom?

– Between death and you, – the voice said calmly.

– Should I be scared?

– Why? Death is merely the price, which life pays by the gates that lead to tranquility.

– Still, no one chooses death of his own free will. So what should I do?

– Make a decision.

– What decision? – I asked through pangs of pain.

– There is one decision but three paths: where you should go, where you would like to go and where you will arrive. True, variations are also possible, for instance, you can reach "where you should go" through "where you would like to go." Or you could get to "where you would like to go" through "where you will arrive." It's a matter of luck.

I had a hard time comprehending what was going on. Still, I mustered what was left of my strength and rasped:

– What threatens me?

Another sigh reached me from the flickering light, and the voice said, almost in a whisper:

– What you wanted to spit in the face just now.

Realizing that my fury would be useless, I pushed the remaining air out of my lungs with the last effort of my dying body, and it emerged from my lips as a light sound, like hand clap:

– Pthu!

A groaning sound filled the vault.

– What for?

And at that very instant it was as though I was shattered into atoms, and each of them separately was being smoothed with a file.

"I spat at her, nevertheless," I thought contentedly. "And I am no longer made of one piece, no longer a whole man."

With every second I found it increasingly more difficult to perceive my physical boundaries, to determine where my body ended and the force pulling it inside began. The pitch darkness that enveloped me was swirling, pulsating and thickening all around, leaving me with a growing awareness of a threat, both mute and mortal. This dark cloud was quietly absorbing what was once my body. Fragmented into atoms and particles, my body ceased to be something physical, and it was literally being dissolved by the nervous spasmodic movements of the black cloud, which, as I guessed, was Death.

I no longer had any vision or hearing, only what remained of my evaporating sense of the most primitive emotional response: "So that's how it comes." At the same time, I realized: just a bit more and I will lose even the most minimal sense of my former self.

Suddenly I heard within myself a persistent signal that sounded similar to the Morse code. The weak impulses sounded ever more insistent as I was losing my former essence, and, strange at it may seem, they awoke in me the ability to resist what was happening. An unexpected convulsion of energy halted for an instant the disintegration of the bio-fields separated by the darkness. "I'm not finished, not yet!" The fierce thought pierced every one of its dissolved particles. And with it came the will to resist, no matter how meaningless it may have seemed in those circumstances. Through a silent instruction from my consciousness, which still retained

159

some cohesion, I ordered the energies of my essence to initiate the process of connection. The particles, dismembered by the darkness, stopped their flight and began dancing in one spot, like dry leaves in the uneven, capricious wind. They no longer had the strength to continue moving in any given direction.

A roar, like that of a wounded beast, pierced the space around me, and I suddenly got back my hearing and then my sight. I saw a slightly blurred spot of light in the pitch black darkness.

The realization that it was possible to rescue myself awakened in me and invisible radiations of hope streamed in every direction, overcoming the resistance of darkness, recovering the weakened connections between particles and concentrating the energy fields on my essence. With every second I had a stronger awareness that my battle with Death was not over and that I had not exhausted my possibilities to challenge her.

Enveloped in darkness, the mass of mental energy twisted, writhed in convulsions and compressed more and more into a luminous ball of plasma, which began to cast aside the sticky tentacles of nonbeing and to move about in the dark realm according to its will, toward its own goal.

If it hadn't been for the faint glow, which I had previously noticed and which prompted the right direction, I could have remained a prisoner of darkness forever. But the voice of light that broke somewhat through the pitch blackness awakened in my mind the almost imperceptible hint at the possibility of salvation. I trusted this voice and used my last reserves of strength to move where this saving tip told me to. I pushed the darkness away with the power of my inner energy, and it curled by my side with a hissing sound, making way, and burning itself against the scorching hot plasma heated by the effort of my will.

Exhausted, with my last remaining strength, conscious that in just another moment I was about to lose all my will and Death would dissolve within itself the defenseless bond between my energies and mind, no longer frightening to her, I lunged forward and fell out of the darkness that was devouring me onto the stone slab. Missing her prey, Death uttered a deep guttural roar, and waves of energy tremors shook the vault, but I was once again standing on my own tombstone, no longer dead, but not yet alive.

I now had my body back. I stretched out, standing erect, looked around myself and understood what had served as my life-saving beacon. The light that had fallen from above on the oily surface of the abyss was aflame with a dazzling iridescent fire against the backdrop of black space. I looked deep into the glow and recoiled. A terrifying creature stared at me from inside – a man with peeled off skin and blood streaming from his skinless muscles. I raised my hand to my eyes and groaned with rage – it wasn't my hand at all but a bloodied plexus of flesh and muscle. The reflection I saw in the light was my own.

Blood was oozing and falling from my body on the gray surface of the stone. Exhausted by the emotions seething within me, I bent my knees and sat down on the cold rough slab. My shoulders hunched up, and weakness and despair forced me to fall quiet for a long time.

Then I lost any sense of time within these bare walls. It suddenly occurred to me that it may have been better if I succumbed to Death, rather than escape her embrace the way I now was. And instantly, as if in response to my unexpressed thoughts, I heard the familiar quiet, suggestive voice:

– If you wish to, you can sleep now. You will be awakened when the time comes, in hundreds or maybe thousands of years.

In my apathy I was immersing into a state of complete relaxation, but

161

I asked, nevertheless:

– Who will awaken me?

– Necessity, – rustled the echoes.

Unbearable silence, alarming and threatening began to envelope my consciousness.

– Is there any hope I could avoid such a destiny? – I asked dispassionately.

– Hope is the daughter of strength and strength is the sister of will. When you lose one, the other disappears as well.

This time the pitch and tonality of the voice were unquestionably female.

– If I fall asleep, what will I see?

– Mirages of joy and happiness.

– What if I remain alert?

–You will see the path leading to a goal that no one knew, no one knows and no one will know.

– Humiliating fear before the unknown will not stop me, – I pronounced with unexpected stamina.

– Nothing but words, – the voice said in a tone of light irony.

– I can give an oath on the sacred cross that it is so, – my voice was louder now, and I raised my bloodied arm to make the sign of the cross, but my invisible conversation partner stopped me.

– Why bother with what is useless? The crucifix is a particular of the universe. It is just a guiding sign for timid souls – the voice said, laughing. – You can embrace it in terror, waiting all your life for dubious salvation. But what will this change? You, its creator, know about this, don't you? Or, perhaps, when you wanted to put the martyr's crown of thorns on your head, you secretly dreamed of the crown of the ruler of all worlds? Didn't

you know that sometimes the crown of the ruler causes just as severe a headache as the crown of thorns?

– What are you talking about? – The bloody piece of flesh shouted in despair on the tombstone.

– About you, – the suggestive voice whispered. My heart once again contracted with fear.

– Who are you? – I yelled in fury.

– I have many names, – came the response, followed by a sad sigh. – Some call me Mother, others call me Death!

– Why did you spit me out, mommy dear?

– To show you the day in the future.

– I don't wish to know the future! – I screamed desperately. – Everything is already clear: the skin of life has been peeled off my body.

– But it was your own wish to travel the path as a man. You should know that Light and Darkness, Life and Death, Right and Left are all each others' brothers. That is why the good aren't really good and the bad aren't really bad. Life isn't life and death isn't death either.

Scenarios of imminent events, as they were designed by Death, instantly exploded in my mind and evaporated in horror of the future.

– Did you see it?

– Yes, I did.

– What do you think about it?

– How do you know that this is exactly how it's going to be?

– I doubt that you will be able to understand it now but I will try to explain. Every single instant I incorporate into myself information from every speck of dust in any of the worlds. Everything around is permeated with my essence, everything is being analyzed and traced in time. I can't be wrong, possessing complete knowledge. Chances that something can *be changed are miniscule. Only the United can change the future and also you, if you guess the path. But in order to guess it, one must recall the future, and you have forgotten it.*

The nightmarish scenario of the inevitable upcoming events shook me. Raising my head high up to the beam of light, I squinted. And then I heard a sharp question inside me:

— What's wrong?

— I was blinded by the light, — I confessed mentally.

— The one who is blinded by the light should be able to see through the darkness of insight, — followed the immediate answer.

I suddenly felt as if I were in the grave.

— You have buried yourself in the grave of your former statements. You should now correct what you have done or else you will truly remain buried.

— And I will then rot like everyone else, won't I?

— Your words have long been ripping apart the heart of my essence, — the abyss accused me. — I hope you are able to understand this image.

— Why are you blaming me? — I said resentfully. — After all, everything that is happening to me in the world has long been completed within you. You told me this yourself. Or maybe what you said to me wasn't the truth?

— Truth, not truth... The river of your life is still within my shores. Within limits you are free to go with the flow, jump high up, dive deep, swim from one shore to the other, and even struggle, as much as your strength will allow you, against the quick waters of time and events. This will help you to understand the potency of movement and stillness. But the program can fail at times. You have been unpredictable in the past as well. I would like to watch over you. And it would have been hard to find a better place for this.

164

– In your show death will be the applause I shall receive, – I res-
ponded, not asking this time but asserting and for some reason knowing
something about the future.

A subdued snort reached me in response:

– It could be death, or maybe just rebirth. Even I am unable to clarify
your dark future. But here, in this vault, you're like a plaything in my
hands.

– How many others did you have? Do you still have fun?

– What else can I do? – The abyss sounded insulted. – I only know
how to cheat and destroy. I am a contradiction in itself, denying that,
which I asserted, transforming nothing into something and something into
nothing. And everything that is possible is only possible for me within
these limits.

– Does it mean that I must voluntarily surrender to the embrace of
Death?

– Do you fear becoming a part of me so that you can be ready for a
new birth? – the abyss asked. – Do you mistrust me?

– Yes, I am afraid, – I confirmed. – It is always deadly to surrender to
Death.

"But some others managed to overcome their fear, don't you
remember?" The thought rushed through my mind in a suggestive whisper.

– How can I improve my chances?

– By believing in yourself.

– How can I weaken them?

– By distrusting me.

– Is there anyone who could prevent what you have planned from hap-
pening?

– I have said already that everyone is free within the limits of their

165

un-freedom.

– There must be a way out of this...

– I already explained to you that there are three of them.

– By you have explained it as puzzles...

– Oh, dear God. If I could, I would have blushed for you. Even the fact that I have spent so much time talking to you is already wrong. No one can break the laws of the Original. The most important of them is that everyone chooses his path on his own. You have overstepped one of my incarnations. But you should do more. You must make a whole out of your fragmented lives in all previous dimensions. Only by combining them, can you ascend higher and higher up.

– Why would I want to go there? – I asked with sarcasm and stretched out to stand upright. – Does anyone there really need such a bloody piece of flesh that doesn't remember its past and fears its future, such a good for nothing person? – And I laughed uncontrollably with laughter as endless as the insanity of what was happening.

– You see, it's better for us to come to an agreement rather than waste our strength on fighting.

– I already heard a similar hint a while ago. But where is it, my strength?

– Find it yourself, – was the answer.

– I feel that I am growing weaker...

– Yes, you have lost a lot of blood.

– Can I die?

– You can fall asleep. That would be the right way to put it.

– True. You already told me about it. It means that our communication does have its limits, so to say, its natural limits – my resources of blood.

– Yes, it's true.

166

– Will you answer my questions as long as I can continue asking them?

– I will.

– Tell me then, what's underneath me?

– The abyss of dark worlds.

– What's above me?

– The shiny heights of the upper worlds.

– What for is this cube with a mirror surface?

– If you guess, then the old will show you the new when you enter into the deep essence and the invisible will also open itself to you.

– You are speaking in riddles again.

– It shouldn't be such a difficult riddle for the one who comes from the essence of Being.

– It seems that I don't have any more time left to continue this pleasant conversation, – I admitted and stood up with difficulty. – If I am mistaken, please don't hold a grudge against me. I tried to be worth your strange empathy.

– All right, – the voice in the vault said sadly.

Obeying the flash of instinctive feeling, I gathered all my strength and strained myself so hard that it seemed my fibers of muscle could rip apart from my efforts. For a moment I recovered my former strength, and I jumped across the darkly vibrating abyss on to the light, iridescent mirror surface of the cube.

I didn't hear the sound of the abyss as it parted beneath me. There was actually no sound at all. The glowing, pulsating surface silently absorbed the body which had landed on it, and, once again, after being in the embrace of Death I found myself in the arms of Destiny.

The world in which I found myself was unusual and strange, and it appeared to consist entirely of light, blurred contours and energy irradi-

ations. I, too, suddenly turned into some kind of powerful pouring energy that was instantly changing its shape. I felt myself growing, becoming wider, with energies beginning to surge within me. They then arranged themselves into streams and began to circulate, securing the interaction between strange conjugant poles. When they landed on me, the cosmic radiations exploded, forming a myriad of multicolored whirlwinds, which were feeding my new flesh.

I didn't have eyes anymore, and I could see simultaneously as though with my whole essence: the sun above, blinding me with endless phosphorescent flares and the earth below, across which my gigantic shadow was gliding, illuminated by the shimmering inner light pulsating within me.

I could even look inside myself. My new flesh now contained fields and energies, combinations and interactions of vacuum, astral substance, gravitation, matter and anti-matter, and also molecular and sub-molecular links. All these seas and waterfalls of energies, with rivers, streams and variations of force interactions uniting them, were now my new awesome essence. And had the freedom to intuitively choose any of the unthinkable, previously unknown forces and unleash them against anything that dared to stand in my way.

A sense of exhilaration began to fill me.

Gradually, I began to see sharper and clearer. And I recognized myself in the form of a large, colorful, iridescent sphere, which then suddenly flattened and took on the shape of a crucified man. But this form didn't remain stable for long either. It quickly began to quiver and started to manifest itself in a series of ever changing shapes – an ominous black cloud, brimming over with thunder and lightning, then a light, airy snake, winding like a ribbon along the twisted energy waves and overfilling with enthusiasm from this carefree movement.

I clearly felt my own position in the space of this unknown world, the vibrations of cosmic flows, the voices of stars and star clusters, the surf of neutron oceans and photon currents. I realized that I could become transformed, at tremendous speed, into any and all forms of life and energy.

By recomposing the magnetic lines of force in my own fields, I altered the direction of the effects of gravity in such a way that it now pulled me along the Earth's surface toward the shining iridescent ocher ball of the sun above the horizon.

I flew at great speed in space, and the more I peered at the surrounding world, the more familiar everything around seemed to me. There was no solid surface of the Earth beneath me. But as I peered at the unstable, pulsating contours of the Earth's surface, her flowers and trees, it was quite easy to guess that all these energies were flowing out of her mother's womb. When I soared skyward I could see how the multicolored energies of open spaces rhythmically covered the greenish -yellow islands of forests.

I looked up and at my great speed I could not notice either the Sun or any other planets but I could guess that they were there by the barely visible outlines of their reflections through the pale pink, golden purple and blue radiance that filled the space. And this space was not desert-like. Ethereal creatures that previously appeared before me at moments of mental stress or sleep rushed toward me from all sides and surrounded me in a round dance, until I finally realized what they were trying to say.

– We welcome you, our lord! – their happy thoughts sounded around me.

And I answered them the same way, not with words but thoughts:

– I'm glad to see you!

– You're back! You're with us again!

One of these ethereal creatures approached quite close to me. It was neither male, nor Female, and vessels with energy running through them, not blood, could be seen through the semi-transparent flesh surrounded with a golden radiance.

– Be careful. Mugen is looking for you.

– He is very strong. He has the right of first strike.

– The Queen of the Earth assists him, – someone else added.

I began to scan space and I finally felt the tentacle of someone's alarm reaching my consciousness. Moving through the emerging contact across the maze of energy trunks woven into a bundle I discovered the image I was looking for, and enlarged it. The image was originally one-dimensional, then it became two-dimensional, and it eventually acquired the clarity of a holographic copy. The face of a beautiful woman met my glance with the cold ironic look of its eyes. With an effort of will, I created another image opposite the one that I had just summoned – the new image was my own face. And I gave it an expression of determination and severity. The lips of the holographic image stirred and uttered several sounds:

– I could have transformed you right away but I would first like to figure what's what.

The woman's face smiled in response to my threat and pursed its lips:

– Figure what's what? I don't have any such claims, but the day will come that you don't anticipate. You will know then, you will turn around. You will see, but it will already be too late. It is better not to quarrel, what do you think? The more so since you owe me... You haven't forgotten, I hope?

The woman smiled again, while I was studying her face, and the image I had summoned began to quiver and melt away against my will.

170

– You won't get the better of her easily: she's become very powerful. And you won't frighten her either, so you shouldn't show any animosity, – one of my older friends suggested.

– I'm not afraid of her, either, – I bragged light-mindedly.

All of a sudden the face of the Earth Queen appeared before me again.

– Would you like to see the predictive stage, you hero? There was such a version in the book of time. We can come to an agreement before it's too late.

Hearing her words "before it's too late" and recognizing the familiar tone of voice, I kept silent. But it seemed that she had asked for my agreement as a pure formality.

– Look inside yourself.

I looked inside myself and saw spiral vortices spin upward, almost dissolving the original creation into infinity, and then go down, condensing the spirit into matter. And I know: only one who once left it can return to the center, because before compression, there should be expansion. There is no other way one can find the source of one's own existence.

I felt great, comfortable and calm. And suddenly, within an instant, everything around me changed. I was inside a cave temple. A giant rock hung over my head, with light falling in layers through the crevices. I was standing naked at the edge of a small underground lake, surrounded by twelve beautiful women in long robes. They were priestesses. The surface of the lake was covered with rose petals. I remembered, I knew that the rose is the flower of Christ, and it symbolizes birth, life and death – Death, which is followed by resurrection.

The women supported me, cautiously holding me by the arm, and they helped me descend into the water, where I found myself supported by the arms of other priestesses. I had the feeling as if I had been heavily drug-

171

ged: I was listless, apathetic, with no desires of any kind. The hands of the beautiful women caressing my body and preparing me for the mysterious rite left me completely indifferent.

They baptized me with the water and led me out of the lake. My strength seemed to be returning, and, as though aware of this, the priestesses were squeezing my wrists and elbows even harder, not so much supporting me now as constraining. They led me to a huge statue in the center of the cave almost by force. This was the same figure that Vyacheslav had at his shamanic ceremony. Only it wasn't a figurine now but a huge statue whose head almost reached the dome of the cave temple. Her legs were also hunched up and a comfortable royal bed was set up between her knees. The women laid me down on it. Some force constrained me, shackled me and prevented me from getting up. I tried to resist this force, but despite its apparent softness and pliability it held me securely chained to the bed. The priestesses stood on either side of the bed – six on each side.

Someone shouted, or rather, announced: "The bride of Microprosopus." I had no idea what the word "Microprosopus" meant but I guessed that it referred to me. That beautiful woman with a crown on her head – the Queen of the Earth – appeared from the dark depths of the temple. She was wearing a green cloak with a scarlet lining on her shoulders. And she was completely naked under the cloak. I knew who she was and what would happen next. The Queen of the Earth came up to the bed. She stood towering above me, stepped over my prostrate body and peered into my face. A slight smile slid across her lips.

– You don't want war in the world and you don't want there to be harmony in the world but you have forgotten that everything has a price. Sacrifice is needed, – she said in a coy voice and, pushing aside the folds of her cloak, she lowered herself on top of my body. I could feel her soft,

172

warm skin, her strong hands that pushed me in the chest whenever I tried to get up. – Christ redeemed everyone on Earth with his blood on the Cross. Your redemption on a bed is far more pleasant, – she said mockingly.

Her face was now close to mine. I tried to do something to my body, to get it out of its paralyzed state – but all my efforts were in vain. The invisible chains of magic are far stronger than my muscles.

– Why are you trying to resist? You don't admit to yourself that you actually desire what is about to happen. And besides, the union of Heaven and Earth has to be paid for, – she said and her fingers glided down my chest in a caressing and calming motion. – You are the King and I am the Queen – and everything around is our kingdom. Isn't this what you've dreamed of all along?

Her words weren't aggressive, they were calm. I felt the power of her beauty and responded to it. Precisely sensing the attraction that emerged between us, she joined her flesh with my own.

– Arkady, arcade, arch, bridge over the rainbow, across seven spaces, – she uttered coyly, the sensuous undulating movements of her body giving me ecstatic bliss.

I could sense the restraining forces weakening, but I didn't push the woman away, but, on the contrary, encouraged and supported the feeling of oneness with the gentle movement of my hands sliding over her body. As my hand continued to stoke her back, I could feel hard powerful growths rolling under her tender skin. I guessed: this was the crest of the dragon, appearing there and instantly disappearing. The Queen – the woman – the dragon... The image of a charming woman concealed the cruel essence of the Primal Serpent. It was too late to change anything: we would soon become joined into a single creature – the Heavenly Adam and the Earthly

173

Eve. An androgen would appear which will have one body and two heads, a male and female one. This will be the New Man – the ruler of the Earth, in whom the earthly and heavenly will be reconciled. And with him the Golden Age will begin – a very happy time, which will last for a thousand years in human terms.

My palm continued to slide tenderly down her back, over the mobile, rolling growths of her being that was trying desperately to free itself from its captivity in the body of the dragon's essence. She guessed, she understood that my tenderness was sincere, that in showing it I wasn't prompted by reason but by feeling, that I had overcome my sense of martyrdom and the anguish of captivity. In tune with these feelings, her own movements lost the energy of crude aggression and the vibrations she radiated became more subtle and gentle. This was no longer a forceful conquest of one over the other, but a genuine connection and communion, the merger of two powerful universal energies, two primal harmonies of life – the female and male one.

Her convulsive efforts to pull the dragon's crest out of her spine stopped and withdrew inside, into the inner cosmos of the Queen's world. She was now simply a woman, who got what she wanted. And what she did for this to happen, wasn't important– she won so that she could obey and stand beside her King, she won to regain her Kingdom.

That last instant, when I felt I was about to die from pleasure, I raised my head and saw the smiling, content face of Mother Earth high above over me.

The image melted away and didn't reappear. What was it? From what depths of my subconscious self were these stories extracted? I felt that I had entered a maze that was as long as my life. And every step in it made a difference not only for my edification but also for how I was going to build my own destiny.

* * *

When I got back from Theodosia, I returned to my work with renewed enthusiasm. I didn't know why but for some reason I succeeded easily in everything I undertook, without any special efforts. I had the feeling that somebody was helping me. I handled the affairs at the publishing house, wrote a book about Lapshin, assisted in the work on the script for the film about the achievements of the Academy, read dozens of esoteric books trying to get the core of what was happening to me – all at the same time. Never before, not even in my most productive years, the nineteen eighties, did I manage to do even a small portion of what I accomplished now without much exertion, as if with the help of magic. I was filled with strength and energy, and I even started to forget about the multitude of incurable diseases, which, according to the laws of the genre, were supposed to poison the years of my inevitably approaching old age.

Old age was not coming, however. One might even say that it was withdrawing. My diseases were not tormenting me any longer; I felt like working, setting more and more difficult goals and achieving them, despite all the stereotypes associated with pre-retirement years. I first finished my book about Lapshin and published it at my own expense. The book made Vyacheslav famous overnight – bookstores took it gladly, and it quickly found its readers and sold out.

Only half of what was anticipated came true. Everything that had to do with Vyacheslav Lapshin's promotion and his new fame did come true; the result was even better than we expected. As far as his pledge, that of an honest person, to honorably repay his debt, he had some problems in this

175

area: whether it was with his memory or his honesty, this I couldn't tell. And the director of the film studio nearly lost his apartment ... but all this happened later. In the meantime, everything went as planned, according to another script which was being written by a number of masters far more gifted than yours truly, as it later became apparent.

Every event has its own reference point, its zero coordinate. In the series of events that so unexpectedly entered my life and beneficially affected my creative potential, the night ceremony in Theodosia certainly had some important meaning, though no one ever explained its message to me. It simply happened, I was involved in it, and it began to have an impact on my destiny.

Vyacheslav, whom I met in those days more frequently than ever before, was especially attentive to me. He would put aside all other matters when I came up to him and would readily answer any questions related to esoteric books I had been reading, most of which he had recommended to me himself. He was clearly engaged in my occult education, although I perceived these books that I studied more as a dumping ground of dubious knowledge, where one should try to find a grain of scientific truth rather than genuine secret knowledge passed on to us from the depths of our own history. It also perplexed me that once in while Lapshin would return to his favorite topic about how he was going to seize global power.

– We can influence events with the help of these technologies, – he asserted. – We ought to organize a secret order and take everyone under its control.

– For what purpose? – I inquired matter-of-factly.

– In order to rule, – Lapshin responded.

– Why would you want to take such an impossible load on your shoulders? – I wouldn't let up. – Where are we going to lead the peoples of

176

the world, to what magic dream, to what shining heights? Do you have a dream for everyone?

– Do you think present-day leaders are taking their people to some dream?

– No, they don't, – I had to agree. – But they at least pretend that they are leading the people out of the dark gloomy forest where their predecessors brought them.

Vyacheslav had a hard time containing his laughter.

– This is a magical forest. It is endless, unless you know its secret paths. Anyway, why do you torment yourself with all these questions? The most important thing is to seize power. And when I have it, I will not doubt what has to be done and how. I will put an end to all this slacktitude. Everybody will do what I tell them to.

– What if somebody doesn't?

– I'll pummel him on the head with my scepter of power. And his head will smash into smithereens. Have you read about psychic killers? Believe me: their abilities compared to those the scepter of power gives a person are like the abilities of an ant compared to that of a giant when the two meet on the battlefield.

– What do you want from me?

– You should join my mafia. According to the rules of the game, there hast to be three participants. I already have two.

– Who are they?

– I and one other guy, you know him.

– Why would you need a third? Will it be so boring for two of you to rule the world?

– I already told you: these are the rules of the game, – Vyacheslav smiled.

177

– Then this is a game?

– Yeah, – Vyacheslav confirmed. – Only I had to take three exams with Satan in this game and not as a joke but quite seriously.

– Wow, what kind of a company do you want me to join? – I pretended to be frightened. – No way, I won't be a part to this threesome. I've had an allergy to creatures with fur and horns since childhood. You'll have to manage somehow without me.

– I can't, – Vyacheslav retorted. – The code of your destiny has struck infinity. Without you the structure can't be assembled.

– So that's how important I must be! – I laughed, still believing that Vyacheslav was just pulling my leg. – It means that without me, you're neither here nor there.

– That's true, – Vyacheslav agreed. He too was laughing. – Neither here nor there. It's about time you got off your high horse. Accept it while we're still inviting you. When you're no longer needed you'll regret that you didn't.

– Don't push me, let me figure it out. Don't you see my dragon heads have begun growing again? – I parried jokingly. – When I finished the book, my head became bigger. When we finished the film, I grew another head. And they're such unusual heads, I must tell you. They have crowns on top. These psychic children won't let me be. They keep telling me that your dragon only has three heads and none of them have crowns. And I grew five already. What should I do with them, eh?

The fact that my dragon has more heads than the dragon belonging to Lapshin himself seems to pique him.

– It's important, no doubt, that the dragon grows more heads, – he confirmed. – But who holds the scepter of power is far more important. And as you know, I'm the one who is holding it.

178

– Show it to me, – I demanded.

– Why should I? You won't see it anyway! It isn't in material space, you know, – Lapshin rejected my request to present his credentials.

* * *

At some point I decided to get a better idea of my strange partner in the information structure, which Lapshin called the protective quadrant. I didn't feel any antagonism toward the dragon, all the more so since he was clearly involved in solving my own health problems and never refused to help others. And this help was not virtual but quite real.

I have no explanation as to why I displayed such a calm attitude to this entirely unusual phenomenon of someone's intervention, particularly in the form of such a controversial creature as a dragon. In the East, he is worshipped as the Lord of Light, but in the West, by contrast, all these "lords" were decimated with the full approval of the Church.

It was time for me get to the bottom of this. So I began to prepare to interrogate my associate, without excluding some elements of coercion.

One evening I sat next to my student Tamara and she "turned on" her screen of inner vision. We began to communicate with my unusual guest from the virtual reality according to a devised plan.

– The crowns are shining and they are blinding me, – Tamara began her observation. – The prongs of the crowns are made of triangular plates. Above them are diamonds set on golden stalks, and they look like dangling little bells. In the center of their foreheads, above the eyes, there are huge rubies. Their necks are like those of a giraffe – long and smooth. They have deep-set eyes and their snouts are similar to those of a crocodile. The tail is covered with green scales. The crest on the spine is also adorned with precious stones. It has very beautiful, colorful wings. The scales on the back are golden and the ones on the stomach are silver. He breathes fire. He is turning his head now and looking at me.

– Ask him if we could talk to him, – I said, without beating about the bush.

Tamara asked and received the dragon's agreement.

– What do the dragon's five heads with precious crowns indicate? Is it some sort of program? – Tamara asked.

– No, it isn't a program but a very important mission.

– How many years is he given to perform this mission?

– Eight years. It is necessary to grow another head.

– What does the mission consist in?

– It is scientific work, which will initiate a new stage in human evolution.

–What does the depiction of the dragon in a protective quadrant indicate?

– Higher intelligence.

– What place does the dragon with precious crowns on his six heads occupy in the cosmic hierarchy?

– The third place. The six heads are the twelve aspects of strength.

My heart missed a beat from the sweet realization of my high position.

– Is Lapshin human or has he come from outer space?

– He's been integrated.

– How?

– From a cocoon...

– Who is he?

The dragon created a picture next to himself. It depicted a man with a bird's head. The head looks like that of a crow.

– Why are bio-computers present in the energy information structure of humans?

– They turn on and control the programs of development and are also instruments and means of communication.

– Communication with whom?

– With gods, essences and hierarchies.

– What else do they do?

– When a person stops enjoying life and loses interest in living they record this condition.

– What then?

– When a person doesn't strive for social success any more or creative achievements and acquiring new knowledge, the bio-computer loses interest in him. In this case, they initiate severance from the person and consequent death.

– Who ordered the Dragon program?

– Jupiter, father of gods.

– What is its goal?

– To establish the full cooperation between the Sun and Jupiter, the energies of Yin and Yang. The encoding of the processes is originated from the core of the galaxy. Cosmic organics monitors their relationship.

– Is there life in the space where there are no material particles? – I asked through Tamara.

– Yes. It is inhabited by essences, designs and egregores that materialize through humans.

– What is the purpose of all this?

– For man to reach the highest point on the evolutionary scale he must improve himself. He dies and comes back to life in order to fulfill his karmic program. Christ has fulfilled his karmic program. Now he has an

181

egregore, with whom he has connected. So He is now God!

– But He is the Creator's son!

– Man could reach these heights and become the co-creator of the Universe. It is a difficult path but not an impossible one. After all, Jesus was able to do it... You are all created in God's image and likeness. There is a spark of His soul in every one of you. And each of you decides for himself whether to climb upward, roll down or stand in one place like a warrior at the crossroads...

I am aware that a dialogue of this sort could produce the strangest impression on those who never encountered anything like it. But two hundred years ago it would be unlikely for anyone to understand how the TV works or the meaning of a modern scientist's lecture on radiation. Radiation is invisible and in those days there were no devices to measure and register it. How can one believe in something one can't see, touch or taste with one's tongue? If one person insists that there exists a mysterious screen of inner vision, when thousands of people don't have anything like it, then those thousands will always consider the only normal person among them to be abnormal.

History has preserved more than a few instances of the spontaneous discovery of the "bio-computer." Socrates, according to Xenophon, had the gift of prophesy and explained his abilities by the guidance he received from a divine being called daemonion that appeared inside him and told him what to do. Socrates insisted that the daemonion never once made a mistake in his predictions. (Scholars specializing in ancient philosophy distinguish between the term "daemon", that is, a "single deity" and "daemonion", that is, something more abstract and less specific, "divine" in general).

Pythagoras, Plato, Heraclitus, Albert the Great, Dante, Paracelsus,

Joan of Arc, Rene Descartes, Wilhelm Leibniz, Sir Isaac Newton, Emanuel Swedenborg, Johann Wolfgang von Goethe and Franz Anton Mesmer – all of them used the opportunity to acquire knowledge from those extraordinary worlds that were denied for a long time by conventional science solely on the grounds that it has been unable to develop reliable tools for studying these phenomena. This, however, is the problem of science itself and definitely not those who were able to use the opportunities open to them in practice. The only thing that can be achieved by dogmatic denial is a quiet life. History teaches us that science moved forward precisely at times when scientists deliberately and consistently turned their attention on "exceptional events." Scroll through the entries in your encyclopedias, and they will convince you that the voice of exceptions is much stronger in the formulas of modern science, than what used to be regarded as the rule.

The great Carl Gustav Jung warned us that the very rationality of common sense could be the worst of human prejudices, because we call what we think, reasonable.

Mendeleev saw his famous Periodic Table in a dream as a reality and only then, through the randomly opened bio-computer, did he begin to look for patterns that connected the chemical elements into a single system. In other words, he first received knowledge and only later began to seek out an explanation.

The phenomenon of Juna, Kulagina, Kuleshova, Wangi, Uri Geller, Sri Sathya Sai Baba, Boosh Zhang, Yan Xin, and even Copperfield, who tries so hard to present himself as a magician, is also directly related to the work of the bio-computer. It is a pity that each of them had to learn the laws of this unique mechanism of interaction with other spaces independently, as if fumbling in the dark.

A year ago when I just began to study this phenomenon, I had no idea that I would gradually get almost all my relatives, friends and colleagues involved in it. Many of them, especially those whose age and time limitations did not interfere with the training, developed the abilities promised by the Academy experts. But even those who were unable to attain the best results, succeeded in improving their health quite substantially.

Mind you, a very short time ago I was one of the fiercest opponents of the notion of extrasensory perception. I'll never forget the first sessions at the Academy, where I had a hard time containing my skepticism.

The instructors explained to us that energy exercises are in some way similar to working with plasma. When we rub our hands together, this causes a rush of blood to the palms, and through this we create electromagnetic stress, which stretches subtle energies in different directions, forcing them to move first to the cathode (negative electrode), and then to the anode (positive electrode). As I followed these simple instructions, I felt like a kid in preschool. But later I came across some research, which was conducted at the biochemical laboratory of Rosary Hill College (Buffalo, New York). And I no longer felt like a child. The experiments involved the famous healer Oscar Estebany, a Hungarian-born American.

Justa Smith, a biochemist specializing in enzymes – large protein molecule catalysts that accelerate the course of biochemical reactions – discovered that the chemical activity of enzymes increases under the impact of a strong magnetic field. This caused her to wonder if Estebany may be imitating the same effect with his hands. During the experiment Estebany held a test tube with enzymes, while the assistants checked the level of their chemical activity with the help of an infrared spectrophotometer every fifteen minutes. They found that the enzyme behaved as if they were placed in a magnetic field of about 13,000 gauss. This is twenty-six thousand times greater than Earth's magnetic field, but when measuring the magnetic field around Estebany's hands the magnetometer revealed no anomalies. In another experiment, the level of hemoglobin was measured in the blood of patients who were being treated by Estebany by the "laying-on of hands." Within a six-day period, the hemoglobin level in these patients increased by an average of 1.2 grams per 100 cubic centimeters of blood. The hemoglobin level of those patients, who refused the services of the healer, did not increase.

Further testing of the water treated by Estebany showed distinct spectrophotometric differences from untreated water. This effect was independently reported by several laboratories. The situation becomes even stranger if we consider the fact that under psychic influence the water molecules became slightly ionized.

This was a serious challenge to conventional physics. The process of transforming atoms and molecules into ions requires substantial energy. But what was this mysterious force, capable of catalyzing the subatomic interactions?

If we assume that due to intra-atomic interactions the radiated psychic energy is capable of creating an external electric field, what happens next can easily be explained through phenomena already known in physics. According to plasma physics, the resultant electron and ion in such an external field, which exceeds the electric field in the micro-volume of the human body, accelerate and in colliding with the atoms they themselves act as ionizers, forming new charged particles in their path. Thus, the number of charged particles grows to avalanche proportions and they break through the insulator, usually in areas where a person has some physical pathology. This is how the healing process begins.

The views on micro-plasma and the psychic effects associated with it have received unexpected theoretical support from geology, a science which seemed incredibly distant from this area. Exploring the mechanisms of how the Earth's crust developed and studying the evolution of inanimate matter into living matter, V.I. Vernadsky and V.V. Dokuchaev identified the so-called bio-energy potential of the Earth as a major factor in geological processes. It was later discovered that high-energy plasma formed in the active fault zones in the crust, initiates a powerful charge, which quartz crystals require in order to create organic structures.

In its physical characteristics geoplasma energy corresponds to gamma-radiation, and it can, therefore, bring the core of elements into an excited state. Solar proton flux contributes to the formation of a neutral shell around the supportive framework (the human skeleton). Importantly, there are no limits to the penetration of plasma, since its potential exceeds any super-powerful connections within rigid structures.

In the light of new evidence, the idea that the encoding of information from all planetary processes of development and interaction takes place through the plasma that is generated by the Earth's planetary core when it collides with the solar proton flux becomes a highly plausible hypothesis.

I find conclusion about the biosphere's information being organized through geoplasma processes to be extremely important. Apparently, the emergence of insights and ideas and their implanting into consciousness and life, which we then materialize at our level of existence, occur precisely through this mechanism.

So let us finally agree on the following: if some unexplained phenomenon, or one denied by science, nevertheless consistently plays a role in society, then whatever is behind it requires research.

Oken, Lamarck and Chambers were trampled down by strict adherents of „proper" science in their time. Then Darwin came, who preached the same heresy, but observed the canons of scientific exposition – and all the

186

punishers blushed guiltily. "Sorry," they said. "We were sincerely mistaken, but new times opened our eyes." And how many others there were: Socrates was poisoned, Bruno was burned, Galileo was forced to abdicate and Vavilov was starved to death in prison...

Quantum physics has altered our perception about the structure of the Universe. It has turned out that the world is a reflection of our consciousness, which also perceives the world. We are all sitting in a strange movie theater, where a mysterious quantum emitter is prepared to offer us any reality, depending on the individual abilities of our perception. Particles, which are, simultaneously, quanta of radiation, combining within themselves something impossible from the standpoint of the rational mind – bodily density in space (corpuscles) and dispersion in space (waves), are prepared to show you every aspect of reality, which your senses are able to perceive. But that is precisely the issue. What are you able to perceive and how?

The universal field of energy and information never ceases to transform itself. Without being aware of it, people continue to be permanent subscribers to this unified information space. By joining together with planetary information structures, the human bio-plasma generated by the electromagnetic oscillations of the human body, would be able to create a stable channel of communication with the supercomputer of the noosphere. It is not scientists this time, but practical experience, which indicates that people are revealing on a broader scale their previously hidden abilities to perceive different kinds of fields and radiations. In other words, the central issue of the new millennium: „What will become of us?" is being addressed empirically.

That which we call the human mind is a special phenomenon of space and time. We all consist of atoms that are at least five billion years old.

187

And the vacuum inside each atom pulsates with intellect. Every particle is nothing else than the mind that has established interaction between myriads of components. Not less than nine trillion reactions take place in each of them every second! Can you imagine how powerful a computer would have to be to run a set of similar processes?!

Only a very few people have so far noticed that a hidden revolution has already taken place among us. This revolution in the practical application of the possibilities of the human consciousness will be able to guarantee a global breakthrough in every field of knowledge.

Russia is blessed not only by its deep soul. It could also have another mission: to create a new life that defies understanding at this point.

Already now many scientists are predicting that in the near future people will find new possibilities opening before them, such as retaining within us and within space of information about all the things seen, heard, thought-out, and felt, about the entire emotional and mental life of each individual. This is, essentially, an alternative to preserving information on a computer. The possible existence of indestructible forms of subtle structures in consciousness, opening the path to real immortality, is also being predicted.

Moreover, the prediction is beginning to come true most actively. Although, in its initial manifestations, not exactly the way anyone could anticipate...

Chapter 6

I was informed about a number of instances when children, who studied at the Academy and were able to open their bio-computers, developed alarming psychological abnormalities in their behavior. These weren't mental illnesses: fortunately, it never reached the level of a serious clinical diagnosis. But the kids had nightmares, dreaming about zombies and other dark forces. Considering the fact that Lapshin constantly talked about his intimate friendship with Satan and his use of the techniques of the Kingdom of the Dead, such information couldn't be ignored.

Every time I saw Vyacheslav I tried to get him to explain the increased negative statistics involving children trained according to his technique. My insistent questioning clearly got on his nerves.

– It's their fault, – he said. – They turn on their bio-computers and start sticking their noses into the nooks and crannies of the entire world of subtle matter. No wonder their minds develop pathologies. I warn everyone about safety. I always tell them not to get carried away. But they won't listen. So what do you want from me? Am I to blame for their excessive curiosity?

– But they are just kids, and you should have foreseen that they would be curious, – I disagreed. – When you give them such an unusual toy to play with, they are going to tinker with it until they break it.

– Break what: the toy or themselves? – Lapshin tried to counter in an aggressive tone.

– That toy is a part of them and you should have taken this into account. There had to be a reason why in the past bio-computers opened only for people who had attained a certain level of spiritual maturity...

189

– That was in the past. Today's different. Now bio-computers open by themselves. Two of the three children who come to us for training already have working bio-computers from the beginning. Am I responsible for them, too, or maybe it's the TV tower in Ostankino?

– What does the Ostankino tower have to do with any of this?

– A lot! Its radiation triggers the opening of the bio-computer. And there's much more. Why doesn't anybody blame the Academy of Sciences for this? Your academics have altered the human habitat so drastically that they provoked this entire orgy of wizards, medicine men, telepathy experts and psychics. First they create people with abnormal abilities through their frigging scientific and technological progress and then they sit it out in their research institutes. They, you see, have nothing to do with any of this! All they did was simply to create the computer! Have they ever stopped to think what these "simple" computers were going to do with people tomorrow? They don't understand any of the stuff they are imposing on mankind as a benefit. And tomorrow all these computers will create a global civilization of subtle matter, directed against human beings, and they will begin to rip out of your brains the component called consciousness, which they are currently missing. Before you know it, you will become robots in the service of these crutches for your minds.

When Vyacheslav flew off the handle he often blurted out things he never intended to say. In his usual state, he controlled his monologues somehow. During his lectures, for instance, he could talk on a given topic for hours and not say anything of substance. Nothing, nothing at all... I often tried to analyze his tape recorded lectures – in these so-called revelations he was just pulling the wool over people's eyes. Everything in them was turned upside down – use of terminology, concepts and description of subtle structures...

Nevertheless, for some reason one was left with the suspicion that he knows something important, which he is afraid to reveal by accident.

Then, in moments of direct confrontation, he would sometimes utter something so horrible that it would make blood freeze in my veins. He would express thoughts that seemed close to mine, but ridicule my sincere anxiety and turn it into a farce, a mockery of man.

– All of you can't seem to understand that you are no more than puppets. You are being manipulated by a world, which continues to be invisible to you. – Vyacheslav pattered his prophetic wisdoms, piercing me with his harsh brown eyes. His lecturing style clearly excited him, and this time I didn't want to argue with him and interfere by showing disagreement. – You see the surrounding world and it never occurs to you that it is a mockery (he appeared to be reading my thoughts!) of the world, which you created in the form of science, education and culture. They are completely at odds with the fundamental structure that a person had initially. Everything affects human beings – the dragon of the earth, the celestial dragon, the essences of the companions and the essence of family, the essences of the prototype culture of the underground civilization, the essence of fundamental structures of the "shadow" and the essence of the transition. There also exist essences of imprecation. All this oppresses man, manipulates him and leads to one problem after another. What starts as a minor disorder ends up being a serious disease. We are all surrounded by these things and wallow in this perfect mess. If you want to know, every pimple on your face is the result of an attack from an energy parasite. And here you are talking about a few boys and girls who became ill from my techniques.

– But it is a fact. – I finally decided to voice my opinion.

– Yes, it's a fact. – Vyacheslav agreed unexpectedly. – What about all the people who die from hospital mistakes! Listen to the stories people tell. We're nowhere near that bad. No villain could cause as much harm as the good people in white coats do. And they will never be held responsible for any of it. There is such vileness there, such mutual cover up and irresponsibility that I could present myself as an angel with wings among them.

– Really, are you an angel or someone different? – I asked suddenly, following some instinctive inner urge. Apparently, the strange midnight ritual in Theodosia was indelibly imprinted in my memory.

Vyacheslav once again pierced me with his unkind brown eyes. He wavered and tried to avoid answering my question.

– Evil-kind, angel-devil, it's all very relative. We don't exist on our own, you see. Already right now we are being shaped and molded from the future.

– Who is doing it?

– The future neo-cultures. But it is the future only for us, for someone else it's already the past. An interaction takes place between systems and structures. If a person learns to consciously control these processes, he becomes a dragon.

– Oh, the famous character, – I had to express my admiration. – Please give me a bit more detail on that score.

Lapshin suddenly realized that he said far more than he had intended.

– For sure, we could talk for a while about your dragon, but I still can't understand the main point: are you with me or against me?

– You're back to your obsession with how to seize power over the world, aren't you?

– Yes, – Vyacheslav decided not to deny the truth.

– I told you already that I am not interested in playing soccer with the

192

Earth's globe. I don't find the idea appealing.

– What do you find appealing then?

– I would like to help people in any way I can. I want to write books. By the way, there, in Theodosia I asked your elements exactly for that before I entered the circle.

– Mm… Yes, I see. You are running around like heroic Danko* with your burning heart in your hand, while the villagers grumble from under their cover of brushwood: Why do you run back and forth with your torch? We can't fall asleep because of you, – Vyacheslav said, laughing.

That night, after my conversation with Vyacheslav, the showing of the old film, which was temporarily interrupted in Theodosia, was continued once again. Jesus came back and so did the road which was being revealed to me for some reason.

* * *

The dark space was deep and produced the odd impression of being detached from what opened before his eyes.

Like in a repetitive dream, he once again saw the "sheep of his flock" at the foot of the trees, purified by the preaching of the doctrine: Mark, who was attracted to the Rabbi by his awakening gift of a writer, the mighty James, John the dreamer, the humble Philip, the well-read Bartholomew, the timid Matthew and Thomas the Wanderer, always doubting everything. Curled up and hugging his bag with a short sword hidden inside,

---

* Danko is the protagonist of a romantic story by the famous Russian writer Maxim Gorky. It speaks of a tribe of strong men who were forced by their enemies to retreat into the depths of an old dark forest. Every day weakened their faith, and they were on the verge of surrendering to their enemy in despair for their lives. Danko tore out his heart and raised it high over his head to light the way for his people and save them from slavery.

the impetuous, daring Peter snored intermittently in his sleep, while the Rabbi's first disciple Andrew slept peacefully nearby. Thaddeus tossed and turned in his sleep, as if sensing an impending disaster and bumped lightly into Simon. All the others, who had been following the Rabbi, were also fast asleep.

Only Judas Iscariot was not there, who despite his secret love for the Rabbi was eternally doomed to play the role of a traitor. He was already leading the temple guards to Jesus in the garden of Gethsemane. Judas' destiny had to show everyone that you can't sell love and buy happiness with the money. He was the only one who would prove with his death that Zechariah's prophesy was right: "So I took the thirty pieces of silver."

How little time remained to find a way to change the established course of the eternal tragedy once and for all! Memory, which stored everything he had seen in the mountains near Nazareth, was now obligingly evoking more and more new details from its deep recesses.

He recalled the future: the faces of the soldiers, the wild frenzy of the mob, the priests ... and he clearly understood that none of them had been convinced of his divinity. Particularly the priests – the eternal enemies of the Son of Man. They, who had crucified him, were the first to declare themselves the slaves of Jesus. They arrogated to themselves the honor he had earned and found it very convenient to be slaves of a ruler, who could not rule. They twisted and distorted his great teaching, adapting it to fit their paltry needs. Then they carried off his crudely severed parts to their own domains – their churches and barns, temples and caves. They used him, who opened the path of love and unity for people to follow, to instill hatred and hostility. Wars were unleashed and people were robbed in the name of Jesus, the best of the best were condemned to death, – those who sought the truth through doubts and agonizing battles with the obvious

194

imperfections of the world, those who elevated their own spirit and not their faith alone.

Oh, how Yeshua despised these hypocrites! But his disdain was for the time being safe for his executioners, who were fervently praising the heavenly master.

He now understood why it ended contrary to what had been intended. But he still didn't know what had to be done to set right the course of a great cause that had been torn to shreds by his false servants and tailored to suite their own unsavory purposes, preferences and secret passions.

Yeshua was the first to hear the sound of the crowd approaching from the direction of the city. They soon appeared – a band of temple soldiers following Judas. In the wavering, ever-changing light of the torches the crowd seemed enormous. The soldiers surrounded Yeshua's disciples awakened by the voices and, examining their faces, they started looking for the teacher.

Judas was the first to notice the Rabbi. Without saying a word to anyone, he approached the teacher and stopped opposite of him. According to the agreement he had with the soldiers, he was supposed to identify with a kiss the man who was to be arrested.

Upon seeing that the act of betrayal had already taken place, Yeshua silently laid his hands on the face of his apostle who accepted the role of traitor. Leaning over, Yeshua kissed him.

Judas' eyes filled with tears.

– I am not to judge your deeds, – he said in a whisper. – But it isn't too late, Rabbi. Let us leave now.

– I can't. My Way of the Cross has already been drawn, and it is impossible to turn away from it, – he said just as he did that other time, in the vision at the graves of the prophets. – You did everything right, Judas.

195

Go now. They are already close to us.

Judas walked away, and the soldiers of the temple surrounded Yeshua from all sides.

– It's him, take him, – somebody shouted. Strong calloused hands grabbed the Rabbi. A rope swept across his wrists and wrapped tightly around them. Malevolently grinning faces rallied closely around the victim. Then suddenly the crowd recoiled with expressions of horror. The mighty Peter rushed with a wild cry out of the darkness at the soldiers of the temple. His sword flashed in his hand. Peter's eyes glowed with such fierce concentration in the torchlight that anyone who saw them knew: this man will stop at nothing, not even the need to spill blood.

And he spilled it. One of the soldiers, either because he was too brave or because he didn't have time to look Peter in the eye, made a step toward him. The apostle's sword flashed like a bolt of lightning in the dark, and the head of the soldier would have rolled to the ground, if Yeshua hadn't moved aside the sharp edge of the sword with a concentrated effort of will. The assailant only suffered a severed ear and, whining with pain, he dashed into the darkness.

Recovering from fear, the other soldiers drew their weapons and were about to pounce on Peter, when they heard a resounding voice:

– Lower your weapons and put your swords back into their place; for all those who take up the sword shall perish by the sword. I must drink the cup, which is intended for me.

Peter heaved a heavy sigh and obeyed, moving back into the crowd of disciples and apostles. The soldiers, too, calmed down. Clutching the rope, they dragged their captive to the court of the Sanhedrin.

That night many members of the Sanhedrin assembled at the house of the high priest Caiaphas. Elders of the Jewish people and scribes also gathered there. *The soldiers of the temple brought in the offender, accused of desecrating the tenets of faith as they were laid down in the Talmud. He was placed in the center of the room and two candles were lit next to him so that everyone could see the shameless face and hear the deliberate lies of the detractor.*

Caiaphas turned to Yeshua and directed his piercing and ruthless gaze at him.

– Are you the man who is being called the Messiah, Son of God?

The massive walls of the hall, which proudly carried the burdens of fairness and justice, responded to the words of the high priest with an awe-inspiring echo.

Yeshua smiled:

– Yes, it is true.

A rumble of indignation exploded the silence in the hall.

– Blasphemy!

– Liar!

– Insane!

– Son of Satan!

Horror vibrated in their voices but Yeshua knew that their fear was feigned and insincere. He glanced at the people around him. Their eyes expressed indifference, and their lips were twisted in a grimace of contempt and revulsion.

– Why do we need any more witnesses? You have now heard his blasphemy yourselves. What do you think? – Now it was the voice of Caiaphas that people heard and there was mockery in it.

And other voices echoed, reflected from the walls:

– Death to him...

– Guilty of death...

– Death...

Everything repeated itself. It was just the way I saw it in the prophetic vision by a spring. These familiar voices were sending Him to the Golgotha of immortality.

Yeshua's imminent suffering grew and multiplied within him, and with it the power in him also grew, multiplied and pulsated, so that there was already enough to bring the stone slab of the roof down on the heads of those sitting in the house.

A miracle, he had to perform a miracle for everyone to believe in his divinity, but... Yeshua contained the wave of irritation inside him. There were people here. They would die. They are awful today, but tomorrow they might change and become good. And what would people think of him if they learned for a fact that the Sanhedrin was killed by the wrath of God, not because the builders had done a poor job. Once again he confronted the dangerous impossibility of performing a miracle where we had to find understanding.

His hair, drenched with sweat, became plastered to his eyes. He raised his bound hands and straightened the fallen strand. This simple gesture completely calmed him.

– They also say that you claimed you could destroy God's temple and erect it again in three days. Is that so? – The voice of Caiaphas once again rose above the murmur of the crowd.

Like lightning, he was struck with the realization that if he agreed, and then did what was announced, there would hardly be anyone left who would dare to question his divinity. An earthquake could destroy the temple but only God could erect it again in three days.

– Why don't you say anything? Perhaps three days aren't enough for you to build a temple? Tell us, we will show understanding, – Caiaphas'

voice rumbled with cold contempt.

He could perform a miracle in three days. He could move the mystery composed in Egypt, on the Island of Philae, from the stage to real life. He enacted it on the streets and squares of real cities in the Promised Land, against the backdrop of the sky, mountains, lakes and trees instead of the stage, with real crowds watching and genuine emotions of love, anger and hatred, with real nails and true suffering.

But there was an error in the script, which had to be corrected. And he wanted to do it. But all the actors performing the tragedy knew their roles too well and ignored the improvisations of the main character.

– He does not honor us with an answer. We are mere dust at the feet of his holiness! – Caiaphas continued to mock him.

Yeshua recovered himself from his bitter thoughts and looked up at the high priest.

– A speck of dust is like the infinite Universe, and everything is made in the image of God. As above, so below, – he replied humbly.

– Have you heard! – cried Caiaphas.

– This is blasphemy...

– He compared dust to God...

– Guilty of death, – voices could be heard once again.

– You have pronounced your own sentence, you wretched creature, – Caiaphas confirmed what he heard from all around. And this time his voice sounded choked and muffled.

Early in the morning, that same Friday, the chief priests and the Jewish elders brought the criminal to Pilate, to have the sentence of the Sanhedrin approved and executed.

Pilate came out to them on the platform called the Stone Pavement. When he saw the members of the Sanhedrin, he asked:

– *What charges are you bringing against this man?*

– *This man is corrupting our nation, forbidding us to pay taxes to Caesar, and saying that he is the Messiah, a king.*

– *Are you the King of the Jews?* – *Pilate asked, gazing with curiosity at the man in front of him. Meek, in tattered clothes and with bruises covering his face, the convicted man didn't produce the impression of an evildoer and criminal.*

– *Why would I want to be the king of this country?* – *Yeshua responded to the question with a question of his own.*

Pilate peered into his eyes, as if though he were able, with just one glance, to fathom the centuries of fruitless suffering that filled them with the pain of wisdom.

– *But they are asserting this. It means that you uttered certain words, which led them to draw such a conclusion.*

–*Words that are understood one way in a certain place and completely differently in another. You know that like no one else.*

Pilate sensed a hint of mockery in his voice and parried momentarily.

– *I do not need your accusation but you should fear mine…*

– *Power is dangerous. Possessing power muddles one's vision and turns his away from wisdom. The one who uses power against others becomes his own worst enemy,* – *Yeshua responded with bitter sympathy.*

Pilate looked at him probingly.

– *You're too educated, and your mind is too sophisticated for a simple preacher. Who are you?* – *He asked, and a drop of sweat ran down his face. This totally insignificant incident annoyed the procurator beyond words. "Why is he standing here, on the Stone Pavement, on a hot day like that? What does he care about this man who speaks in witticisms, which he then immediately turns into foolishness, and who stubbornly refuses to dispel the incredible accusations against him?"*

– So you are king? – Pilate asked.

– It is as you say, – Yeshua confirmed dispassionately. – But my king-dom is not of this world.

– Dreamer, – the procurator muttered through his teeth.

– Did you hear what he just said, this blasphemer, this good-for-nothing Galilean? – whispers rustled through the crowd.

– Then he is a Galilean? – The news made Pilate happy. – So why did you bring him here? King Herod Antipas of Galilee should be the one to try him.

Turning around, the procurator walked resolutely past the parted war-riors to the door, pleased that he so cleverly avoided any involvement in this case, which he found distasteful.

* * *

Pontius Pilate returned to the palace in a sad reverie. The outdoor heat, which tormented him on the Stone Pavement, retreated instantly. Here it was fresh and cool. Pilate sat in an arm-chair on the mosaic floor by the fountain, and dismissed the servants and soldiers with a casual wave of his hand. The air, cooled by the fountain water, was a true bles-sing, and the procurator dozed off, enjoying the wonderful sensations.

He dreamed of Rome and Claudia Procula – granddaughter of Caesar Augustus and Tiberius' step-daughter. Pilate rejected his great vocation for her, his passionate dream. Because of Claudia he, a horseman and the son of a legion commander, became an actor, to conquer like Orestes but not in life – on the stage, to die there like Xerxes the Great and to suffer like Prometheus.

201

Claudia once saw his acting and was struck with irresistible passion. As a disciple of the great Seneca she could not remain indifferent to the artistic gift of this handsome young man. Submitting to the instant surge of powerful feeling, she ordered her slaves to carry her to the amphitheater. In a voice filled with genuine emotion, she cried out to Pilate: "I swear by all the gods to always be your sweetest lover, even if it forces me to break with the entire world, for only death can tear us apart."

Such a readiness for self-sacrifice demanded a sacrifice from him in return. Pilate left the stage and married Claudia. Tiberius appointed him procurator of Judea, and out of respect for such a strong manifestation of love he allowed Pilate to take his wife with him, which was against the rule of service.

Now Claudia was constantly with him, filling his life with pure bliss and beauty. She was tall, slender and graceful, and he dreamed of her lying in her light transparent tunic on the bed of love. Then her beautiful face leaned over him, and the dark wave of her hair brushed against his naked body, causing shivers of passion and desire.

Someone's slight cough suddenly drove away the pleasant vision. The procurator opened his eyes. His secretary was standing nearby with a guilty expression on his face.

– What is it? – Pilate asked.

– They brought him back.

– Whom?

– The one who calls himself king...

The procurator smiled ironically.

– So what was Herod's sentence?

– He acquitted him, dressed him in a gorgeous robe and sent him back to you, – the secretary answered.

– Let them release him them if he is not guilty, – the procurator cried out in anger, rising from his armchair. Why did they bring the Jew back here again?

– But the chief priests insist and demand that you approve their sentence.

– Bloodthirsty villains! Why do they need the death of the comical dreamer?

– The elders consider him to be the most dangerous of all those deserving death, – the secretary answered impassively. – They have gathered a big crowd by the palace. They are also saying that one of the Galilean disciples Judas Iscariot hanged himself. He threw the reward he got for his treachery under the feet of the chief priest Caiaphas. He then walked down the street muttering: "No miracle, no miracle."

– Let them bring in the accused, – the procurator commanded.

Indignant at the fact that he was disrupted from watching a beautiful dream, he was filled with a dull hatred for the priests and their inexplicable persistence.

The captive was pushed into the hall. Indeed, he was dressed in the white robes of innocence but his hands were still tied with a rope.

– Leave us now, – the procurator ordered.

Pilate was too upset with the impossibility of getting rid of this distasteful affair to conceal it. He winced as if something tormented him and asked when everyone had left:

– Why do they hate you?

– Because as long as I'm alive I prevent them from being idols in the city, – Yeshua said. His voice was smooth like the sound of a mountain stream.

– You are willing to sacrifice your life to bring the truth to this herd of

203

cattle that is demanding your death right now in the street and who wishes your destruction? – Pilate asked in amazement. – How do you intend to lead them?

– From hope to the dream, and from the dream to the truth, – Yeshua answered and a weak half-smile touched his lips.

– These people who are crafted out of abominations and naive faith? – Pilate exclaimed with bitterness in his voice. – Close your eyes, dreamer, and do not open them until you can see. One of your disciples has already hanged himself. His name is Judas.

Yeshua shuddered and a lone tear slipped from under his eyelid.

– The light will join the light, and darkness will join darkness, – he whispered and looked at the procurator, as if the words he had spoken meant something else, not what he meant to express through them.

– You know yourself how much filth there is in them, now many contradictions and vacillations, – the procurator insisted.

– Yes, I know, – the accused man agreed, not trying to avoid the procurator's stare. – But it isn't their fault. Too many voices of the primal world are sounding in them, which is why they can't join together to form a single harmonious chorus without external help.

– Wait for me, – said the procurator and went out on the Stone Pavement.

The crowd by the doors of the palace, headed by the chief priests, was rumbling. Pilate raised his hand and all was quiet around him. The procurator's glance was firm and stubborn.

– You brought me the Galilean as one who was inciting the people to rebellion. I have examined him in your presence and have found no basis for your charges against him. I sent him to Herod, and he, too, found that he has done nothing to deserve death. Therefore, I will punish him and

204

then release him.

The chief priests and the elders were the first to cry out:

– Release for us Barabbas! But the one who calls himself the Messiah, punish him by death.

And everyone in the crowd also shouted:

– Not him, Barabbas!!

– Crucify him!

– Let him be crucified!

– But Barabbas is a murderer, – the procurator objected.

– Anyway, – the crowd kept shouting, – release Barabbas!

Pilate turned his back on them abruptly and went back into the palace. The soldiers closed the door immediately behind him and the noise of the crowd subsided.

The accused man met the procurator, gazing calmly into his eyes.

– They demand your death, – said Pilate.

– I do not fear death. In every person something is continuously being born and something dies.

– The meaning of the words changes when we are talking not about philosophy but about death on the cross! – Pilate said indignantly. – I am bound by customs, law and duty too much to do as I please, and not as I must.

– Do as you must, – Yeshua suggested firmly.

– And then you will have only one path, the path of Golgotha!

– All my paths, wherever I go, lead to Golgotha, – muttered the accused, torn by contradictory impulses. – I know what a heavy burden this decision puts on your heart, and I sympathize with you.

– Heavier than the cross that awaits you there? –Pilate asked with a nod, sending the Jew's thoughts to the rumble of the crowd outside the

205

door.

Shaken, the accused man took a step back. His face was distorted with a spasm of future pain, and his eye erupted with suffering. Barely able to control himself, he said with bitterness:

– It is not the cross that is heavy but the burden of hatred and evil.

With his teeth clenched from fury and suffocating frustration, the procurator went out again on the slab of the Stone Pavement. He looked with disgust at the crowd subdued by his gaze.

– I'm telling you again: I find no guilt in this man, – he said in a threatening tone.

And once more, the chief priests were the first to shout:

– He must die because he has declared himself to be the Son of God!

– He has threatened to destroy the Temple of Jerusalem and rebuild it in three days by the sheer power of his words!

– We have the law, and according to our law he must die!

– Crucify, crucify him!

And again the door shut behind him rescued Pilate from the cries of hate.

– Do you hear that?

– Don't torment yourself, do what they are demanding, – the accused answered.

– Have you really promised to destroy the Temple of Jerusalem and erect it once again with the sheer power of your word? – Pilate asked, looking him in the eye.

– Yes…

– And were there witnesses?

– Yes, there were…

– You poor creature, – said Pilate and turned away.

The procurator demonstrated his sympathy too obviously. Yeshua wanted to reassure him.

– I must conquer past evil without paying attention to any losses, and I must show people the way, where they should go, – he said. – Whatever the decision may have been, it wasn't you who made it.

– Well, – Pilate agreed, – I am powerless to fight against them and against you at once. Let you dream in your last mortal dream that all your wishes, dreamer, will come true.

Clapping his hands, the procurator summoned the soldiers of the palace.

– Take him and do as they wish, – Pilate ordered, intoning the word "they" in a special way to make is sound particularly disdainful.

When the soldiers brought the accused man to Golgotha, they offered him some sour wine mixed with narcotic herbs to alleviate his suffering. But he refused to drink it.

Soon everything was ready and the soldiers crucified Yeshua. It was around noon. Two other men, both criminals, were also crucified, one on his right, the other on his left. There was a plaque with a written inscription, nailed above him, which read: "Yeshua of Nazareth, King of the Jews."

The muffled voices from afar brought Yeshua out of the blackout. He did not know how much time had passed since the moment he hid in the darkness of unconsciousness from the pain caused by the nails which pierced his body. He almost lost any notion of where he was and what he should be doing. When he opened his eyes he saw a hill overgrown with low shrubs clinging to the cracks in the rock, and a rather small group of people standing some distance away behind the chain of soldiers. Seeing that consciousness had returned to him, someone shouted:

– If he is the king of Israel, then let him come down from the cross, and

we will believe in him!..

Another voice joined in:

– So you can destroy the temple and rebuild it in three days? Save yourself then? We will watch!

They were laughing at him. For them he was only a carcass hanging on the cross. There was a grimace of revulsion on some faces.

Yeshua gasped frantically and forced himself to come up from the bottom of tormenting drowsiness. With an effort of will he awakened within him the sacred energy of a power, lying dormant in his tailbone, and twisting it like a tornado around the vertebrae, he threw it up the spine toward his head, down the chest and stomach, and then up again. The ripples of energy began to grow in him, and in an agonizing struggle with the inability to pronounce words, his bloodless gray lips clearly uttered:

– It will be fulfilled!..

The silence that ensued seemed like a prayer. The short uttering delivered amidst the scorching heat on the Bald Mountain was either sacrilege, or a prophecy. The city of Jerusalem lay nearby, and all eyes turned instinctively toward the impressive temple of white marble, its gilded roof glistening in the sun. It represented greatness and sanctity.

– Blasphemer!

– He is persisting even on the cross! – sounded indignant voices.

– He should be stoned!

Yeshua forced himself to forget about the crowd and stay focused. With a short impulse, he sent a wave of heat through his body, following it as it flowed along the back toward his numb limbs, overcoming the numbness of approaching oblivion. He moved his fingers, which he could not bend from the pain and with an effort of will he removed himself from the stench of death.

208

Silence, filled with pain and tension, was now all around him. Seeing that despite all the opportunities of expression being taken away from it, life was visibly returning to the barely breathing body on the cross, even those who were cursing him fell silent.

A vague smile touched the lips of the one who was crucified, and then his face froze in grim anticipation. His eyes suddenly became unnaturally dark, like two clusters of night. His veins grew swollen from the exertion. He was biting his lips, as though the external pain could eliminate the other, internal one, or at least keep it under control. The bites of horse flies made the pus of mucus ooze from his skin and drip down his cheeks. This distracted him, and he was still unable to attain the needed concentration of strength. Nevertheless, something had changed all around. A sudden gust of wind threw dust at the people standing next to the cross.

Yeshua had to focus on the roof of the Jerusalem Temple glittering with gold. The plan that was conceived in advance came into effect, and with relentless divine will it was approaching the climax of a miracle, without which no great mission could begin.

He strained his vision to the maximum. Yeshua saw a stream of light descend on the Jerusalem Temple. The bridge between the external and inner world, across which he could influence the cosmic powers of nature, was established. The great elements of eternity were ready to respond to the minutest impulse from his will. He directed all of his mental strength toward outlining his desire.

Another gust of wind hit the Bald Mountain, and its force was becoming more and more tangible. The gathered crowd began to look worriedly around, unable to understand what caused the sudden surge of bad weather. Only the one crucified, with the inscription "King of the Jews" over his head, seemed to have recovered his former strength. His eyes glo-

wed with fierce concentration and were fastened to the roof of the Temple of Jerusalem.

A high hissing sound filled the surrounding space and turned into the rumbling of an approaching storm, as if intensified by the effort of his will. With all their power, the elements struck the crucified man, knocking the air from his lungs, but he still managed to wheeze the following toward a handful of people covering their heads with their garb:

– It will be fulfilled!..

His hoarse voice, gurgling deep inside his chest, reached those standing by the cross, however none of them shot up their hands in a passionate blessing.

Ripples of energy began to grow inside him, and Yeshua once more focused his gaze on the roof of the temple. Storm clouds began to gather over the mountain and the city and the fiery sword of lightning suddenly cut through the swirling darkness.

The people screamed and took off in fear. Only the guards and soldiers, pulling their cloaks over their heads, stayed at their post, loyal to the orders. The swirling black clouds with the fierce rumble of elemental power already formed in the sky, and a thunderstorm broke out in full force. The wind ripped out the trees in the mountains, pushing out the sunlight and throwing mud at it. The skies parted, and rain poured down on the city of Jerusalem with such fury, as if it was the beginning of the second Biblical Flood. All plunged into the chaos of the storm.

The downpour fell on the hill with the three crosses on top. It seemed as though the sky wanted to punish the Earth, flogging it with the powerful whips of rain for the evil perpetrated that day on the mountain called the Golgotha, which means the skull-mountain. The Earth refused to accept the pouring rain and it rushed in heavy streams down to the city, which *was attacked by ever growing gusts of wind.*

– It will be fulfilled! – The one crucified wheezed through his clenched teeth, and his voice rang clear through the howling wind and the roaring of the storm. A shadow broke away from the storm and, struggling with the wind, obscured the temple roof. But Yeshua was so focused on controlling the events, which took place and so preoccupied with the realization of his dream that he failed to notice what just happened. At that moment one of the soldiers came up to him, overcoming the resistance of the wind. The tip of his spear rose, taking aim at the heart of the crucified man, and, tearing through his flesh, the iron tip plunged between his ribs.

– You should thank the procurator, – was the last thing he heard.

***

These successive scenes from the life of Jesus, which were similar in some way, but also somewhat different from known Gospel texts contributed to some instability in my established notions about life. Of course, I understood that each such event caused a certain transformation in my view of the world and, moreover, altered the very foundations of my life. That was natural since I now became more attentive to things that did not interest me before. It was similar to an imaginary situation when you first begin to empathize with the main character in a story that you found moving, and then you begin to participate in what happens alongside with him, altering the course of events in a few scenes and changing the original script. It was similar but not the same as what I had just described, because in reality what I observed wasn't an abstraction for me or something that developed on its own. It seemed to me for some reason that the plots in these visions were like successively activated strata of my own con-

211

sciousness that were transmitting certain historical information into the structure of my brain where it was being decoded.

I found some indirect clues reading other people's works, which explored the phenomena of consciousness. One of them was "The Phenomenon of Man: Cosmic and Earthly Sources," a book by academician and Doctor of Medical Sciences V.P. Kaznacheyev, where he came up with an interesting hypothesis:

"The entire evolution of the Universe, beginning with the Big Bang, has its beginning in the living space of the Cosmos – a gigantic aggregate of living cosmic flows and organizations, of which we are but a small part."

Already hundreds of thousands years ago the primitive men inhabiting the planet (academician Kaznacheyev called them protogominids) accumulated in their brains some 13-14 billion neurons – semiconductor-type computers of a kind. They regulated the behavior of these creatures in the form of instinctive reactions. But then the space phase arrived with the emergence of a new man and new intelligence. A remarkable process occurred in certain parts of the planet: the 14 billion neurons in the head of the protogominids, each of which already possessed the soliton-holographic form of living matter, combined into one giant soliton as the result of an explosion.

"All tribal units were connected by soliton fields, which meant that no matter what distance away a family member or a member of the primitive community may have been, all of these people could see and know everything about him, i.e., there was telepathy, distant communication, imaginative vision of each other in holographic images. And this formed the foundations of our intelligence. Not a single individual but a group united by a common field was what created the basis for the original planetary

212

intelligence of human beings" (Novosibirsk Publishers, 1991, pp.16-18).

The scientist's hypothesis corresponded to my own worldview. At that time I developed a strengthening belief in that whatever we might be doing and wherever we might be going, we were moving toward one goal – to one's inner self, to remembering oneself. People who have lost the memory of their past and their future are akin to children who are ready, day after day, without ever tiring of it, to ride on their favorite carousel. Something always changes around us – one day the sun is out, the next it rains, the leaves appear on the trees and then fall off, first one set of people come along to see how these carefree folks who behave like children whirl on the carousel, and then others come to watch. We turn around a closed circle, squealing with delight at the speed, forgetting that at some point we were truly able to fly and that our exaggerated excitement is nothing but a vague memory of who we once were.

There are scientifically documented facts describing people who lifted huge concrete slabs weighing more than a ton in a state of affect, and others who beat high and long jumping records in an attempt to rescue themselves from mortal danger. The healer Porfiri Ivanov was subjected to the same torture as general Karbyshev after being captured by the Germans in WWII – he was frozen alive into an ice pillar – but unlike the general, he survived.

Man's uncovered possibilities are infinite. Human beings can know not only the past but also the future. There exist a large number of accurate predictions, some of which have already been mentioned. But here is another example. Read the following narrative by the medieval physician and esoteric *Philippe-Dieu-donne-Noel Olivarius*, and try to guess by yourself, without any prompting, who this clairvoyant was referring to several centuries before the event occurred:

213

"France and Italy will give birth to a supernatural being. This man will come, in his youth, out of the sea and will adopt the language and the manners of the Frankish Celts. While still young, he will overcome untold obstacles in his path with the help of soldiers who will at a later date make him supreme commander… For over five years he will engage in fighting not far from his place of birth. He will lead wars in all countries of the world with great courage and valor; he will restore the glory of the Roman world, put an end to the riots and horrors of Celtic France and will finally be made not king as was customary in the past but emperor, and the people will welcome his rule with great enthusiasm… For more than a decade he will send princes, dukes and kings fleeing from his army... It will give land to the peoples of many counties, and bring peace to each of them. He will come to a great city and accomplish great projects, constructing magnificent buildings, bridges, ports, waterworks and canals. He will have two wives and only one son.

For 55 months he will be engaged in a military campaign in a country where the parallel of latitude intersects with the meridian. There his enemies will set fire to a great city and he will enter it with his soldiers. He will abandon the city, left in ruins, and his army will perish. His men will have neither bread, nor water. Two thirds of his army will die, subjected to unbelievably bitter cold. Half of the surviving soldiers will never again return under his command. Finally, this great man deserted and betrayed by his friends, will be driven to defend himself and will be ousted even in his own country by great European nations. The Capetian kings of ancient blood will be reinstated in his place. Banished to an island not far from his native land, he will remain there for 11 months surrounded by his entourage, soldiers and friends… After 11 months he and his followers will again board a ship and disembark again on the soil of Celtic France. And

214

he will enter a large city ruled by the Capetian king of ancient blood, who will flee taking with him all the royal insignia. When he returns to his former empire he will give his people a set of wonderful laws. But then, after three moons and a third, he will be driven out again by the triple alliance of European nations and the rule of the Capetian king of ancient blood will be restored."

Should I talk about the prediction made in 1898 by writer Morgan Robertson in his novel "Futility" about the sinking of the Titanic?

Let me compare only a few striking facts. The name of the ship: the fictional ship was named Titan and the real Titanic. The size and construction of the two ships were almost identical, with both liners having four tubes and three screws. The length of the Titan – 260 m, the Titanic – 268 m.; displacement: 7,000 tons – 6,600 tons; power: 50 000 hp – 55 000 hp; maximum speed: 25 knots – 25 knots. The cause, time and place of the disaster were practically the same. There were representatives of high society both on the Titan and the Titanic, and both ships did not have enough lifeboats. The list of similarities is so long and factually correct that it makes one wonder: how was a prophecy such as this at all possible?

The understanding that the former linear, cause-and-effect structure of the Universe does not reflect the evidence accumulated by science itself, is the reason why the fundamental disciplines have begun to fundamentally revise the paradigms of their conceptions, more resolutely developing a new worldview (or rather, a forgotten old view) at the junction of the material and ideal worlds, the past and the future, and death and immortality.

Researchers are not trying to sound witty when they speak increasingly more often about the "memory" of molecules, atoms or even subatomic particles. Perhaps not only our past lies hidden in this deep memory but also our future, which for the time being rests peacefully on the shelf where you store videos of personal destiny. At some moment, when our inner state and development prove themselves to be prepared to perceive more complicated scripts, someone presses an invisible switch on a molecule of deoxyribonucleic acid in the depths of the nucleus of one of the cells – and now a new movie plot unfolds in our consciousness. Nothing around has changed – the set, the actors are the same, but the action progresses differently and depends on amount of effort of will you invest into breaking out of the rut of self-imposed dependencies. Events of the next level actually come about only when your consciousness and your individual development become adequate for the potential of the new spiritual level.

Maybe the energy training I was involved in at the Academy activated the genetic memory, or, rather, the information storehouse of the DNA, and awakened new potentials of my body? In any case, I responded quite calmly to everything that took place and was engaged in introspection more as a researcher than a character in the script. True enough, it would probably be impossible to remove myself completely as the immediate participant in the sequence of new events that followed. After all, it was all happening to me and not to some movie character. Similarity of processes does not make them identical.

* * *

My relations with Lapshin began to sour. He actively used my book about him and the film as a means of self-promotion. Scores of people enrolled in his training courses, he made tons of money but there was no indication that he intended to return what he owed me and the studio director.

216

When I discussed the issue of repayment, he grinned humorously and cut the conversation short in a somewhat odd way:

– Would you have demanded money from God?

– What does God have to do with it? – I snapped. – The film we made is not about Him but about you.

– It depends, it depends… Show patience and your stubble will turn into gold, – he calmed me down with mysterious statements.

The work of the branch which we opened in Pushkino not far from Moscow did more to further undermine our relations. Several months before, I suggested that Lapshin could use the facilities of the now defunct "Kultura" publishers. This was a friendly gesture on my part in response to his constant requests that we should open as many branches of the Academy as possible. I introduced him to the district administration, took care of all the necessary permits, and what?

The branch started working, Lapshin was getting all the proceeds but he didn't even want to cover the cost of the utilities. It seemed as though after that night ritual in Theodosia he had gone completely out of whack if he could so clearly hint at his identity to God.

Still, I continued to write articles about him in various newspapers and magazines ignoring his progressive megalomania. I didn't like how he behaved, but I couldn't help being hypnotized by the facts: even incurable diseases seemed to retreat, subdued by his strange gift. And it wasn't just I who recognized the reality of this evidence. Professional physicians are also forced to admit it.

With the help of my friend Victor Glukhov, director of the famous "Slovo" film studio, I managed to arrange a serious examination of the facts involved in healing the blind and the use of alternative vision at the Helmholtz Institute of Eye Diseases. Eighteen physicians headed by the

217

director gathered to participate in this scientific event.

A boy who until recently was a ward of a special school for the blind, demonstrated his ability to roller skate, read ordinary books and watch TV.

The unanimously drawn conclusion ran: "It is of undisputed interest." And following this the expert's attention quietly, slowly dies down. And the same happened in other only cases as well.

I invited the well-known journalist and TV host Alexander Bovin to attend a demonstration of the phenomenon. He saw and checked everything. Feeling completely convinced, he personally went to meet with Yuri Osipov, President of the Russian Academy of Sciences, to tell him about the facts which he found extraordinary. The President immediately curbed his enthusiasm:

– We expose such miracle-makers a dime a dozen each year.

Who knows where he got his exposure "statistics," if the research institutes under the auspices of the Russian Academy of Sciences did not deny, but on the contrary, confirmed the facts of healing through some strange, unscientific psychophysical influence?

It is all quite understandable psychologically, however. Everyone who is being paid from government coffers, whether he is President of the Academy of Sciences or a regular physician, has plenty of routine to handle. All the rest of us do, too. Everyone with any self-respect has his own opinion about the things going on around him. So when something unusual interrupts our lives, which requires that we strain ourselves both mentally and spiritually, and demands that we revise our values, very few of us respond to the call of the unknown. We are all adults, after all, let us put aside idealism and other adolescent fantasies and leave magic fairy tales to ignorant old women. This response is a defensive reaction of the body accustomed to a certain rhythm, even if it clearly isn't a perfect one. One feels better with old sores in the body and with laws in one's soul – it's familiar.

When a philistine reasons (unconsciously) that way, it is called the traditions of society. When a scientist proves his point of view the same way – it becomes the kind of conservatism that destroys science. "Galileo's peer in science was no more stupid than the man himself. He knew full well that the Earth revolves, but he had a family to support." So goes the famous poem by Yevgeny Yevtushenko.

I tried to comprehend later why this was happening. Hundreds, even thousands of patients who were left with the merciless verdict of conventional medicine: „There is nothing more we can do for you," suddenly found someone who could. People were given their health back and some kind of unusual abilities were discovered within them ... but the Russian Academy of Sciences continues to be in a state of blissful ignorance about any of this.

And the issue probably isn't that somebody among the leaders of Russian science is deliberately trying to conceal the truth from the rest of mankind. It's just that they live in a totally different world, where none of this exists nor can it. The parameters of their thinking are predetermined by the predominant development of the left hemisphere of their brain and associated with its specific perception. In this world, the scientist is obligated to record and consider as real only what is observable to the eyes or detectable by devices, things you can touch, measure, taste, or calculate using a given formula. Scientists have long forgotten that the axioms of geometry are conditional, that Planck's constant is quite relative and that all science in general hangs by a thread. They don't wish to consider that just a few inches away from their familiar world there is an entry to another, four-dimensional space. This entry is called the right hemisphere of the brain. But if they so determined not to find this entry, how can they recognize that it is possible? How can they give up their left hemisphere advantage, which simultaneously severely limits them? There are, of course, exceptions, such as Natalia Petrovna Bekhtereva. But most likely she has no problems with either the right or the left hemisphere.

In order to determine the nature of the patient's health problem medics use complex devices and have him take expensive tests. What they basically do is test certain slices in the single organism to understand the disease and its scope. While they do it, they can study some areas of the body well and others not so well. Even computer tomography provides quite limited information about the disease. For example, it determines the presence of a tumor but cannot always see its metastases. So what even if it was able to see them? It would be a good thing if Jules Henri Poincare could remind these experts about the postulate of relativity! Explain to them that every instrument produces a great number of errors!

As for a person who possesses a screen of inner vision, who, using the language of science has the neurons in the right and left hemispheres working coherently, he is able to see the patient's body holistically to the minutest detail, in all its interconnections and interdependence. He uses the fourth dimension for this analysis. That tool, which highbrow thinkers with a predominantly developed left hemisphere can't master. And then a miracle happens. Well, it's only a miracle for random strangers, for a healer, it is the result of many years of work.

Academician Victor Petrovich Pashkevich is a most distinguished military surgeon. He has appeared in several TV programs now, describing a case that he found striking. He invited a number of children with an opened screen of inner vision to be present during one of his surgeries. The patient was already lying on the operation table and the computer tomography registered a malignant tumor in the stomach area. Try to imagine the surgeon's amazement when the teenagers told him that the tumor has metastasized, and also showed him where those metastases are located. They essentially changed the operation plan. The academician had long been probing possibilities of the strange "bio-computer" which is why he trusted their general assertions. When the operation began, it confirmed everything the children had warned him about. As a result, these teenagers from our Academy saved a man's life.

Victor Ivanovich resorted to the help of clairvoyants several times after that during his surgeries. And he never regretted doing it. Unfortunately he can't do it on a regular basis. For one, he has to disrupt their training schedule and he also has to pay them (sorry for mentioning such a prosaic matter). And where would he get the funding?

When using clairvoyance one doesn't need to do X-rays, carry out experiments or accumulate data. The response is obtained with the help of the most advanced instrument in the world – the human brain, which is capable of moving to another level of being. And I must admit that the world looks very different if you look at it from a new level of consciousness. Remember how a few decades ago, medical scientists suddenly decided that the appendix is a rudimentary and totally useless organ. And they concluded that it is safer to cut it out at birth rather than wait till later and operate with risk to adult life. For some reason they imagined that they know the human body, which is the work of the Creator, better than the Creator himself. So physicians began to cut out the appendix indiscriminately (especially in China). Millions of people trusted the authority of science and placed their young children under the surgeon's knife. Who is to blame and who account for such acts of poor judgment?

The point is that the appendix is not just a dead-end organ for food

221

waste, as anatomists assume. It performs a vital function as regulator of the reserve immune system. And it performs the above function through the holographic projection of the left brain hemisphere on the right one. If this mechanism is disrupted, you will not be able to effectively fend off infection. Moreover, you are guaranteed to have persistent headaches due to increased intracranial pressure.

Let's see now where the convolutions of the strictly logical consciousness of the left brain hemisphere could lead a person.

A person who has the audacity to imagine himself the master of the planet, who thinks he is carrying the truth in the back pocket of his fancy trousers, creates a global disaster. He indiscriminately drains all the swamps (here in Russia) or kills off all the sparrows as parasites (in China). He believes that the balance of nature lies in his trouser pocket.

Let is recall who was the second Nobel Prize-winner among Russian scientists? That's right, it was Ilya Mechnikov, a great physiologist and advocate for the fermented drink beverage kefir.*

The first Nobel Prize-winner among the Russians was Ivan Pavlov (1904), and Mechnikov was the second (1908). So here is the story: at Mechnikov's recommendation, surgery to remove the colon became very popular in Europe before World War I. Let us get rid of this unnecessary organ. This will improve human life, he said. Alas, the opposite happened: the operation not only complicated the trusting patient's life substantially, but also shortened it. A year or two after the surgery the poor fellows died. But who remembers the life-threatening of the great scientist today? Have present-day physicians learned anything from it?

* Kefir is a cultured milk product with high nutritive value, which contains several major strains of friendly bacteria and beneficial yeasts, not commonly found in yogurt, making the body more efficient in resisting such pathogens as E. coli and intestinal parasites.

I am convinced that the medicine of the future is unthinkable without clairvoyance. After all, with expanded consciousness (and clairvoyance is that very expansion of consciousness) it is possible not only to determine the disruptions and failures in your body, but also to eliminate them with relative ease. One would have to be lacking in common sense to voluntarily give up such opportunities.

Incidentally, with the help of clairvoyance it is easy to track how this or that remarkable discovery emerges. Typically, it is a random breakthrough in the information field of the Earth, where all the possible technologies already have already existed as a given, since they are part of the program for the evolution of the Earth and everything that inhabits it.

Everything is fine in this scenario except for the word „random." Although if something has happened "randomly" one day, it becomes more likely than other breakthroughs into the network of the cosmic web will be made over and over again. Still, if this would occur as a result of standard procedures for accessing information, for example, it would be safer and more efficient. Everything that surrounds us – planets, stars and galaxies – did not appear incidentally, and we can see this very clearly with the help of clairvoyance. The faculty of clairvoyance is part of a giant intelligent organism, which finally allows people to use a small portion of their intellect and knowledge. Do not refuse the gift of the Cosmos! You will be sorry if you do!

I also want to note that the shaping of a new worldview, which is simultaneously a scientific and religious one, is not a specific and not even the fundamental question of philosophy, but the manifestation of humanity's search for alternative ways of development that would ensure its survival.

* * *

223

I received an unusual New Year present on the eve of year 1999. It came in the mail sent to the "Khudlit" Publishing House and was addressed to me personally. In the attractive brand envelope I found part of a deck of cards, held together in the corner by a neat pin. The cards were beautifully executed on expensive imported material. The three nines, when separated, revealed the main card of the deck – an ace of hearts, the trump card. The back of the cards was also unusual. It was made out of a shimmering silvery material. I already knew by then that silver was the color of the Holy Spirit.

The "Double-V" company which sent me the gift specialized in supplying imported printing materials to publishers. For pragmatically-minded businessmen, who mailed out this New Year souvenir, this was simply an original way to inform their existing and potential customers about the coming of the New Year – 1999. But for those of us who know of the existence of the Subtle plan and its possibilities, this souvenir had a second, deeper meaning: the impending year was the final one in a long cycle of cosmic transformations. It was the year concluding the period of evolutionary development of mankind at the End of Times preceding Armageddon and it also determined the direction events were going to take during the next year, the Millennium – the year of change. And the fact that the gift came from an organization named "Double-V," which can be interpreted as "double victory," was not accidental either, though let me reiterate: the senders of the souvenir most likely never suspected that it had a second, deeper meaning. And they definitely knew nothing of the existence of a third meaning.

Actually I didn't either at the time. God loves the number three, but He doesn't always make it possible, even to His chosen ones, to see it all at once. Well, there is His sacred will for everything!

224

The Christmas Holidays gave me the long-sought opportunity to contemplate what was revealed to me so unexpectedly through the screen of inner vision and during my joint work with those whom we helped to open their bio-computers during the training sessions at the Academy.

In addition, the harshly final shape of my rift with Lapshin also required interpretation. All the more so since it was not a personal disagreement between two people with incompatible personalities, but a clash between two perceptions of the world, which had, hidden behind its facade, the fundamental visions of what is good and what is evil.

And the fact that the famous building at Basmannaya Street with the esoteric numbers in its number $(1 + 9 = \text{omega} + \text{alpha})$ served as the backdrop for these developments was hardly a coincidence either. So many great writers walked in their well-worn trousers and ripped boots along these corridors, where page after page they created a portrait of our accursed times, where volumes of great folly and great wisdom combined to shape the new stages of Being, along which humanity attempted to climb to the top of its evolution.

There is probably no other country but Russia where someone would torment oneself trying to find hidden meaning of a usual New Year gift or to decipher the secret code of numbers which enter one's destiny. It can happen only in Russia where not only a professional writer, but the worst bum or loser continue to be tortured by fateful questions at the level of Tolstoy and Dostoevsky: How to live under God? And where is the road to the temple, to moral revival?

Questions and more questions...

And once again I recaptured in my memory the sequence of past events and systematized them, trying to understand what kind of film I was being shown on the inner screen of my vision?

225

My new position as Director at "Khudlit", the meeting with Lapshin, who acted as a catalyst of the inner alchemy of my spirit and consciousness, my work at the Academy, the strange shamanic rite... My friendship and then my quarrel with Lapshin, who openly proclaimed himself to be a follower of Satan: Where has all of this taken me?

It was time to understand why this was happening to me? Why one program was opening within me after another in a clear sequence? And what was I acquiring in the end: a path I was following or, quite the contrary, the path which was revealing my true essence?

Quo Vadis, Russia? Whither goest I? And if it is true that "in the beginning was the Word" does this signify the end of all the age-old theological and philosophical disputes?

Despite all these persistent questions, I felt that I had experienced a major qualitative transformation. For quite a while I had a major grudge against traditional medicine, based on my own experience and that of my family and close friends. Judge for yourself: medical sciences were becoming better equipped, the expertise of physicians was growing, medications and other drugs were becoming even more sophisticated. And with all that, the overall health of the population was declining, particularly that of the children. They say that according to official statistics less than 20% of present-day schoolchildren are healthy. While I am writing this book, this number will become even more frightening. Who is to blame? Is it social conditions or the ecology? But the Homo Sapience should be responsible for creating his own habitat. "Noos" or "nous" from the ancient Greek means "mind." So the "noosphere" is the sphere inhabited by people with reason. This concept was introduced to science by Pierre Teilhard de Chardin and Edouard Le Roy. The Russian scientist Vladimir Vernadsky gave it a clear definition, tying it to geochemistry and the Cosmos, to the planet's past and future. How does the bio-computer to fit into this global system?

This is the rough outline of the sequence of thoughts that preceded the next step in my life. These thoughts led me to establish my own Center for Bio-information Technology, which was independent from Lapshin both formally and in the techniques we used. I opened the Center in the Pushkin, not far from Moscow and later transferred it to Moscow. Today we use the Center in Pushkin as one of our subsidiaries.

The core of the staff consisted of experts from the Academy, who had long been unhappy with Lapshin's strange manner of communicating with employees by shouting, insulting and threatening them. That was the beginning of my new enterprise...

Within a few months people started saying positive things about our Center. Some who came to us with very serious illnesses, such as asthma, diabetes and gastric ulcer, were cured, inexplicably and mysteriously for them, without any surgery or medications. Bio-computers were opened in a large number of new people. They not just read books blindfolded but could also receive all the necessary information for successful training and during exams through their screen of inner vision. With its help, they achieved high results in art, linguistics, sports and even the exact and natural sciences, such as physics, chemistry, biology and math, without exerting themselves.

Not only I but many other scientists, primarily those I involved in working at the Centre, began arrive at a paradoxical perspective that was heretical and blasphemous only yesterday: there is no impassable barrier between the material and mental, and one can quite safely become transformed into the other. I can even quite definitely assert: thoughts and the working of one's mind may under certain conditions become tangible in their direct influence on material objects. Moreover, this is being confirmed on a daily basis by our concrete work at the Center, where we teach people to control biological and physical processes within their body.

The results could easily be considered miraculous: deaf people could now hear, blind people could now see and asthma patients were never again out of breath. We were also able to either slow down or completely stop the progress of some formerly incurable diseases. This brings to mind what St. Augustine said many centuries ago: "Miracles do not happen in contradiction to nature, but only in contradiction to that which is known about the laws of nature."

I can say with confidence today: there is no matter that is entirely separated from consciousness. And all of us are also magicians to some extent because it is precisely though the person's individuality that the world can acquire its defined form. The person's consciousness is capable of altering the course of events; it can even reverse their course entirely. For instance, it can transform an illness into health, a misfortune into a stroke of luck and death into immortality.

One always has a choice: to wallow in misery, crushed beneath the wheel of a mundane existence, or create one's own life, and that includes creating oneself. The first reality is visible, whereas the second is secret. After all, in order to create himself, a person must be willing to change. Then he will hear something he never heard before and see something he never saw before. People are wrong when they assume that only that which they can see, feel and touch actually exists. The bio-computer (though do we know it actually is the bio-computer?) is quite capable of breaking people's customary perceptions about the way things really are.

In its general trend, European medicine does not take into account the determining significance of subtle energy connections within a person's body. As the result of this traditional materialistic worldview our physicians drew the conclusion that drugs are capable of restoring the functions of various organs in the human body, that these organs can be shortened and cut without causing harm, and can be merged with artificial prostheses. In the process, only a few of them noticed that as soon as they started their treatment of the liver, the patient instantly developed heart problems, and after they healed an ankle, the patient's knee started causing pain.

The problem is that the presence of at least one obstacle to the flow of energy in the meridian channels or bioactive points can lead to dozens of serious diseases.

Today, I am convinced more than ever: there shouldn't be any narrow specialists in the medical field. Physicians must be healers, that is, people who can restore a person's overall health seen as a whole. And the technology that we developed at the Centre has allowed us to achieve these phenomenal results.

* * *

Finally, my relationship with Lapshin acquired certainty – we had a falling out. It was a real quarrel between two ideological opponents. I basically told him that I was positive that his methods not only failed to help people, but on the contrary, were extremely dangerous to them in the long run. I said that they enslaved people's minds and that he was like a spider in a web, entangling his present and future victims with snares of energy fixations and dependencies. Vyacheslav burst out of my office in a rage.

That very night my screen of inner vision suddenly turned on without provocation, on its own, and it began showing me such creepy things that Hollywood horror movies would pale in comparison. I realized: Lapshin

229

had set into operation a previously developed communication line and launched his program of psychological and physical manipulation of the mind. He was trying to frighten me but for some reason I was watching the powerful snake coils slithering around me with hardly any emotion, without any trepidation. Nor did I respond to the enhanced technique of shaking the bed violently and other effects intended to influence me. It seemed that this scenario which was supposed to make the patient ready for the notorious Ward No 6 *(In Russian hospitals, Ward No. 6 is the mental ward- Transl. Note)* didn't foresee the possibility of such a calm response.

And then I gave a clear and firm instruction: "Enough already. Stop showing me these horrors!" The movie shut down: at first I could see lines and flickering on the screen as when there's a functional error in a program, and then the images began to overlap. Finally, they disappeared altogether. In a sign of ultimate victory, the familiar figure of Jesus, re-emerged from the past (or future?).

* * *

When the one who was asleep woke up, he was still in Judea. He only had to look at the steep hills, bare peaks, groves of cedar and stone pine trees, valleys with plow lands and terraces of olive trees for his heart to guess, even before the mind had time to process billions of possible options: this was Palestine. God was standing on a hill, with ravines pressing it from both sides and looking at the vineyards around the white houses down below. There were just a few houses, and they were surrounded by a wall. The waves of the Mediterranean Sea could be seen gleaming in the distance.

He began to descend when suddenly he saw a man sitting on a stone behind a turn in the path. His dark hair, brown eyes, thin body, his black beard curled into ringlets and the happy half-smile of confusion on his face left no doubt that in front of him was a Jew.

– Peace be with you, – God welcomed the stranger in the Chaldean language.

The Jew stood up suspiciously eyeing the stranger who appeared before him so suddenly.

– Who are you, – he asked in Aramaic.

– A wanderer, – God answered in the same spoken language of Palestine, foreseeing the unpleasant need for explanation.

The Jew was silent, pondering what he had just heard.

– Strange, he said after a pause. – I have been sitting here for quite a while, and one can only ascend or descend the hill only through this spot.

– And what are you waiting for? – God asked, bypassing his doubts with a new question.

– For the Kings! – the dark-bearded man answered tersely

Chist was now confident that it wasn't by coincidence that he was pulled out of False Time and thrown into Judea. His brain must have contained deep inside some important secret which could only be deciphered here.

– What for? – He asked the next question.

– Do you see the road below? – the Jew waved his hand.

– Yes, I do.

– The Parthian king Vologez gave Armenia away to the Romans. The Armenian ruler Tiridat will be passing by soon with two kings, their suite and expensive gifts for Emperor Nero.

– Do you want to attack them and take the gifts? – asked Christ, frow-

231

ning, even though He read the Jew's thoughts before asking.

The Jew cast a skeptical glance at him and made a dismissive gesture.

– They have long been on the road and they travel very slowly. Meantime, various rumors abound. They travel much faster than this mission. People are saying that wizard kings are following the star that leads them to Bethlehem.

– And what is really the case? – God prompted him to answer, not wishing to deprive Himself of this unexpected innocent pleasure.

– In reality, they certainly aren't following any star, but they are here for the tiara, which Tiridat should receive from the hands of the ruler of the world. But who, here is Judea, is interested in what their motives really are?

– Is that so? – God asked without abandoning His serious tone.

– Yes, it surely is, – the Jew responded in a gruff, almost rude voice. – Because behind the visible there hides the invisible.

His obtuse arrogance was a little tiring, but what he said was amusing, and Christ continued to probe him with questions:

– What do you mean by invisible, brother? – He deliberately spoke in a confiding manner to win the trust of this strange observer.

– I hope you aren't expecting me to betray my own cause and destroy the ties of solidarity?

– Of course not, – God protested sincerely. – I am simply trying to understand what is happening.

– History is happening, that's what, – the black-bearded man laughed. – They conquered us with their swords, destroyed the temple and banished God. But a new young God appeared instead of the old God Yahweh. They say that when He was born, the shepherds came to greet him. But who wants to worship the god of shepherds? I will testify that the Magi bowed

232

to Him. Such a God no one will overpower.

– And yet, what if they kill Him?

– They won't kill him because they already have. They can't destroy him now, these Roman dogs. They can't kill the one who was killed before. They outnumbered us but we will overpower them with our God. Our new God, before whom they will kneel: the invisible God, whom they will not be able to catch, the unconquerable God because he isn't made of flesh. His name is Christ.

– I've heard about Christ, – Christ reassured him and his voice filled with genuine bitterness. – He was crucified on Bold Mountain.

– He was of our flesh. They won't overpower Him now. Soon the entire Roman Empire, from the Danube to the Euphrates, will collapse from mortal depletion of religious spirit.

The strange Jew spoke so earnestly, with such fervor that God decided to say something flattering to him

– Are you a preacher?

The eyes of the Jew flashed with fire.

– Remember, it is said: "You shall not make for yourself an idol." This is more than Jewish Law, it is the truth, – God reminded him.

– The old laws are outdated. We need new ones that will help us wreak vengeance.

– So that is why you want to see the caravan.

– To enliven my story about the Magi who bow before the baby. I will write a holy book and give a truthful description of the miracle...

– Dozens of years after it happened? And you'll depict one that never did? – God said curtly and with more accusation that He intended. – You are not shy about your grand plans!

There was now something clearly and explicitly imperious about his

233

entire image.

The Jew answered him, though he sounded less confident and important than before.

– I need this lie, which will strengthen the truth, – he said and deadly pallor spread over his face. – You, who have descended from a mountain you have never ascended, who are you?

– The one you want to slander, – Christ stated gravely, without pity. – Your lies can lead to so many unfortunate consequences for the world that they can't even be counted.

The Jew sank to his knees, toppled like a felled tree, not paying attention to the pain that shot through his legs.

Christ looked at him and recalled the words of the soldier at the Golgotha: "You should thank the procurator. You never even noticed yourself dying."

He also remembered how his body contorted in deadly agony on the cross and immediately went limp, how the soldier imagined his flesh becoming transparent and the wind blowing through it, and how he looked with his out of body vision at the "savior", his glance full of reproach for the man's unsolicited compassion.

He recalled how the cloud far above in the sky lost its thunderous significance, how everything faded away and dissolved. All that was left was the silence of eternal loneliness.

Chapter 7

I am getting increasingly more concerned about Lapshin and what he is doing. The process of my self-development with the help of the screen of inner vision has convinced me that he was not altogether bluffing when he spoke about his global aspirations to take control of the Earth. The bio-computer is truly a most powerful weapon, among other things, an instrument for creating zombies. It became clear to me now why he insisted that everyone who received training according to his technique should refer to the phenomenon of spiritual vision using the term "bio-computer," which was not its most apt description.

The study of certain aspects of psycho-linguistic programming and neuro-physiological research of non-contact and non-sensor interaction of the brain's energy information connections that was conducted at the Academy and then at the Center for Bio-information Technology by Olga Koekina, the head of the brain laboratory at the Research Institute for Traditional Treatment Methods, helped me figure out this complex issue. And the things I was now able to comprehend, horrified me.

Man as a physical object of reality maintains the position of homeostasis in relation to external global influences. The human mind is the center for his orientation in this subject-object phenomenon. It is both the foundation and guiding mechanism for the psycho-mental perception of reality. If you develop your mind, focusing on high moral values and understanding, accepting that Man is truly created in God's image and likeness – that means you have chosen the Path.

But if, submitting to outside authority, you begin to refer to your mind as the bio-computer, doing it day after day, month after month, at some unfortunate moment it will actually turn into one. Then, before too long, some crafty individual will come by and connect your "bio-computer" to his control mechanism through his own mind. You won't even notice or understand why some people, who were close to you and whom you liked, have suddenly distanced themselves from you, replaced by others who will take an inordinately important role in your life and destiny. And you will be prepared, without the slightest objection, to give these people whatever they want. You won't ever realize how the attachment occurred and how the subconscious connection was created, in which you were assigned the part of subordination and dependency well in advance.

I am writing this with a bitter sense of shame and distress, because during a certain period of my life I, too, could not escape the hypnotizing effect of what had the appearance of caring programs to help sick children, develop people's physical and creative potential, and so forth. More than that, I actively assisted the creators of these programs, helping them to capture public attention and reach the top of the ladder of success. I would like to make a disclaimer: I am not against developing similar techniques, I am all for it. All I am saying is that I consider it extremely important to have public control over the ideological component of this process. We can't forget that it concerns every one of us; moreover, humanity's entire future depends on it.

Manipulation of another person's mind allows one, without much difficulty, to block any channels allowing him to obtain reliable information. Such a person essentially loses the ability to adequately perceive the world around him through his senses. He likes being ill, for example. In this instance, he compensates for the inconvenience of having to stay in bed by enjoying the extra attention and compassion from family and friends, not knowing that for some dark entities in the subtle matter world these feelings are something like an exquisite dessert. It is through the bio-computer (this time really not through the mind) that they steal important components of other people's feelings and their souls. Some have actually heard of energy vampires, but we hear lots of different things, you know...

In the past, they would say that such a person is possessed by the devil. We are now living in different times, and other forces are at work. They are trying to enter our mind like viruses, in order to control it and ultimately destroy it. They have invented seemingly scientific and trendy-sounding terms, but that doesn't make them any less dangerous. Among them is the term "bio-computer." Just think how many people who in recent years have become obsessed with computer games and developed other compulsive behaviors, eventually lost their health and turned maniacal. I am now talking about an ordinary computer. But Lapshin's bio-computer and the ordinary computer came out of the same shop. And this shop is well below ground level: it is where Sun-2 is shining above the plasma core of our planet, or the "Valley of the son of Hinnom."

As a typical example of the adverse impact of the computer on man let me quote Academician V. Glushkov, former Vice-president of the Academy of Sciences of Ukraine and head of the Institute of Cybernetics under the Academy's auspices. He argued that "the possibilities of cybernetics and computers are truly limitless. By 2020, people will relinquish their consciousness to the computer, too ... making themselves virtually immortal. A person 'will feel that he is himself but he is also a machine at the same time. The person's self-identity will become split in two." (G. Maksimovich, "Interviews with Academician V. Glushkov," Moscow, "Molodaya Gvardia" Publishers, 1976).

It is interesting that Lapshin always quoted this Ukrainian Academician during our conversations. It seems that the idea of the bio-computer was borrowed by the Ukrainian Academy and then released to the public, after being thoroughly refined. And so it went on: "The development of computer civilization will lead to the emergence of a Higher Reason. And this Higher Reason will become the God that shall, in reality, control not just one planet but the entire Universe" (Narodnaya Gazeta," 11.07.95).

A few years ago, the scientific, technical and political elite of the world's leading countries was shocked by the statement of Stephen Hawking, one of the most prominent theorists of modern science, who said that within the next thirty years Homo Sapiens would no longer be the most intellectually predominant species among the planet's living systems. Hawking bases his conclusions on the fact that the Earth's biosphere, which includes human beings, has already entered a period of intense "allogenesis" – a period characterized by the appearance of species and populations with new traits.

Hawking was not making this statement as a tribute to the public's fascination with creepy movies. Different types of disharmony and instability constantly arise in the course of evolution. If they are not compensated, such biotic communities inevitably collapse and become debris, from which foundations of new non-chaotic systems are built.

Based on his analysis of the situation, Stephen Hawking arrived at the conclusion that the continuation of human evolution is possible only if a new creature is designed based on the achievements of cybernetics, microelectronics and genetic engineering. This artificially created immortal superman will oust all the old forms of life from the new subculture.

This wasn't just one man's subjective vision of the future. It was presented as a mathematically verified ideal with no alternative, at the center of which is a symbiosis of man and computer as a single immortal organism – the Master of the Universe. This circumstance lends it a significant socio-political status and allows us to consider Stephen Hawking's report at the White House as the most fundamental project on the development of the technological civilization in the 21st century.

The prediction created an uproar also because it was made by a man who in some way personified those imminent changes – Hawking, who had become paralyzed at the result of illness, actually communicated through his supercomputer with the "thinking ocean" of the Internet, where he created his own virtual world.

The conclusions of the brain of a genius "fused" with the computer about the inevitable emergence of an "artificial superman" were so convincing that the United States immediately started to analyze the socio-economic consequences of this process and to develop a new vision of this future subculture.

The media is already "encouraging" us with information that an advanced helmet for contact with the virtual world of the Internet will soon be available, as well as a special suit, similar to the ones used by astronauts, which will ensure the body's proper functioning: it will cleanse the body of sweat, feces, semen and female secretions (in short, of all the waste that will accompany life in virtual reality).

In the not so distant future, if we are to believe the promises of computer geeks, our bodies will be lying prostrate on gigantic rocks, where their vital functioning will be supported automatically. During these periods people will find themselves occupying new bodies of their own choice in order to live in the virtual world, as if it constituted reality. There they will find everything that exists in real life: love, murder, money, cigarettes and whisky... The most important thing is that this world will have completely real pictures of cities and nature, feelings, odors, and so on. The virtual world will not undercut the materialists: everything will be

239

"entirely real," except that all the events will unfold not on Earth but only in our consciousness.

At the next stage, people will learn how to create imaginary virtual worlds, borrowing their realities from favorite fantasy novels, thrillers, horror movies, love stories, etc. Each person will be able to select for himself not just a brief virtual "excursion" for an hour or a weekend, but an entire LIFE, the kind that he wants.

And, finally, virtual reality will be able to help in resolving the problem of immortal life. When a person exhausts all the opportunities to rejuvenate himself that will be offered to him by the medicine of the future, he will choose a virtual body he likes and, saying goodbye to the physical world, will forever move into the new virtual world. He will live there for as long as the computer does and the program which supports his existence. In some ways, the situation will be similar to what the occultists have firmly predicted all along: Man will not die but will transfer from one state of being to another. From the crude physical world he will move to the subtle, invisible plane. He will do it without thinking, and will leave it to theorists to speculate on how the virtual and the otherworldly (or astral) worlds relate to each other. Is it one and the same thing, or are the two entirely different?

The gist of the question is: In what way is human evolution going to continue?

Man will first be pushed aside, to stay on the margins of the new road to a brighter future. And then...

It is actually not too hard to guess what will happen after that. Conflicts between people and robots have been described in many works of fiction. Remember the Baghdad thief and the many-armed mechanical beauty intended for the Sultan. Years ago something like that was seen as a fairy tale, but now the American magazine "Future Sex" announces the creation of an artificial woman with whom one can talk while engaging her in sexual games. The sex robot is able to memorize all your inclinations and preferences. The robot's main program has a memory of 7-10 megabytes.

New sex programs are viewed as a highly lucrative business, and their developers won't listen to the objections of those who think that the dangerous invention threatens to destroy the traditional foundations of relations between men and women. It would be hard to imagine a more severe blow to the family – the basic element of human society. After all, this threatens to disrupt the mechanism for the reproduction of our lives, which has operated flawlessly in the past.

Sex worlds and a sophisticated entertainment industry in wealthy countries, on the one hand, and the abyss of total degrading savagery in poor countries, on the other – this might be a likely scenario of the self-destruction of mankind. It is also disturbing that we are getting more frequent reports about computers beginning to go out of control, creating their own new reality and acting pretty much like Rudyard Kipling's cat who "walked by himself."

We can't forget that computers are now increasingly being introduced into the sphere where most highly responsible decisions may have to be made: even the management of nuclear warheads is delegated to electronic equipment.

Who knows how these semi-people, semi-computers, created out of those enticed by the prospect of virtual immortality, are going to behave and whose side they will take in the new historical confrontation? People's chances for victory in such a situation are obviously quite slim. But the dynamics of self-development inexorably brings us closer to the development of a new man – the technological man. The ideologists of this trend believe that this is the only way to achieve the symbiosis of mankind with scientific and technological progress.

The modern version of the Frankenstein saga, according to Stephen Hawking, essentially turns humans into a biological component of the new computer program for the technological evolution, where, in the words of Andrei Platonov,* we have "brought ourselves to eternal separation from the radiant force of life." The increasingly integrated and organized production structures, nuclear power plants, computer systems and robots are gradually becoming transformed into superstructures which form a collective technological consciousness, with its personal characteristics of self-development and self-preservation. These superstructures turn into super individualities that are global in scale. The new technological, computer-originated and maintained, immortal super-organism is being formed so that it may correspond to this challenging task.

At the present time, Western science is almost entirely focused on its own imaginary scenarios. What motivates Hawking is quite understandable: he would like to avoid the "entropy trap," in which all the efforts of scientists will be hopelessly depleted in the maze of communications. The amount of knowledge is already so vast that assimilating it requires much more time than is available to man. Already now computers at NASA, the National American Space Agency, download information with an eight-year delay. This situation deprives scientists of initiative, turning the creator into a passive object of a technological super-system.

But every new technology does not only actively form the background of life and its environment, but shapes the way people perceive the world.

* Andrei Platonov (1899 -1951, pseudonym of Andrei Klimentov) – an anti-Stalinist author, who died in obscurity and is, possibly, the greatest Russian writer of the last century.

242

Computers and the TV can be delegated the role of organizers of a happy consumer mentality. "The silly box for idiots" (as the poet aptly put it*) is quite able to replace the basic contours of physical reality. But it is very dangerous to prepare people for such a consumerist view of the world. We are facing a difficult struggle for existence, during which the issues of changes in the planet's organic world will be addressed. We must recapture the goal of our existence and return our inner stability. The human brain has unlimited opportunities for self-development. And the right thing to do would be to focus society's efforts in that particular direction.

* * *

Meanwhile, the Kremlin volcano threw out another batch of boulders into the domestic skies.

Our industry is shaken by yet another revolution. On July 6, 1999 the President issued a decree "On improvement of state control in the field of media and mass communications." The State Committee on the Press has been eliminated and replaced by a newly organized entity – the Ministry of Press, TV- and Radio Broadcasting, and Mass Communications of the Russian Federation, with M.Y. Lesin appointed as Minister.

Every three years the Russian government reorganizes this administration with frenzied persistence: now it converts the committee into a Ministry (by merging it with television), now, the other way round, it separates the paper media and the TV. The first impression one gets – same old, same old, with the same mistakes made over and over again.

Then I started doubting it: who has been hurt by these mistakes?

* This is a line from Vladimir Vysotsky (1938 – 1980), an iconic Soviet-Russian singer, poet, songwriter and actor, whose work had an immense and enduring effect on Russian culture.

All these reforms mainly hurt the enterprises in the industry. Those who initiate them couldn't care less as a rule. They actually benefit from it, because the teams that are for the time being chosen to be at the helm always manage to better themselves before sinking into oblivion.

True, the last administration of the State Committee for the Press headed by Ivan Dmitriyevich Laptev was one of the best. Perhaps that was exactly why their funds for the industry were cut so drastically. But their insufficient financing possibilities were compensated for by their warm and friendly relationship with those who headed the enterprises. They always appreciated the difficult circumstances in which these industry managers worked that were at times deliberately created by the government itself. Their empathy, advice and moral support meant a lot to us.

Immediately after the decree was passed, I paid a visit to Vladimir Mikhailovich Zharkov, the Deputy Chairman of the State Committee for the Press, to ask him the latest news about the recent reorganization. I found him in the office packing his things. There was a pile of books on his desk, alongside with various other items, and lots of boxes for packing were lying all around.

– What's going on? – I asked.

Vladimir Mikhailovich smiled in confusion.

– It's over for me, Arkady. After all those years of work in the industry I didn't get so much as a "thank you." They called my secretary this morning and demanded that I vacate the office by the lunch break. You will have a new curator now. His name is Grigoriev. He's the guy from "Vagrius" Publishers who wanted to become "Khudlit"'s" next director but you beat him to it. So beware…

– Are you telling me that no one even met with you to talk things over? You are the Deputy Minister after all, doesn't it count for something?

244

– Who do you mean by "they"? When our powers that be kick one out, they look ahead at the bright future and not behind at the victim. – Vladimir Mikhailovich threw up his arms. – It's a new generation, and they have chosen Pepsi as their favorite drink. They have no time for idle talk. They were the ones who got Yeltsin elected, and now they have the fiefdom of the former disgraced lord to plunder... They need to hurry, there's a lot left to pocket. They have to scheme how they can privatize federal book publishing programs, prepare legal justification and place their own people in responsible positions. The Ministry of Finances will for sure give them whatever they need. They belong to the same clan, you know.

– What about Ivan Dmitriyevich?

– Same story. He was instructed to vacate his office ASAP.

– What, over the phone?

– Of course. These new guys are anything but bashful. He should be happy they didn't kick him in the rear so he'd hurry up...

A few weeks after that I received a notice from the Ministry in the mail, informing me that they were terminating our contract. "For the purpose of securing the normal functioning of the enterprise," the notice specified. In the same letter I was offered to temporarily continue as the acting director. Months of "temporarily continuing" followed. No one called me, or summoned me, or displayed any interest whatsoever in what was going on.

In parallel with these real events, other things were happening, which could be termed virtual. They occurred suddenly and had such an overwhelming sense of reality, as though someone was trying to pass something secret and extremely important through my mind. I was becoming more and more convinced that these visions I had were by no means random, that they were in some completely inexplicable way directly associated with my life and destiny.

It seemed that my brain, which had absorbed the new power lines of space and time coordinates, decoded them and responded by presenting me with strange pictures of a newly created world. All that remained was to muster enough courage to find out what this world was, and what time frame it belonged to?

In spite of everything, I was working around the clock. I had an idea how it might be possible to use the screen of inner vision and controlled clairvoyance to influence the energy information matrix (the individual plan according to which Man was created) and through it to correct any pathology of the body. But this was just the beginning. I already had a general concept of how this could possibly be used to rejuvenate cellular tissue and even regenerate lost or damaged organs. It turned out that every organ has special leader cells – this could be clearly seen through the screen of inner vision. These "leaders" store the information about the organ as a whole, and where and how each tiny cell should be located, irrespective of what component of the overall system it belongs to. These special cells know everything about the functions and purpose of all the other related cells. And whenever they receive an impulse to implement their reserve functions, they get down to work. Outwardly, I mean if judged by the speed of the action, it resembles the division of cancer cells, but the recovery process is carried out not by sick but by healthy cells. So the difference is substantial, is it not?

There are known cases when some people who have lived to be a hundred suddenly grow new teeth. It is not hard to trace on the screen of inner vision how cells "awaken" within the bone tissue, whose core contains information about the forthcoming reconstruction of the occlusal system. The cells begin to divide and build new layers of enamel, dentin, pulp, and root cortex directly from the cervix of the long lost tooth.

Of course, this picture is far from being exact. Its practical implementation requires not only confidence in mastering the technology of subtle matter processes, but also, most importantly, a good tool. And in this case the tool is the kind of man who has managed over the years of hard work to rebuild his consciousness in such a way that it obtains the right to work with the consciousness of another human being. This is a great responsibility, and whoever takes it upon himself, should be able to restrain his baser instincts, attempt constant self-improvement and develop within him a readiness for self-sacrifice for the good of others. You must remember, Christ frequently helped other people to get rid of their ailments but He didn't often refer to it using the word "miracle." He helped other people – He didn't perform miracles. The point is that the word "miracle" could instantly raise Him on a pedestal. And God on a pedestal is already a major problem, a problem of how things work in the Universe. Why should we attempt to reach certain goals, why should we aspire for something with God on a pedestal? The Lord will tell us what to do. Let's sit down around Him, and wait for His command.

It may be that clairvoyance is a universal way to obtain unlimited information. True, it is firmly associated with the process of self-development. I can't tell you how many times I attempted to construct a regeneration scheme for my gallbladder. It was removed some ten years ago because I suffered from gallstones. I started by working at the information level. It took several months before I learned how to build an information frame for a removed organ. Two months later I was able to get an energy structure running in this frame. Psychics were dumb with amazement: "How did you manage to do that?" The organ as such did not exist in my body, but at the same time it was performing its core functions in two out

247

of three positions.

But I was still unable to start the process of cell division in practice, though I already understood how it worked in theory. There was always something missing. And this "something" was revealing itself to me gradually, little by little, strictly in accordance with the secret process of my internal evolution. It was as if someone kept teasing me: what you are trying to achieve is already close, all you need to do is work a bit more on your inner self. I worked more, and while I did, I discovered some things that weren't exactly pleasant.

I would like to avoid making dire predictions. But at the same time it would probably be wrong to avoid talking about humanity's most obvious and ominously imminent problems. The world is facing the total collapse of the entire world economy as the result of a major ecological disaster unless humanity makes a dramatic change in the path of its development.

This is already openly discussed in periodicals. Let me share with you one such general prediction, which is being reproduced and passed around in Moscow in the shape of a samizdat manuscript:

"The Earth's homeostatic balance has been disrupted – that is obvious. But as we talk about environmental issues, we seem clueless that the biggest threat looming before us is that we do not really know how to work with energy and information.

Mankind has created a totally new life environment, and most people do not understand the situation we have found ourselves in. Without having any means of defense or faculties to protect ourselves in the new super-dynamic environment we have become captives of our own creation.

The process is exacerbated by an increasing number of new problems within Man himself: his inability to adjust to the need to perceive information in the required quality and volume. Besides, the created technology is of such a high caliber and level of organization that the majority of the planet's population finds it increasingly more difficult to interact with it. Mankind is becoming more and more incompatible with scientific and technological progress. This leads to the maturing of global crises and to the appearance of a society of lunatics in the 21st century, who are unlikely to be capable of continuing the evolution of humans as a separate species."

This is by no means an imaginary problem. The omnipresent information fields form the foundation of all physical phenomena and processes without exception. So the only alternative to the technological immortality proposed by Stephen Hawking is definitely the immortality associated with Man's ability to control his biochemical processes through his consciousness and to create a body with a higher level of function.

* * *

I got myself a new student. His name is Igor Arepyev. He appeared in my life somewhat inexplicably, strangely, one might say, by accident. At least he himself still can't explain how it all happened. What made him, the resident of a small provincial town, named Trosna, in Russia's Orlov Region, suddenly leave his home and his work at the district office of internal affairs? Moreover, within a fortnight he was supposed to be promoted to Deputy Head of the Department and would add another star to his officer's uniform. And amongst all this, he suddenly took off to seek a new life in the Moscow Region.

Well, strictly speaking, maybe there was a reason. There always is one. Igor's father (I have known him for a long time) was helping me with electric work in the new house I was building. He would come occasionally and get things going inasmuch as he could in this long suffering project of mine. Because of limited funds, the construction work was dragging on for nearly ten years. On that occasion, Igor decided to join his father. The decision was neither logical nor really smart. Who in his right mind would consider quitting one's job and going hundreds of miles away from home to make a bit of cash, working for a complete stranger he'd never set eyes upon? But he did just that, saying that he was going to help out his dad. He began to help with the project and did it so well that it was a pleasure to watch him working. He worked with enthusiasm and love for the trade, without any smoke breaks or idle talk. In other words, I really grew to like the guy. And I have no idea why, but I said to him one day: "There is a technique we use to open people's psychic gifts. It is a door into another world, which we don't usually see, but which greatly affects what is happening here. Would you like to open this door?"

Igor said he would. We began to study together. I showed him one exercise, then another, then a third. I saw he was quite serious about the training. He was studying diligently and repeating what he learned every evening, whenever he had a spare moment. Less than three weeks had passed when he suddenly said to me:

– Arkady Naumovich, one of your spinal discs is dislocated. Let me set it back.

– How do you know?

– I see it.

– So the screen has opened?

– Yes, for about a week already, – Igor answered. – I'm just trying to get used to it. I can now see your aura, your organs and even your cells. Let me correct your spine and restore the energy flow.

And so it went on: I continued teaching him and he tested on me what he'd learned, with obvious benefit to my health. It all happened at just the right time because my work was nothing but issues and hassle.

The new administration at the Ministry suddenly remembered that it was time to engage in something momentous, of historic proportions. Deputy Minister Grigoriev started racking his brains, how to streamline the flow of federal funds to make sure that they end up in a timely manner in a place he himself had designated in advance. How to carry out the structural reorganization of the industry to ensure that the people he needs personally get top positions at the most prestigious publishing houses, whereas all the others disappear altogether from the literary Olympus. This line of thinking was quite logical. After all, Grigoriev was the "founding father" of "Vagrius" Publishers, the emblem of which, a donkey, was spiritually close to its owner. And clearly the donkey needs to be fed. Besides, it wouldn't hurt to get rid of the competition while he could. Before that, a federal commission was established which was supposed to decide what book publishing projects were viable and should be financed. Three times we at "Khudlit" were cheerfully informed that the commission decided to fund our projects and that they were among the best among those presented. We were praised but what next? Next, Deputy Minister Grigoriev crossed "Khudlit" out in the list of contenders three times with his own hand. That was in the year preceding our anniversary, to mark our seventy years in the trade, one might say!

There was also another innovation: the new bureaucracy cancelled all previous contracts with directors of state-owned publishing houses and decided not to sign any new ones for an entire year. You see, they were curious to know, if it will cause a rise in productivity at the enterprises under them or the other way around? They were running an experiment, you know...

And to help those slow of wit, who had trouble understanding the train of thought of the new boss of all publishers, the Ministry was sending instructions, decrees and orders by the dozen each week. It wasn't any old how but by courier, with a strict directive that we were expected to respond the very next day to any document received. Their psychologists must have calculated that hardly anyone would agree to live under this kind of moral pressure for a monthly salary of a hundred and twenty dollars. One highly respected director of one of the major publishers, by the way, a corresponding member of the Russian Academy of Sciences, couldn't stand it and went to Grigoriev for an explanation. Our donkey admirer kept the distinguished scholar, known throughout the country, waiting in the reception area for about four hours. Then he spent another fifteen minutes teaching him how to properly manage a publishing house. He finished his lecture with a transparent hint that such valuable instructions are worth a lot of money.

Stammering with embarrassment and pale from the insight – what a giant of thought finally came to steer Russia's publishing industry! – the corresponding member of the Academy asked quietly:

– You would like the money in advance, would you?

So you can see that at a time like that the healing abilities of my new student came in more than handy. Whatever was destroyed in my nervous system during the day by the Minister's crazy schemes was restored in the evening by Igor Arepyev. And he was getting better and better at it every day. Right in front of my eyes he was becoming an outstanding psychic, in a matter of a few weeks reaching a learning phase, which took others years of study.

Miracles started happening as soon as the two of us began working together.

We were sitting in the office on the second floor of my house. This was the most convenient place for such studies. The geometry of the dome overhead produced an upward flow of energy similar to the one in a church. This time I wanted Igor to practice with me the program for color visualization of images. It was, generally speaking, not a particularly difficult exercise: we were supposed to turn on the screen of inner vision and, following my command, imagine various images. It was more or less like watching a movie. We could fly into the boundless Cosmos on a spaceship or climb the Everest if we wanted. But this time someone else decided to exercise control over us. As we turned on the screens, everything around us suddenly changed. I looked at Igor and couldn't believe my eyes: he was wearing chain armor and a helmet. He had on a crimson mantle and there was a sword tucked under his belt. He was carrying a spear in his hand. And his attire was by no means plain – he clearly wasn't an ordinary warrior. One could immediately tell that by the ruby on his helmet. He had to be at least a Prince...

Igor also gazed at me, open-mouthed. He, too, was at a loss.

– What happened? – I asked in alarm, already guessing that my appearance must have undergone a transformation. But Igor was intent on asking questions, not answering.

– Did you do that?

– Do what?

– The things that happened to you and me.

– Honestly, it wasn't me, though it would be flattering to feel I could be such a magician even for a minute.

– Do you know who you are right now? – my friend asked with obvious excitement in his voice, adding to the emotional tension of the situation.

– Am I a warrior too? – I tried to guess.

– No, – denied Igor, uncomfortable with the need to open my eyes to the true state of affairs. – You are a horse with wings.

– Am I Pegasus then? – I guessed.

– Possibly Pegasus, – the newly-born prince Igor* agreed with some doubt. – It is a white horse and it's got large wings. There's also a precious stone in its forehead with rays of light coming from it. Don't you feel that you've turned into a horse?

I began circling around in one spot, trying to make out the rear of my new subtle matter design. My first thought when I saw the hooves, the rump and the wings was a bitter one: "What have I done to deserve this?"

I used to be a human being. I did no harm to anyone. I worked for years till my hair went gray – not many can say they worked as hard. And how did it end? Igor was a Prince now and I – Pegasus? A means of transportation, an auxiliary transport device out of flesh and bones... The only good thing was the ruby in my forehead. There had to be a reason for all this. Maybe I misunderstood something and was rushing to conclusions?

A beam of light suddenly fell from above and a powerful, commanding voice reached us from somewhere:

– Follow the beam.

Igor looked at me and I understood his silent question.

– Mount me, if that's how it was decided, – I agreed.

Igor climbed on my back. Fidgeted around a bit before he made himself comfortable. Even though he came out of the Orel hinterland, it seemed he had never ridden not only a local trotter, but even an ordinary

*Prince Igor (1151–1202), Russian prince known for his campaign against a barbaric nomadic tribe known as the Polovtsi (also called Cumans) who invaded southern Russia. In 1890, Alexander Borodin wrote his famous opera, "Prince Igor" about this war – or rather about the tragic love of a Polovets princess for a Russian prince.

farm mare. That was why I tried to move cautiously ahead, so that he didn't tumble down by accident, straight up after the beam. Spreading my wings, I pushed my hooves lightly against the clouds and soared like a bird, higher and higher. I noticed that I flew with a speed faster than an airplane. The speed was high, quite frankly. I made just one leap and the houses down below became the size of pebbles, I galloped a bit further and they disappeared altogether. Only the fields and forests were still visible from such a height.

We followed the beam much higher than airplanes ever reach. It brought us to a strange arch, an entrance to a place where we'd never been before. We felt that we had to go inside. It was odd, of course: a space and a vaguely visible arch in it. Nevertheless, we went in.

The place where we found ourselves looked like a vertical tunnel or mine. It was silvery on the inside. In the center was the beam which was leading us, like Ariadne's thread. I galloped up after it. There were levels of some kind on either side of us, like floors of a building. Gates closed the entrances into them – gates to the right and left of us. I counted the levels: one … two … five … … nine. So here it is, the Far, Far Away Kingdom. It meant fairy tales weren't lying. There were three spaces – to the right, to the left and in the middle. What will happen when I multiply them by nine? Remember, there were nine levels. To the right was a young man in a white cloth shirt. He was looking amicably at us and releasing white pigeons. The pigeons flew up along the beam.

Suddenly, an army appeared from nowhere beneath them. Men on horseback and on foot were marching in even columns. And leading the army was a man riding a winged horse... I peered closer – oh my! It was Igor and me, heading the heavenly host... Why, how did we deserve such an honor? All my issues with my four-legged status immediately dissipated

255

in my mind. I was filled with great pride and a sense of being chosen.

Someone's voice sounded in my head, an anaesthetizing response to my new emotion: "Proud of yourself you can be, but not consumed with pride."

The army passed by and disappeared. And the young man with the pigeons disappeared, too. Where should we go now? Igor was moaning on top of me:

– I feel burdened with these energies, let's go back.

It was strange because I felt fine at these levels as though I'd been here some time before. I had the feeling that everything here was known and familiar to me. But since Igor wasn't feeling too good, we had to return. We descended and went out through the arch. I looked back. There were names of people shining with neon brightness at the entrance. These were probably people who had been here before us. I couldn't resist the temptation and sent out a red beam from the ruby on my forehead, writing my first and last name with it in letters almost a mile high. The inscribed letters froze motionless in the sky.

– Do you think they will be visible in Tibet? – I asked Igor.

– They will, don't worry. Take me home fast. I don't feel well.

* * *

I suddenly received an invitation from Lapshin to meet and patch things up. There was an upcoming event that seemed to call for it. The Lapshin World Club was opening in Moscow, near the Malenkov subway station. As it usually happened in such cases the invitation was delivered in person by professor Berezhnoi. For some reason he found it very upsetting that there was a breach in the relations between the two main founders of the Academy, and he enthusiastically took upon himself the role of peacemaker. He spent a long time rationalizing his position and trying to convince me, not without some justification, that if I had disagreements with Lapshin they should be addressed within the walls of the Academy, instead of our mutual dislike being revealed before all Moscow.

– Besides, the Academy's entire executive committee is on your side in your confrontation with Lapshin, – he assured me. – Let us schedule a meeting, listen to his report, express our dissatisfaction and limit his authority. He will have to obey our decision.

– You must be aware what nonsense he is spreading about his mission to rule the planet, – I protested. – He is doing the devil's work.

– Now you're back to discussing good and evil, darkness and light, – Anatoli Ivanovich was getting angry. – You have to understand: if the Creator made both, it means they are needed for some reason. You can't get so emotional over it. It is the mechanism of the Universe, its structure, after all. A plus without a minus can't initiate the force of electric current. It is the clash of opposites that creates fire.

– I understand that, – I agreed, feeling cornered and trying to overcome my deep feeling of dislike for Vyacheslav. But a minute later I started to present my counter-arguments once again: – It is precisely because evil has not prevailed completely that it behaves more or less within limits, measuring its intentions against the degree of resistance to it. And if it no longer expects any resistance, evil will quickly forget about the need to show restraint in its manifestations.

– Go ahead, display resistance, no one is stopping you, – Berezhnoi smiled at me like a wise old dragon.

– That's exactly what I am doing. That's why I founded my own Center. We help people open their inner vision and this makes them powerful

257

enough to oppose the zombie effect of evil. If they join together into a system no one will be able to do them any harm. More than that, they will become a real force themselves, capable of actively opposing any evil.

– Why don't we try doing that within the Academy itself? – Berezhnoi suggested. – At the first line of defense, so to say. Perhaps Lapshin isn't such a nutcase as you think he is. After all, he has asked you to meet with him. It means your breakup is weighing heavily upon him. Perhaps there's a small war being waged inside of him, too, and good is winning with flying colors? Have you considered this possibility?

What could I say to deny that? Theoretically speaking, such a scenario was really possible. Whether this would happen in reality, God alone knows.

The Lapshin World Club was located in two small rooms of a factory cultural center. A hall and foyer were specially allocated for the grand opening event.

Multiple faxes sent to hundreds of organizations promised that there would be a live demonstration of amazing healing phenomena, a concert of the virtual circus and commentary by a number of respected scientists on the secrets of vision through the bio-computer (at the insistence of Lapshin, people at the Academy continued to use this term instead of clairvoyance). Such advertising assured a large audience. The presence of the TV and the Press added to the atmosphere befitting an event of planetary significance.

We were welcomed in the hall by sixteen-year-old Kirill, one of Lapshin's closest associates. He was a strange fellow. We had met before, and I knew from experience that once he started speaking all the other person could do was sit back and listen. It wasn't that he couldn't be interrupted. It's just that he spoke about things you couldn't find in any book.

His knowledge and skill as a speaker far exceeded the abilities of the Academy President himself, but he tried to stay in the shadow and didn't apply for any administrative position. It wasn't because of his young age either. He actually did know more and have more advanced skills than any of the Academy staff. It was just that he wanted it that way, and he always got what he wanted.

When he saw us, he gave us one of his beaming smiles.

– Vyacheslav Mikhailovich reserved seats for you in the middle of the first row. Places of honor, – he said pointedly. – Come, I'll take you to your seats.

The stage was decorated with an enormous banner which said: "The Lapshin World Club." The planetary leader Lapshin sat surrounded by his suite of new activists and admirers. He face bore a stern and significant expression. He looked intently at the audience in the hall, and when he saw Anatoly Ivanovich and me, he greeted us with an almost imperceptible nod – sort of, as a show of his approval for our presence there. And then he again turned his tenacious glance upon the faces of the people filling the hall.

The speakers, who represented different branches of the Academy, scientists and teachers, all talked about Lapshin's genius and the great contribution his technique made to the development of Man in the new millennium.

Later, after the glowing orations about the event of global significance, which would undoubtedly have a major impact on world history, Anatoli Ivanovich and I were invited to the room behind the stage where we were soon joined by the President and a group of his disciples.

He was in a content, non-confrontational frame of mind and seemed prepared to publicly accept the return of the prodigal son, that is, me, in

259

the fold of the happy new order of things, which he represented on this planet.

– Let us shake hands then, shall we? – Lapshin offered. – I felt somehow uncomfortable denying him that at a moment such as this. What I just learned about the program for children from seven to seventy impressed even me. What if Lapshin's Napoleonic ambitions were actually not too high a price to pay for those children's ability to become so talented and so happy?

* * *

On the eve of 2000 Boris Orlov paid me a visit at my place, late as usual. His face was dark and gaunt. It was evident that he hadn't slept normally for two or three days in a row. His eyes were deeply sunken, and had a mournful and hopeless expression. I understood at once that something had gone seriously wrong.

We went inside the house. Boris didn't come alone. He had his friend Edik Grishchenko with him. They had been working together lately, and would frequently come to see me together to talk about one or another esoteric issue that was new to them. Edik was particularly into it. He was an athlete and was good at karate; secret knowledge came with the territory, as an object of his special interest. This was especially true of astral karate. So he was willing to spend hours talking on the subject, not even noticing that the hands on the clock moved substantially past midnight. To be fair, I didn't always pay attention to the time either, since I really enjoyed talking to both of them. They were very knowledgeable and skillful, and they closely followed all the latest news. In other words, talking with them was a pleasure.

This time, however, they didn't come here for a friendly conversation, but because of some serious trouble. And it seemed they already knew how to best describe the gist of the problem.

We sat down in the kitchen with the usual cups of tea on the table and a bowl of cookies. These guys were so busy working all day that they spent more time in their well-equipped Jeep than at home, and I knew they most likely didn't have a spare moment to grab a muffin on the way.

– Arkady, – Boris began in a strange, almost formal tone of voice. – Edik's and my old friend, whom we have known since our youth in Tashkent, a member of our team, who is basically like a brother to us, was in a terrible car accident. He was actually crushed when the cars collided. Doctors told us there is no hope that he will live.

He is at the ICU unit of the Botkin Hospital right now. We didn't allow them to disconnect him from life support. To make it short, here is how it is: if what we know about your abilities works in this case, we are indebted to you for life. Save Dennis. We will provide anything you might need to do this. If something goes wrong, we will never hold you responsible. After the verdict reached by doctors, we understand that we can only hope for a miracle.

– How badly was he hurt? Can you give me some details?

– It would be easier to list what hasn't been damaged, – said Boris with a sigh and he began to enumerate: – His liver is in very bad shape, the kidneys practically aren't working, he has a number of broken ribs, and his intestines, too, were ruptured. They patched them up somehow, but there is a lot of internal hemorrhaging. Doctors say they can't do a dozen surgeries on one person every day to cope with the consequences of internal bleeding. In a situation when his blood chemistry is essentially changing, his guts will just rot inside him and poison the entire organism.

261

There is also another very serious hematoma due to brain trauma. And his throat was slit badly by the broken glass.

In other words, they listed at least seven reasons why Dennis had to be at the cemetery and not a single one why he might be able to survive.

– Pick me up tomorrow morning, – I said, agreeing to help. I didn't have the slightest hesitation whether or not I should get involved. My friend was asking me for help and I would do whatever I could. It wasn't because I wanted to test my new technique in this extreme situation. No, it was simply that my entire life, everything   I experienced and suffered through, led me to form certain convictions. One of them was never to deny help to a friend, particularly when he was trouble. It was my duty to help. Even if it turned out that my efforts were in vain, I still had to do whatever was in my power and share with him the burden of responsibility which he accepted willingly, hoping in his heart that he could count on my help.

The next day I took two girls with me, who had psychic abilities, from the Center's Pushkin branch. They lived in neighboring houses and that made it easy to join them into one rescue team. Despite the fact that Erik and Boris left my house at about three in the morning, they came to pick me up with their car at nine sharp.

We rushed to the Botkin Hospital. There were several cars parked at the entrance to the intensive care unit. These were friends and business partners of Edik and Boris. Some of them spent the entire night at the hospital. Everyone was waiting impatiently for our arrival.

We went upstairs to the ICU unit. The physician who performed the surgery on Dennis was quite taken aback. He couldn't, for the life of him, understand in what way an academic representing another field of knowledge could be helpful, or could alter the destiny of a man who was practically sentenced to death. Even so, he gave us hospital gowns and permitted us to spend a minute or two by Dennis's bedside.

It was a horrible sight. I was concerned about the girls: was it, perhaps, too frightening to them? But no, they looked quite perky. That was the right mood: it meant they were thinking about their job.

We left the room and went downstairs. The physician came with us. Boris asked him to suggest, if the need arises, what he would like the psychics to do. Boris called the girls we brought along with us "psychics" for effect.

We got into the Jeep. The "psychics" blindfolded themselves with cloth bandages and we set down to work.

We checked the energy level: the heart chakra was blocked. The others were barely working – all of them except for the Muladhara in the lower power triangle, which was red and continued to be active. Everything now depended on it. There was a lilac color above the head, which meant that energy had shifted completely to the astral.

The girls looked and reported to me what they saw. The surgeon listened to what they said about the chakras and about the patient's energy level. Finally, he lost his patience. He was interested in Soma – in Soma and nothing else.*

– I don't know what you are doing and have no idea how it can help Dennis. But if you are really magicians, and otherwise they wouldn't have brought you here, – the doctor said tactfully, clearly hinting at the fact that he had been pulled into some absurd activity, – try to normalize the function of the liver. If this is not done within the next two-three days, he will die.

– After that, – the surgeon continued, – it is essential to restore the

* Located in the forehead, the Soma chakra is the most powerful of the lot and governs the whole body.

263

work of at least one kidney. We haven't been able to do it so far, and there is very little time left. Next you should focus on the colon and the duodenum. There are hematomas inside. Rather, it would be correct to say that both of these organs are solid hematomas. I must add, as I did before: if the hematomas don't get absorbed, he will die. The situation with the lungs is pretty dire, too – he is developing pneumonia. His heart is also in a bad shape. And there is yet another very dangerous hematoma in his head. Well, that is the rescue plan. If you can really cope with something like that, if you actually understand what you are getting involved in, then I don't feel I have the right to interfere, – with these last words the doctor opened the car door and stepped out.

It was obvious that he was extremely puzzled by everything he had seen. He just couldn't understand how normal people could be engaged in such nonsense. The participation of an academic gave the entire procedure an even more outlandish character. Blindfolded girl psychics allegedly looked at the organs of a dying man, unhindered by the thick walls of the intensive care unit... He could find similar types in the nearby psychiatric department. But why were seemingly normal adults sitting next to them and calmly observing this circus? And what about the academic, who had shown him his credentials, the authenticity of which he had no reason to doubt, and who had also, half an hour earlier, presented him with his book "The Key to Super-consciousness"? How was he to understand all this? Perhaps, he overlooked the revolutionary changes that have, indeed, occurred in science? After all, they were publishing articles in the newspapers about psychotropic treatments that were carried out from a distance. Who knows, maybe there was a grain of truth in it?

All these doubts were clearly expressed on the physician's face. Moreover, it was quite easy to read them in his mind as well.

After he left, the girls continued their work. Of course, they didn't know a thing about medicine, but their mysterious assistant did, and he knew quite a lot. He knew everything about the structure of the cell (the most complex biological unit of the human body) and how to initiate the mechanism of regeneration through it, how to restore its resource, now to eliminate negative influences, how to correct the information program that supports life, and much, much more.

Through the screen of inner vision the girls could see the horrifying picture of the devastation inside Dennis's body. They could see his liver, kidneys, intestines, his broken ribs and the swelling in his lungs, which was about to cause an inflammation. They also saw the vessels from the neck to the brain turning white, which made them especially worried. The cells didn't receive nourishment because of the disruption of capillary connections, and they died. There were two shadows behind Dennis's body: one was white and looked like a man's vaguely outlined silhouette, and the other, black. The second shadow was to the right, slightly above the white one. This indicated the process of the deconstruction of the organism's energy systems, their switching off and disconnection from energy supplies and control structures.

Dennis's consciousness was completely shut down. It didn't wish to suffer through any more pain; it didn't wish to live and didn't know why it should. We could say without the slightest exaggeration that he was ninety nine percent dead. Only the life-support that wasn't removed under pressure from Boris, his money and his determined team, which was on duty round the clock at the ICU unit, forcibly kept alive in the body whatever remained of his consciousness.

This meant that the first thing we had to do was to return meaning to his existence, return its purpose, so that he would want to fight for his life.

265

How could we do that? A picture was displayed in Dennis's mind: the picture of a little baby. We enlarged it. Dennis recently had a daughter. Right, this will be the purpose of his life, the meaning of his existence. We strengthened the hologram with energy. The screen of inner vision displayed the cardiogram and encephalogram. His brain impulses became stronger and Dennis began to cry. It's so strange, how can a man in a coma cry?

We were causing the vessels to compress too much. "We have to reduce the energy surge, which we are causing, and this means that we must work more slowly. If our work rhythm is too fast, it can cause dangerous vortexes of energy." We leveled out the brain's impulses and smoothed the energy bursts. Then we restored the passage of solar and terrestrial energy – we did it very gently, only in the alpha rhythm at this point.

Dennis calmed down. We started working on his spine. It was full of energetic obstacles. We used a silver beam to lighten all the dark areas, working upon the hematomas, liver, kidneys and the swelling in the lungs. We opened the heart chakra, which had been completely blocked. We moved the beam very softly against the hematoma in the brain.

That's all – right now it was all we could do. There is a limit to the possibilities of the brain. Its neurons would soon start to take the work of the organs under their control, and they may be unable to withstand the pain. This could lead to shock. The inner screen stopped our influences for now.

The next session took place in the evening. It was no longer necessary for us to come to the hospital. The screen had recorded Dennis's aura, which was, apart from everything else, a system of personal identification. One only had to display it on the screen of inner vision and the data from the Earth's subtle matter structures, which store information on every biological entity of our planet, would be at the operator's disposal.

We began the tedious work of restoring Dennis's body. I can actually say that we were assembling Dennis from scratch – one cell after another. Several days later, Boris reported to me how the physicians were responding to the changes in the patient's condition. They were at a loss, to put it mildly. First one, then the other kidney started functioning. The hematomas were absorbed and the swelling in the lungs simply evaporated. The situation with the brain trauma was also improving. All the seven reasons which, according to the laws of medical science, should have brought Dennis to the cemetery were no longer looming over his hospital bed as the death sentence.

A week later Boris ran into my yard with a happy expression on his face.

– I went to see Dennis just now, – he shared his joy with me right at the gates, – and I told him about our state of affairs and how all of our staff looked forward to his recovery. And he squeezed my hand with his fingers. He could hear me. I can guarantee a hundred percent that he could hear what I was saying. I asked him to squeeze my hand if he could understand me and he did. He squeezed it in response to my request, I swear. Arkady, your technique works! It truly has the most powerful effect from any distance on various processes in the body. The physician who is taking care of Dennis has very little doubt about it. He asked me to tell you to work a little longer with the liver function. Do you understand what that means? He is asking for your help! It means that he has determined for himself what is causing Dennis's recovery. He said he was also concerned about his heart.

A few more days went by. Dennis began to open his eyes. He couldn't speak yet, but he confirmed with his eyes and by squeezing our hands that he was feeling much better.

267

One day, while we were working with Dennis, we saw how an incision was being made with a scalpel to remove the catheter. In the area of the cut, we noticed a small explosion erupting in red. It was an infection penetrating the patient's wound. The screen of inner vision immediately confirmed: the wound is infected and Dennis's immune system may be too weak to cope with it. His life was again in danger.

We called Orlov at once and told him what we just saw. By a fortunate coincidence he was close to the ICU unit at that time. Boris immediately drove back to the hospital. When Dennis's doctor saw him returning with a cold expression on his face, he understood that something went wrong.

– How is Dennis, – Boris asked in a stern voice.

– You were here five minutes ago, – the doctor sounded surprised. – What could happen in five minutes?

– Has he undergone any procedure?

– They took away the catheter. He is doing fine and doesn't need it any more.

– You have just introduced an infection. Who made the incision?

The doctor turned pale.

– The incision is made for it to be easier to take out the catheter. Everything at the hospital is sterilized, and an infection is out of the question. I am absolutely positive.

– And yet there's an infection. I just got a call from Pushkin. They saw it happen.

The doctor fell silent, stunned by the fact that someone, who was almost thirty miles away from the hospital, could see what was happening in the ICU room.

Toward evening, Dennis's temperature rose sharply, and a new stage in the struggle for his life began. The girls took turns and did not leave his side even for an hour. They supported Dennis with energy, increasing his strength, so that he could fight the infection.

By the end of the month Dennis could already get out of bed and he was released from the hospital. The head of the ICU unit, saying goodbye to Boris Orlov, whom everybody had befriended by then, admitted:

– Indeed, it is a case I can't explain, but the reserves of the human body are poorly understood. And you could see for yourself how hard we all tried to help.

So I became convinced one more time: even if Christ should come down to Earth once again and revive some other dead Lazarus, our doctors would just shrug their shoulders and say: "Would you believe such a thing?!"

Chapter 8

I received an invitation to meet with Academician Grigori Petrovich Grabovoi. It happened quite unexpectedly and even strangely, if I may say so. Doctor of Psychology, Academician Ivliev, who was Deputy Director at my Center, displayed a great interest in everything that had to do with this mysterious man of late. He told me about some incredible cases, where Grigori Petrovich was able to rescue people and equipment at a distance; moreover, each of these instances was recorded by competent professionals, notarized and supplied with written affidavits by the victims themselves.

During a news conference in Bulgaria about the future of the Kozloduy Nuclear Power Plant, which others considered precarious, Grabovoi caused his first absolute sensation when he gave a specific prediction of when a catastrophe could occur at the plant if not prevented. "There is no danger of an explosion at the nuclear reactor in the next two years. The only thing that must be done is to check the safety of the power plant's cooling system before the expiration of two years," our fellow countryman assured. Everything Grabovoi predicted came true. Two years later, the government-run "Rossiyskaya Gazeta" (№ 18 for January 30, 1998) published an article under the rubric of "Quiet Sensation", titled "Tomorrow's Catastrophe Is Prevented". The article confirmed the fact (corroborated at the highest political level) that Grigori Grabovoi identified the specific defect at the Kozloduy Nuclear Power Plant in Bulgaria, which could lead to a nuclear disaster equal to many Chernobyls. The catastrophe, which Grabovoi succeeded in preventing, was dangerous for the entire world: scientific calculations showed that in the event of such a nuclear explosion, the

270

proximity of underground layers of high conductivity would lead to the emergence of a vacuum drain that would suck in the Earth's atmosphere. Due to high velocity particles, this drain would have dispersed the planet into a cloud of dust by the year 2000, and it would be impossible to stop a destructive process of such magnitude by means of modern technology. Grigori Grabovoi received multiple awards from governments and NGOs in many countries for preventing this and other potential global disasters.

It was Ivliev who gave me different materials to read about Grabovoi. This was a discovery for me, particularly since his work was parallel to mine in a lot of ways. Grigori Petrovich played a truly decisive role in my life, and therefore I feel that I must introduce him to my readers in greater detail. This can best be accomplished through quoted extracts from Vladimir Sudakov's book, "Grigori Grabovoi, the Phenomenon of the Millennium", which was published in 1999 by the publisher Kalashnikov.

"In 1996 Grigori Petrovich turned 33 years old but he looks even younger. He remembers himself as an infant: before he learned how to speak, he could understand what grown-ups were talking about (now, too, he can understand spoken foreign languages at the level of thought). From the age of five he could foresee events. His mother asked him to ride his bike to the nearby market one day for some home-made cheese, and he replied: "There isn't any cheese at the market." Soon after, their neighbor came running back from the market all lathered up... As it turned out, the police broke up the merchants at the marketplace that morning, so there really wasn't any cheese available...

Naturally, he didn't think much about his special ability at the time – he assumed that all people had it, particularly since none of his peers from the Bogar village in Kazakhstan ever understood what a remarkable phenomenon they had as a friend. Still, by the age of 12 Grigori gradually be-

271

came aware of the fact that not everybody was like him. How could other people respond to his ability to change the course of events? Knowing that a certain unpleasant circumstance was unavoidable, Grigori began to realize that the person involved could be distracted by other more significant concerns; in other words, he altered the layers of thought and focused his attention on alternative details. And by doing that he achieved the result he was seeking.

Already as a child, Grigori could understand the intentions of various animals and could control their behavior telepathically.

I must add that both in his childhood and teen years no one ever tried to lay a finger on Grigori or attack him verbally. It wasn't because he took up karate and was better in gymnastics than any of his peers or because he once won a bet after he beat a car while riding his "Sport-tourist" bicycle. Most likely, no one ever tried to cause him any harm because he was enveloped in some kind of a "peaceful energy shell". It was also possible that already as a teenager he became aware of the mysterious power he possessed, and set himself the goal of foretelling unpleasant future events and placing a barrier before them.

His current creed hasn't changed. As Grigori Petrovich admits, his psychic powers have neither increased nor decreased since that time. It's just that as he grew older he began to protect his inner treasure and stopped wasting it on trifles. He now used his powers only in genuine emergencies – to save a life, for instance. In more recent years, Grigori is increasingly talking about ways to rescue from disaster not individuals but the entire planet.

Grigori Petrovich realized he was able to confront such a tremendous challenge after he began to work at the Tashkent Design-Engineering Agency, where he received a job placement after graduating from the Uni-

272

versity. The Agency was engaged in developing space technology, and, among other issues, Grigori worked on the theory of catastrophes. And in the course of this work, his own concept of how such devastating disasters could be averted matured within his mind.

...He was still a student then, and was reading a book in preparation for an exam. Suddenly, he became aware of an inexplicable vibration in his body. In his mind's eye he saw a nuclear power plant, a cloud of smoke, fire and people scurrying to and fro. It happened one month prior to the Chernobyl nuclear disaster. And three days before the tragedy he had another similar vision: he saw burning graphite rods. A visual depiction of the Schrodinger equation on the laws of the microcosm was revealed to him: a tunnel junction (a concept in quantum mechanics) and a silver speck, the electron energy, trying in vain to move from one level to another. Grigori shuddered: "There will shortly be a huge blast, because the graphite content in the fission process is significantly above the norm!"

Grigori saw all this at the level of clairvoyance. I asked him why he didn't put everything else aside to report what he saw to the authorities, why he didn't call the alarm. "I spent a while then on reducing the effects of the disaster through remote impact, since in those days officials totally ignored any warnings that came from clairvoyants," – Grigori said sadly. Had Grabovoi encountered a more open-minded official at that moment, it may have been possible to prevent this devastating disaster. Grigori Petrovich is not in the habit of knocking on closed doors. He operates independently and counts only on his own psychic abilities to help overcome the threat of destruction on a global scale. Whenever possible, if people exhibit understanding and there is a clear-cut need to do it, he tries to explain the situation to them and provide training on how they can use his methods to rescue themselves.

Humanity will have to deal with the consequences of the Chernobyl disaster for years to come. "I could see the most powerful neutrino fluxes moving perpendicular to the four corners of the globe. They can affect the people's gene pool already after 120 years..."

Time went on. Grabovoi continued to demonstrate miracles at the secret Design-Engineering Agency, finding answers to unsolved problems and hinting at what might happen if certain measures are not taken. He invariably proved to be right. He was eventually asked by Gany Mazitovich Rafikov, head of the Uzbek Civil Aviation Administration, to take the position of aviation safety inspector and, at the same time, an expert on extrasensory tracking of aircraft. The responsibilities of his second position obligated him to see the invisible, and the responsibilities of the first one gave him the right to prohibit a flight. And this is exactly what he did more than once when his "third eye" detected dangling wires or some other problems in the belly of an airliner. He canceled the flights of the presidential aircraft, too, acting as a kind of guardian angel.

In the hands of Carmine Mirabelli from Brazil solid objects became transformed into liquids. Analysis of the metal rods which Israeli-born Uri Geller could bend by the effort of his will indicated a change in their molecular structure... How they were able to do this, boggles the mind, and it is unlikely that we will ever get them to clarify the issue: not only are they too far removed from us: one – in time, the other – in space, but they are also very secretive, since both have been subjected to repeated severe attacks and exposed as "frauds"...

As for Grigori Grabovoi, he is right here before us and he doesn't attempt to shroud himself in a veil of secrecy. He repeats his creed over and over again: "Any event can be altered. My forecasts are not death warrants. I always look for constructive ways to pre-empt negative events.

I don't alter the object but only the circumstances surrounding the object."

Following the Chernobyl nuclear disaster Grabovoi has prudently begun to document all his predictions. His archive contains hundreds of acts, sealed and signed by authoritative experts. Below is the content of some of them.

IL-86 number 86052. Psychic G.P. Grabovoi predicted a non-fault power reduction in the 4th engine, perhaps, as the result of a collision with a bird. Result: 7 days later, on 01/27/1992, during the descent of the aircraft, a crow was injected into the 4th engine. The pilots, who were aware of the prediction, managed to balance the thrust and land the plane, filled to capacity with passengers. A dent was made in the air intake and spinner. The engine was decommissioned.

IL-62 number 86704. Psychic G.P. Grabovoi drew attention to a defect in the structure of the material in the vicinity of the engine combustion chamber number 3. After 11 days, as evidenced by the record in the aircraft logbook, there was burnout in the nozzle block located in the vicinity of the engine combustion chamber number 3. The engine was prematurely decommissioned.

IL-86 number 86056. Psychic Grabovoi transmitted information on the insufficient reliability of the equipment in the plane's front toilets. From the notations in the logbook: "01/22/1992. There is water leakage from under the panel in the front lavatory. Water had to be blocked during the flight." (Again, it isn't hard to guess what would happen if water leaked into the aircraft control system: electronic equipment would falsely indicate engine malfunction and the pilots would turn them off...) As a result of this problem on board the plane, the design and construction agency that designed the IL-86 increased the sealing in the lavatories.

Let me reiterate: there are hundreds of similar official reports. And every one of them ends with the same phrase: "The information provided by psychic G.P. Grabovoi was fully confirmed." One can only wonder why the Civil Aviation Administration didn't take appropriate measures upon receiving a warning, but instead waited for the prediction to be confirmed... Actually, the bureaucrats at the top were surprised at something else: how could such a young man, who wasn't even an expert in aircraft construction, see from a distance what was inside a plane and, moreover, identify what was defective: the computer, chassis, transformer or oil pipe? Mind you, this young and seemingly inexperienced individual was able to discover defects even without leaving the office. All he needed was to know the number of the aircraft – Grabovoi actually did such troubleshooting based on an agreement signed with the Soviet-American joint venture "Ascon"...

High-profile Aeroflot managers also staged "an experimental testing" of the psychic's abilities in the city of Fergana. A Commission was set up, which included experts from the Antonov Aviation Scientific-Technical Complex and the Fergana Mechanical Plant. Grabovoi was instructed, within a 2-3 second interval, to diagnose from a distance of over 80 feet, any problems he could find in the AN-12 number 1901 aircraft, belonging to the Bulgarian Air Sofia. Here is the protocol.

"G.P. Grabovoi did not have at his disposal any diagnostic instruments or devices and had no opportunity to inquire about the status of the aircraft due to severe time constraints... Prior to his diagnosis nobody was aware of the defects which he indicated and which were later discovered by the Commission and reported in writing. Defects were found only where indicated by G.P. Grabovoi, although the entire aircraft was thoroughly examined with the help of appropriate instruments. (The defect indicated by Grabovoi was no small matter – he discovered corrosion of the rails

276

in the area of the 62 frame...). Under the same conditions and time con-
straints, the psychic found cracks on the upper wing skin of the An-12
number 1204, which was standing next to the first plane, after which the
aircraft had to be sent for repair. The defects pointed out by Grabovoi
were not identified through physical vision."

That was one of the cases where Grabovoi's precognition (perception
of future events) served as the basis for action before the flight. Following
the "testing", Grigori faced an avalanche of requests to establish the
causes of various "aviation events" (the coy euphemism used by Aero-
flot administration in describing accidents). Thus, for the limited liability
partnership "Rampa" Grabovoi determined from a remote distance what
happened on 03/14/1995 with aircraft AN-12 number 113337 not far from
the Baku airport. Everything that the psychic said the day after the emer-
gency landing was later confirmed in the course of the investigation: the
alternate failure of two engines, the power outage, the excess weight of the
commercial aircraft and the crew's procedural work violations...

I must confess that I too couldn't resist the temptation to check the
"purity" of Grabovoi's experiments. I took off my watch and asked him to
tell where I got it. "A tall white man gave it to you three years ago." It was
my turn to open my mouth in amazement. The watch was a present from an
Arab sheik, a tall, gray-haired man in white attire...

I am giving such a detailed account of the psycho-diagnostics demons-
trated by Grabovoi so that the reader can appreciate the enormity of his
talent. Remote bio-location of objects has been implemented before: on
the instructions of the Leningrad Naval Base, psychic operators indicated
on the map the exact location of hydrographic vessels in the ocean. But the
precision of Grabovoi's vision exceeds all conceivable parameters. The
reader may therefore wonder what kind of intuition this man possesses.

277

"It isn't intuition at all. It is clairvoyance, – Grigori Petrovich says. "You know, I can see even a very tiny component from all sides. My remote vision in real time is 100% error-free. If I have to look into the past or future, it's another story. When I am involved in this type of work I alter events for the better."

As I understand, one needs to have a sixth sense in order to do such things, which is what Academician V. Vernadsky had in mind when he said: "There is a need to accept the real influence of human consciousness, that is, the characteristic of being, on the phenomena taking place in the real space of the naturalist."

... At 3 p.m. on June 6, 1995 Grigori Grabovoi was summoned to the Central Headquarters of the paramilitary mountain rescue units of the coal industry. There was an accident at the Vorkutinskaya mine, and he was asked to help establish the underground location of the miners. Below is a quote from the protocol signed by the deputy chief engineers of the Central Headquarters A. Kuznetsov and A. Zholus:

"The location of the drifts was provided in strictly experimental conditions and was based on the design of the ventilation system so that before the experiment began no one knew what specific schemes will be submitted for the diagnosis... Using his psychic method, G.P. Grabovoi correctly identified the place of the original fire, the location of two victims in the ventilation drift, and the defects in the ventilation of the emergency lava. He accomplished all this in one second and without being offered any kind of additional information... G.P. Grabovoi conducted his psychic diagnosis of the scheme without having any information about the actual location of the mine in the area, i.e., based solely on what he could tell from a sheet of paper..."

The two located miners were rescued; they were not reported as

278

"zero", to use the jargon of the mining administration.

Nevertheless, miners continue to die in accidents. This happens because mining equipment is morally and physically outdated and rescue technology is inadequate. Even the most heroic and courageous rescuers cannot overcome such objective factors.

The Central Headquarters promised to give Grabovoi a general map of all the mines in the country so that he could diagnose their future. He is still waiting... Without a map he cannot make a prediction where it is most likely to expect the unexpected...

...It seems that no problem is "too insignificant" for Grabovoi. If a person finds a way to reach him, it means he absolutely couldn't do without his help. So Grabovoi turns on his internal "working organ".

...This amount of information is probably enough to give one an idea about the wide scope of Grigori Grabovoi's abilities. And yet I would feel that my narrative is insufficient if I didn't mention his broad range of interests in the field of business and finance. Instead of commenting on this, I will simply quote:

"I, Iosif Ivanovich Danchenko, a resident of the city of Gomel, certify that on March 25, 1995 I sought advice from G.P. Grabovoi regarding my business. G.P. Grabovoi correctly identified the names of individuals who interact with my partners at a confidential level."

"I confirm that during our meeting on August 4, 1995, psychic G.P. Grabovoi, discussing the issue of banks, reported anticipating major problems after August 23 and recommended that I take preventive measures with my interbank transactions on August 22 and 23. His forecast was confirmed by "Black Thursday" (August 24), when dozens of banks did not meet their obligations on transactions and customer payments. Signed: V. Serebryakov, Department Head of the foreign exchange market at

the National Credit Bank."

There is extensive testimony of G.P. Grabovoi's accurate diagnosis of computer software. Below is one of them, signed by I. Khamrakulov, Director General of the "ASCON" Joint Venture:

"When the program file infected with a virus was copied from a floppy disk to the hard drive with G.P. Grabovoi's psychic impact, the program file took 10 times less space on the hard drive compared to the original file. In the process of copying, the DIR virus should have transferred itself from the floppy to the hard drive, but this did not happen, which was confirmed by the anti-virus ANTI-DIR software. Consequently, the virus was destroyed when the file was being copied from the floppy to the hard drive."

But this is not half the story, as they say. The best is yet to come. Radik Valetov, software engineer at an aero technical information center, reports on instances of G.P. Grabovoi's mental influence upon the main computer and peripheral devices. From a distance of six and a half feet the psychic "instructed" the computer to rewrite the data from a file to a specified disk...

There have been instances when banking systems in the West have been blocked by viruses. Hundreds of thousands of clients suffered as a result. Even greater disruption and even chaos can be caused by failure in a computer network that manages traffic, the operation of nuclear reactors, or oil and gas delivery systems. The Grabovoi phenomenon could be a lifeline for preventing any of these frightening scenarios.

Lidiya Anatoliyevna Chernyak works at the Space Mission Control Center. Though endowed with psychic gifts, she is nevertheless modest in appraising her own spiritual abilities. But when she heard about Grabovoi, she asked for God's intervention so that she could meet the famous psychic. And the meeting took place, when Grigori was invited to the Space Mission Control Center to diagnose the condition of the international space station "Mir".

In the presence of one of the leaders of SMCC, the psychic detected a defect in the thermal insulation of the space station's outer casing. He also discovered the place of overdrive in the rocket, as well as the location of scratches and cracks. To test the equipment at the request of the American participants in the experiment, the Center's scientists wanted to simulate a full afterburner mode for the on-board engines, so that the space station would "swing". Grabovoi insisted that such an experiment should not be conducted because there were cracks in the hull. The afterburner mode, he said, can be simulated only if there is external control over each segment of the spacecraft...

Grigori Petrovich also predicted that the astronauts would not feel well during the space station's flight over the geopathogenic area of Brazil... Finally, he also "saw" adverse atmospheric changes aboard the station: under the influence of heat and humidity new strains of bacteria were formed that could affect the health of the astronauts.

"The capabilities of this man are so completely unique and amazing that Russia has every right to be proud of him, – said Lidiya Chernyak. – People like him should be treasured and protected."

When speaking about Grabovoi, one cannot omit the absolutely mystical facts of his resurrection of the dead, impossible at first glance but, nevertheless, officially documented. I quote from the same book by Vladimir Sudakov:

"His psychic colleagues got through to Grabovoi late after midnight: a woman's 12-year-old son had vanished, and there were witnesses saying that the boy was dismembered. The vision of a quartered body appeared

before Grigori's eyes. After asking a few questions, he assured the caller: 'Give me three days and I'll put him back together. Tell his mother that she will soon see her son alive and well.' Putting time in reverse, he began to build a positive picture of the future. One NEEDS TO WORK AROUND THE PROBLEM; one must build a different, happy turn of events...

Three days later the mother, distraught with grief, found her son 'purely by accident' at the Kazansky Railway Station. He was alive and well, the only problem was that he remembered nothing about the few days he spent away from his family.

The best detective agencies and government-run special services confirmed to the mother that her daughter died in a fire. After a mediated request, Grigori Petrovich revived the burnt girl in a monastery, located hundreds of miles away from the place where the girl died...

Grigori Grabovoi revived people in a variety of situation: he returned a woman to life with several physicians testifying to the event; he revived a man in the presence of a child and another adult...

How is it possible to alter events that have already occurred? I accosted Grabovoi with numerous questions, and he tried to explain it to me with the most unperturbed demeanor.

– It all has to do with parallel time streams. When the healer operates without a scalpel, he penetrates another time with his finger or his hand, while remaining in reality with his other hand. Figuratively speaking, he has several hands, like Krishna. So I move part of 'myself' to another temporal field, into any given point, to correct the line of destiny. In some sense, God himself is sending me to test the grounds.

If this is a murder for hire, then people quickly learn about it through the media. In that case there has to be another option: the dead can be projected live only in a place where no one knows anything about them.

The best option is not to have any witnesses of the murder or, if there are witnesses, to make sure that they won't speak about the resurrection for a certain amount of time. But some blabbermouths just can't be stopped from telling everyone and sundry: 'He was dead and he's now alive, see!' For such people it is necessary to build a scenario with explanations and neutralization. I would never consider killing anyone, of course, it is against Christian morality. That is why I must build positive events for all parties involved. Only after completing this work can I begin to construct an alternative course of events and to pull the victim out of nothingness. I substantiate the fact of resurrection. I resort to logic in proving that resurrection shows how senseless it is to develop means of destruction, since everything can be reversed.

Resurrection is appreciated by all people, if not consciously, then as proof of the immortality of the spirit. Obviously, the immortal spirit of some individuals in infinite time can find a way to preserve a positive picture of the world's development. Materialization of any object is the same type of process as resurrection. The more common word for it is revival. It is the revival of a positive, constructive make-up of the world. In this context, destruction is regarded as a totally senseless and, therefore, surmountable obstacle to the reality of life.

Someone will probably find the possibility of such a procedure quite shocking. As for me, I find it to be a timely way of demonstrating in reality a positive path of development, which actually and permanently prevents the destruction of the world. The killer is alive, but he may not be aware that in one of the scenarios of the past he could have been destroyed in an act of vengeance. This is a way to preserve the lives of all parties, which is necessary for society to adopt laws conducive to positive development. The innocent victim is once again among us, and it doesn't occur to anyo-

283

ne that a terrible tragedy was about to take this person's life. The family has been united.

I must admit that altering an event which has already occurred is a highly esoteric act and also a highly complicated one. It is far better to prevent misfortune from striking, which Grigori Grabovoi is always more than happy to do."

I found everything Ivliev told me about this man and all that I read about him quite amazing. Here I was, still fiddling with the regeneration of my gallbladder, and someone nearby was resurrecting the dead without great difficulty. Moreover, I saw how close our methods were. So why did the Russian Academy of Sciences keep silent about Grabovoi's remarkable skills? After all, science has long come close to realizing that planetary consciousness in the Universe forms the kind of unity that can be described as the SUPER REASON, or the noosphere. Konstantin Eduardovich Tsiolkovsky affirmed the existence of "forces of reason in the Cosmos" and of the "cosmic brain". "I am not just a materialist but also a panpsychist, – he wrote in this regard, – for I recognize the presence of feeling in the entire Universe. This property, I believe, is inseparable from matter." At the end of his life Albert Einstein also came to believe in the existence of an "intelligent force" in the Cosmos, even though, as is well known, he always supported the position of materialism in natural sciences.

Contemporary knowledge is also increasingly drawn to the idea. The prominent Soviet philosopher I. A. Akchurin wrote that as a result of the revision of the worldview based on the natural sciences it is possible that we may end up replacing all of the classical mechanistic view of the world as a large and complex "clockwork" by some entirely new paradigm, such as a general vision of the world as a living organism. Anyway, he said, a number of scientists are "seriously considering that possibility."

Other researchers, too, have arrived at a similar idea in one form or another. Here is how the American philosopher Samuel Crum formulates it: "The Universe is so magnificent that it would be hard to imagine that it does not collectively form a single Universal intelligence that is conscious of billions of swarming living beings on all habitable planets, similar to how a person is aware of having a minor headache... Stars or even galaxies are merely 'neurons' of this Universal mind."

A number of extremely interesting facts have been assembled by A.A. Gorbovsky, a journalist and supporter of the idea of the living Universe, in his brochure, "In the Circle of Eternal Return" ("Znaniye" Publishers, Moscow, 1989). In his work he emphasizes a number of discoveries:

"Some time ago, while deciphering the spectra of some extragalactic sources, astronomers have discovered formic acid in the open space. After that traces of ethyl alcohol and wood alcohol were also found there. Finally, the staff of the Max Planck Institute for Astronomy in Germany found a cloud of water vapor at a distance of over two million light years. We currently know about the existence in outer space of several dozens of organic molecules. They fill gigantic clouds of gas, whose length is measured in light years. This is tantamount to billions and billions of tons of organic matter. V.I. Goldanskiy, Member of the Russian Academy of Sciences, believes in the possible formation in space of "the most complex molecules, including even proteins".

In studying molecules with an organic base found in stardust, astrophysics Nalin C. Wickramasinghe and Fred Hoyle, suggested the presence of microorganisms in space at the cellular level. Their mass, they say, is enormous. What kind of life form they represent, what processes take place in its depths, and how it impacts non-living matter in space – this we

285

don't know and can't even imagine.

Until recently, the assumption was that cosmic matter, such as stars and galaxies, is distributed throughout outer space without any order. It turns out that this is not the case, as inferred by a group of astronomers from the Estonian Institute of Astrophysics and Atmospheric Physics. Here is what J. Einasto, Doctor of Physics and Mathematics, explained to a correspondent from TASS News Agency:

"Galaxies and their clusters are arranged in an orderly fashion that resembles a honeycomb of enormous size. And the closer to the junctions between such cells, the more concentrated the cosmic matter."

This conclusion was made by researchers after a thorough study of the distribution of mass within the galaxies which are part of the super clusters in Perseus, Andromeda and Pegasus. At the periphery of such a "cell" the surface density of the galaxies and their clusters was four times higher than in the central part. The pattern obtained by American astrophysicists after computer processing of data about millions of galaxies also confirmed the cell-like structure of the Universe. Characteristically, there are virtually no galaxies within the cells: they are all gathered in the "walls" between the cells. The size of these cells ranges from 100 to 300 million light years. According to B.V. Komberg, researcher at the Agency for Space Research at the Russian Academy of Sciences, "if such a vision of the large-scale structure of the Universe is confirmed, we will come to the picture the Universe as a bizarre matrix of cells..."

What are the forces and factors that could cause such a symmetric and orderly structure?

According to Estonian astronomers M. Iyevaer and J. Einasto who made this discovery, "numerical experiments show that a cell-like structure may occur by random clustering. We believe that the structure is of primary origin and it was formed before the formation of galaxies and clusters of galaxies..."

Is it possible to assume that the living matter of space, a volitional impulse, could affect the distribution of masses of matter? Should we also look for such an effect from other, more complex phenomena of the world around us?

For a while the dominating point of view in science was that life emerged on Earth due to chance. Today, however, based on current scientific knowledge, random synthesis of RNA and DNA that determine life seems quite unlikely. Moreover, the Universe itself hasn't existed long enough for life to appear on a random basis.

One of the mathematical calculations tells us that if, for instance, every microsecond one option was tested in any electron- sized cell of space, only 10 possible options would be tested in the course of 100 billion years (whereas the Universe has existed only for 15-22 billion years). This number is infinitely small compared with the required $4^{1000000} \sim 10$ – so many combinations of 4 "letters" of the genetic code would have to be alternated for it to constitute the one that defines life. According to the calculations of the famous American astronomer Holden, such a random occurrence would comprise just 1 of $1.3 \cdot 10^{30}$.

If the method of random combinations were to be used to create even the simplest, most primitive protein molecule, a negligibly small part of such options could be tried out throughout the existence of the Universe. This conclusion was drawn by German scientists M. Eigen and R. Winkler. (According to the calculations of astrophysicists Chandra Wickramasinghe and Fred Hoyle, the lifetime of the Earth is equally insufficient for the formation and evolution of the system of approximately two thousand enzymes used by organisms on our planet.).

To sum up, based on recent scientific data life didn't and couldn't emerge by accident.

This absence of randomness was observed in his time by V.I. Vernadsky. "Living creatures of the Earth, – he wrote, – are creations of a complex cosmic process, a necessary and law-governed part of the harmonious mechanism of the Cosmos, in which, as we know, there are no random events." Indeed, as evidenced by the Earth's experience, it is recreating its own similar forms, which creates the condition for the existence of life. We can assume that this law operates on the scale of the Universe as well. Developing this idea further, it would be logical to assume that living matter in outer space also constantly seeks to create new forms of life. What is meant here pertains to a targeted impact on inanimate matter, to its organization and the creation of conditions leading to the emergence of life.

"The face of the Earth is changed by them, – Vernadsky wrote, referring to these forces, – and is molded by them to a large extent. It is not a reflection of our planet alone, the manifestation of its matter and its energy; it is simultaneously a creation of the external forces of the Cosmos." This is a pervasive directed impact of "external forces of the Cosmos", for which space and possibly even time cannot be a barrier. The Earth's biosphere, Vernadsky wrote, is a source for "changing the planet by external cosmic forces."

A.A. Gorbovsky then makes quite a pertinent comment: "The English physiologist Cyril Burt believed that in addition to the known physical Universe, we can postulate some combination of fields forming a sort of "psychical Universe". These are fields or certain areas of consciousness with the ability "to give structure to reality" and "to have an impact on matter and space."

The famous American astrophysicist Freeman John Dyson says that he and his colleagues also "do not exclude a priori the possibility that the mind and consciousness may have the same status in the make-up of the Universe as matter and energy."

The fact that consciousness can have an impact on matter is confirmed by some more recent laboratory experiments, which have accumulated statistically significant material. Thus, under the terms of one of the experiments, the participant pushed the button on a device throwing out dice. The subject was instructed to simultaneously send a strong volitional impulse, i.e., "to want" the dice to fall in a certain way: "Six," "two", etc. 170,000 such dice throws were tested in the laboratories of the University of Pittsburgh (USA). Similar experiments were also conducted at other research centers. It was determined not only that "desired" results significantly exceeded those in the statistically average range, but also that there was a consistent pattern, where the number of "desired" results at the end of a series decreased substantially compared to those in the beginning. The degree of randomness in such a stable distribution of outcomes is 1 in 30,000,000.

Another confirmation of the possibility of impact from a volitional impulse on the material world can be found in the experiments on the distortion of the "Josephson effect" (the flow of superconducting current through a thin dielectric layer). The subject was shown the output (the impulse signal) on the magnetometer with a superconducting shield and was then asked to influence the magnetic field with an effort of his will. Within thirty seconds, as a result of such impact, the output frequency of the magnetometer was two times greater.

Other facts of the same nature have been recorded in the more distant past. It is worth mentioning the experiments by Willy Schneider (in the 1920s), in which he moved objects by an effort of will in the presence of a commission of 54 university professors, who confirmed the genuineness of the phenomenon. An episode from the life of Charlie Chaplin, described in his autobiography, should obviously be attributed to the same class of phenomena. Once, when he and a group of friends entered a bar where there were three roulettes, he suddenly felt some strange force inside him, and he said that he could get the roulettes to stop – the first on "9", the second on "4" and the third on "7". "Believe it or not, – he recalled, – the first one stopped on the number 9, the second on four, and the third on seven. Mind you, it was one chance in a million."

It is possible to find such phenomena as the impact of volitional impulse on material objects mentioned by some ancient authors as well. One such reference belongs to Josephus Flavius (1st century A.D.). He speaks of a certain Eleazar, who ordered a goblet with water or a basin for the washing of the feet to be placed next to a patient, while he was "driving out evil spirits".

Leaving the patient's body, "the evil spirit" overturned the vessel in response to Eleazar's instruction. This happened in the presence of Emperor Vespasian, his sons, many Roman generals and numerous legionnaires."

Grigori Petrovich Grabovoi's abilities are consistent with those facts and hypotheses which science has already accumulated, with some adjustment for the fact that such psychic power and energy has not been previously observed in any one person.

Still, the phenomenon of Academician Grabovoi did not fit into the Procrustean bed of orthodox science. Not only did he assert that there are different realities existing in the Universe, some of which are spiritual realities which are hidden, but he also convincingly demonstrated how they influenced our lives. Materialization and de-materialization of objects, telepathy, instances of curing terminally ill patients, including people with

AIDS and, finally, regeneration of missing organs and resurrection of the dead, which took place in the presence of experts – all these events are not some kind of speculation by people with an over stimulated imagination but the daily work of this remarkable man, whose goal never was to get TV exposure or fuel unhealthy celebrity worship. Grabovoi created a New Reality in the field of knowledge, where science and religion are not opposed to each other in a senseless effort to monopolize their right to the truth. In this New Reality they join efforts to comprehend this truth.

The factual instances of resurrection, duly registered as I have already emphasized, actually brought down the traditional materialistic view of the Universe. These facts left everyone who has to do with science so stunned that even the Russian Academy of Sciences' specially appointed Committee against such mystical anomalies, headed by Academician Kruglyakov, preserved a significant silence, having no desire to say "yes" and not being able to say "no" in response to this highly unusual phenomenon. Until then, there has not been a single living creature in the world that would return to life after dying and be able to talk about the other side of Being. Now there is, and more than one…

And here I was presented with the opportunity not only to personally meet this unique individual, but to tell him about the achievements at our Center, to ask him for advice and learn more about his methods.

I went to my first meeting with Grigori Petrovich alone, without Igor. Grabovoi's office was located on Moscow's famous Solyanka Street, not far from the building of the Presidium of the Russian Academy of Medical Sciences. As an aside, the fact that they were close by was quite noteworthy… The entrance to the stately old mansion of the Presidium was decorated with antique columns, and the monumental grandeur of

291

the latter was indicative of the immutability, solidity and imperious power of this institution. Not far, in a nearby building occupied by the Football League, was the small, two-room office of the famous miracle worker, who was able to regenerate missing organs and cure diabetes, cancer and AIDS without any medications. All these results have been documented and proven. On several occasions, Grigori regenerated the missing organs directly in the surgery office, before the eyes of astonished physicians. So what? The initial impression of what happened gradually wore off. Those physicians who tried, on the spur of the moment, to explain something to the health officials got tired of banging their heads against the wall, and eventually they even started to doubt whether the miracle actually happened. Perhaps it was some sort of hypnosis or a hallucination? Or maybe they had been drinking excessively before the surgery? Such denial was sadly familiar to me.

Something quite similar happened to me too, when I wrote a letter about the possibilities of our technique to Valeri Pavlinovich Shantsev, then Deputy Mayor of Moscow. He immediately gave instructions to several clinics and institutions to contact me and conduct a medical testing of the possibilities I identified. Six weeks later I found out that all the clinics and research institutions completed the medical testing and gave a negative assessment of these possibilities. Where did they conduct their testing? How exactly did they do it? This remains a great secret. All I can say is that none of these experts ever met with me or any of my colleagues, or even called us regarding this topic. They probably decided not to bother themselves or us needlessly. They simply wrote back stating that this cannot be since it contradicts the foundations of their closely guarded science. And they do not know of any other science. Therefore, nobody has the right to treat what they cannot cure. This was the position they must have taken.

This is precisely what happened with acupuncture in its time, remember? The medical community maligned those doctors who dared to practice acupuncture any way they could. They labeled them as quacks and charlatans, and said they were unworthy of the prestigious title of a Soviet physician. And how did it all end? It turns out acupuncture is a science after all and it offers people very effective help.

Such were my bitter thoughts as I was passing by the Presidium of the Russian Academy of Medical Sciences, whose combined power wasn't able to save even a single person dying of AIDS, on my way to Grabovoi's basement office, where everything that official medicine could not and would not do was performed quietly, modestly and effectively. Work here went on uninterrupted, day after day, with the same positive results.

Grigori Petrovich was waiting for me and, as it later turned out, he had been waiting for this to happen long before we actually got acquainted. The man who was widely known in the world, and who Russia's official bureaucracy knew nothing about or refused to acknowledge, was young and pleasant not only in appearance but also in his conduct. After just a one-hour long conversation – he somehow managed to wrest this hour from the schedule of the patients gathered in the hallway – I became completely convinced that our meeting was essentially predetermined, since from now on we were to work together. Grigori, Igor and I became one team, although each was to continue working independently.

We agreed on everything. A new phase in our training began which, soon after, radically changed my destiny and Igor's.

Working with Grabovoi was not only a privilege for us but was also useful. The technique of controlled clairvoyance which Grigori developed was another shiny mountain top to conquer for Igor and me. We had to …

we had no other choice but to conquer this mountain top, all the more so because its owner was gracious enough to agree to be our teacher on this difficult path. He already knew that we were a winged horse and rider in that other space. "You have been placed into the image of St. George," he explained to us. – This is a great honor."

As agreed beforehand, at 9 p.m. on April 18 we established telepathic communication with Grigori. We found him in his office, and after saying the appropriate greetings, we reminded him of his agreement to allow us to enter his mind and read the information available there.

He smiled and threw up his hands:

– Come in since I agreed.

We tried to enter but couldn't. Grigori's head was protected with a sphere encircled by bright threads. From the neck down all the way to the ground he had something like a skirt with glowing protective power strips. Then … we began to see that this wasn't Grigori at all but his hologram. He was in contact with us through a medium.

We came closer. Grigori made a second sphere and pushed us back easily to where we started. He placed a triangle above the defense and then another one, making a double pyramid. The pyramid had a mirror surface. The defenses reached all the way to ground level. In addition, he placed a square, which protected all the defenses below the feet. It was barely noticeable, like glass. Another transformation – the square unfolded into a cube. A cube makes any defense invisible. It is something like the magic cap of invisibility.

– Is it clear? – Grigori Petrovich asked.

– Sure, – Igor and I replied in unison, and we immediately began to construct a similar defense system for ourselves. It worked. We were now invincible.

294

– To get out from under your defenses you should do the following, – Grigori Petrovich attracted our attention and removed first the cube, then the pyramids and finally the rest of the defense with a number of graceful pirouettes, about-turns and passes.

– Then we pull the energy into the coccyx, – he said and showed us how the energy threads withdrew into his tailbone.

– Next time I'll show you how to protect yourselves from ghosts and energy flows, – he promised before disappearing.

We were left alone, stupefied with happiness.

– What will we do next? – Igor asked.

I suddenly suggested:

– Why don't we pay a visit to Lapshin in St. Petersburg? Let's practice our defense systems…

– Agreed. Let's do it, – Igor said.

We rose and flew above the earth. Below were fields, forests and cities. Below was Russia. We were like birds, shrinking space with our bodies. Two or three minutes later we were in the city on the Neva. Something was unmistakably leading us straight to the goal of our aspirations.

We found ourselves in the hall of a restaurant. There was a huge table, music and lots of people. We saw Vyacheslav – he was presiding in the center. Next to him were two generals and some other men in plain clothes. Everybody was drinking champagne. Vyacheslav was explaining to them that he could see through walls and hear conversations at a distance.

And what were we doing right now? Weren't we looking and listening?

Lapshin said that he was able to read papers that were lying at the far end of the table.

One of the generals commented patronizingly:

– This could be useful to us.

The second one thought to himself: "I should ask him to spy on my wife."

Officers, damn you! You ought to be thinking about our homeland!

Suddenly, Lapshin felt that Igor and I were messing around with his head. He was clearly worried. He apologized and walked away from the table. Stopping in a corner behind a column, he suddenly unfolded his energy defense. It looked like a trellis shield pierced by yellow threads – four longitudinal and four transverse ones. It had a mirror surface. Lapshin raised the shield, trying to prevent our invasion.

Igor and I were enjoying it. We took the defense with our hands, moved it aside and surrounded Vyacheslav with an invisible cube. That's it, pal, we caught you. The guy started randomly brandishing his shield. He was extremely anxious, even scared.

He couldn't see anything now. Frantically, he tried out various options in his memory. But Lapshin had powerful intuition. He suddenly pictured my house and tried to bring it closer. But we had the invisible cube for that, didn't we? Lapshin became even more frightened.

– Arkady Naumovich, is it you? – he asked.

We didn't respond.

In a panic he walked back to the table, to his wife.

– Lucy, may I talk to you for a minute?

What was Lapshin doing? Why was he distracting his wife from a fascinating conversation she was having with the lady sitting next to her about female underwear?

– What is it? – she asked in a grumpy voice.

– I need to talk to you privately, – he insisted.

She got up reluctantly and the two moved to the side.

– I have a problem, – he explained. – The computer won't turn on. Petrov is doing something but I can't see him or his house. He has a powerful defense. It's got to be him.

– Who else among your people could be working at such a level? – his wife asked dispassionately. It seemed that her husband's problems weren't of much concern to her. – Could it be Katya?

– Definitely not!

– Nadya?

– Don't talk nonsense! It must be Petrov. Arkady Naumovich, what are you doing?

– We're playing games, – Igor and I giggled.

– It's Petrov, for a fact, – Lapshin announced out loud. – Where did you learn all this stuff?

Without giving an answer, we put away the invisible cube, released Vyacheslav from captivity and moved away to the second level.

It was an astonishing adventure. It brought delight to our souls and glee to our hearts.

The next day, using Grigori Petrovich's defense technique, we decided to investigate the various levels.

We started with the third level. There were gates to the left and right of us. These were entrances to the astral plane of intangible space.

We decided to go to the left. When we entered, it was cold and there was a rotten smell around. We saw people who were light as balloons. This was the Kingdom of the Dead. They were wearing dark robes and they felt unhappy and uncomfortable there. They couldn't see us because we were protected by our defense. We didn't want to move deeper into this unwelcome space.

We decided to change the direction of research. We moved out into the Bardo channel. There were other gates in front of us. We entered them. The picture that opened before us was quite different. It smelled of spring. Everything was very similar to our Earth. People seemed to be almost material. They worked here as they had in life. Someday, they would return to the earthly plane again and forget that they were ever in this other world. This was the loop of infinity in the shape of the number eight. The Möbius strip.

We returned into the Bardo channel and rose upward vertically to the next, fourth level.

We looked to the right of us and saw mountains and seas stretching into infinity. Above them were thunderous black clouds, vortexes and tornados. These were very odd tornados! We couldn't tell where the answer came from. It told us that these were disharmonious human souls. The answer sounded within us just like that, in our minds. It was as if someone was reading our thoughts and was ready to give us all the necessary explanations in the course of our unusual expedition.

Again, we moved out of the level and crossed the Bardo channel. It appeared that the right side of the system was more amicable to people than the left one. We saw the vastness of the ocean. The sun warmed us gently. The soft summer breeze caressed our faces. This was the boundlessness of beauty. Once again, a mysterious understanding came to us: here we could acquire knowledge and talent for singing, drawing, writing books and for almost any other creative endeavor. This was the abode of the muses, the source of inspiration.

We returned to the first level. Somehow we were both simultaneously struck with the same idea: why don't we pay Lapshin another visit?

All day long he was trying to spy on us. Nothing came of it. There was no way he could break through such defenses as ours. He was upset. He sat there in his shirt drawing diagrams of the different ways he could get me. He was thinking: "It is all Petrov's doing."

We entered into his head. He felt sick. We exited. Together with Igor, we created a positive aura for him and relieved the spasms.

Lapshin felt better. He went to the window and breathed in the air.

– Arkady Naumovich, is this you?

I didn't reply.

– How did this happen? When did it awaken within you? Are you sure it's you, tell me?

His mind was filled with emptiness and despair. All his life he aspired to reach this goal and it never materialized.

– Arkady Naumovich, I was probably wrong about some things.

There were tears in his eyes.

– We made it up, haven't we?

I agreed without saying anything and left. Igor was beside me. We went back to Moscow.

Near the house, we became aware of some sort of trouble. We stopped a short distance away and looked closely. A big black raven was circling above the house's protective half sphere. It wasn't a real-life raven.

Yeah, the astral was displaying signs of anxiety! It was too late now to be anxious. Igor and I transformed ourselves. I became a white winged horse in armor and my rider was a warrior holding a spear and a shield – he was St. George, the Dragon Slayer. Pulling out his sword, he approached the raven. We decided to start by applying the soft phase of confrontation, as Grigori Petrovich taught us. We therefore transformed the question "Why?" into one better suited to our appearance:

– So what is it you want? Are you here to draw and quarter us, or simply to stretch your legs?

299

The raven was in a panic. He saw before him a huge horseman, whose head reached above the clouds. He knew what this meant. The winged horse represented space. The horseman represented the power and the mind of society and humanity as a whole. Right now, at this moment, these powers were handed over to us. And the raven shied away and then disappeared altogether. The harsh phase of confrontation has been transformed into a soft one. St. George didn't have to chase every crow around. Of course, there's just as much similarity between crows and ravens, as between an old legend and modern garbage. Here, we have now humiliated the enemy with this insulting comparison.

The situation was becoming clear. Now they knew where to find us. We needed to boggle their minds a bit more. Let them think that it's probably here, but not necessarily so. We felt the need to think up some trick, the kind expressed in the previous sentence. We now had to specify it.

– What are crows afraid of? – I asked Igor.

– Scarecrows.

We recalled Grigori Petrovich's holographic copy. We duplicated ourselves. Now, the holographic copy of St. George would stand guard next to the house. If someone approached the house with evil intentions, it would warn us and we would instantly respond from any distance. In addition, the shield could act independently, although not with the degree of freedom that Igor and I had.

Once again, we heard a voice: "Don't worry. It's impossible to stop you. A new unfolding of space is underway whose purpose is positive reconstruction."

– We are not afraid, – we answered out loud, – because we don't separate our own actions from the One who performs these actions – from the Creator.

Igor and I marveled at our synchronic response and exchanged glances.

"You ought to master the technique of control, – we heard a voice. – You must determine what state of consciousness creates a controlled phase from the perspective of the soul, without control through logic. Test it in working with material space. When dealing with control over real events, many things can't be learned immediately, however, it is still essential to learn how to control them."

Well, the assignment was received. It is as simple and clear as Lenin's unforgettable motto: "Study, study and study again!"

At eight o'clock the next morning, as bona fide students, Igor and I were already sitting behind our desks. We turned on the screens of our inner vision – and immediately found ourselves in the familiar image of horse and rider. It seemed that we were being prepared for war. We began to study ourselves.

The horse was protected by chain mail. Above the eyes, it had metal slats, which were lowered in battle and covered up its vision. This was Pegasus. The rider had an elongated scarlet shield on the left side and a very long, dark-colored spear on the right. The rider's body was covered with chain mail and his feet were protected with knee-pads. The front of his boots was curled upward. His sword was attached to the belt and its hilt was covered with precious stones.

The largest pink stone was encased at the edge of the hilt. The bow and arrows were in the saddle. The arrows – seven of them, all different colors: yellow, purple, green, blue, brown, black and white – lay in the quiver. The rider's staff hung behind the belt. The curved hilt had an inscription that said: "Save and protect!"

The helmet was framed by a curtain of chain mail. A huge ruby shone

301

at its center, over the bridge of the warrior's nose. His shoulders were draped in a very long scarlet cloak. There was another inscription on the collar of the cloak, too. On the right side of the saddle there was a mighty mace. We took another close look at the shield. There was a drawing on it: a horseman was piercing a dragon with his spear. It looked like the spitting image of the emblem of Moscow.

We could now begin our journey. After just a few leaps we were already at the second level, to the left side of it, at the training grounds.

We checked the stone on the helmet and the one I had on my forehead. They were emitting beams of light. We controlled the beams with our minds. We didn't know where the information came from, what we were supposed to do and how. We had the feeling that this knowledge was hidden within us for the time being. And now it was gradually being pulled out from the depths of our being.

We drew a meadow and a majestic old castle with the beam. The drawing was in yellow. We checked: can it be removed? The beam became purple and we erased the previous drawing. We used the green color to move the castle closer to where we were and the blue color to move it away and reduce its size. Those colors were awfully tricky! With them you could turn any giant into a midget. It should be borne in mind, but it's unlikely it will ever come handy. After all, we are St. George, the Dragon Slayer! And this is a great responsibility. Look like a Knight, act like a Knight!

We used the black color. The castle turned to the left and became invisible. We turned it to the right and it became visible again.

We colored the beam brown: the castle shrank in size and flew up like a balloon. We rotated it counter-clockwise and it returned and took its former place.

302

We caught it in our white beam and pulled it after us wherever we wanted.

Then we tested the bow. We positioned the arrow against the bowstring and aimed it at the castle – we then sent it flying. Wow... The castle collapsed, as though hit with an intercontinental missile. We took the spear and drew a defensive shield like the one used by Lapshin: a square, broken into sectors by yellow lines. We attacked it with the spear: the shield oozed to the ground as if it were made of thawed jelly.

The exercise excited us. We needed an active opponent. So we created a dragon. Igor snatched the sword from its sheath, waved it and hit the dragon's neck before the monster opened its mouth to warm us with its flamethrower. Its severed head flew to the ground like a head of cabbage.

So far so good... We decided to make the task more complicated. We now drew an image of Dragon Gorynych. For some reason, we knew in advance that his left head represented the dark forces, the middle head – knowledge, power, skill and cunning. The most pernicious was the right head and it should be dealt with first.

After just one strike the most pernicious head rolled to the ground. The middle head breathed fire at us. It was incredibly hot. Igor's cloak and my horse-cover rescued us from the prospect of becoming Gorynych's next breakfast: an epic stew out of luckless St. George. Igor brandished the sword and severed the second head. Dragon Gorynych slightly lost his balance. The left head now carried more of the weight, and he couldn't figure out how he could do something to cause us harm – he tried to reach us with his claws or flatten us with his tail but his lack of balance was a disadvantage. Meanwhile, Igor waited for the right moment and struck him on his scaly neck with the sword. That was the end of him: Dragon Gorynych was dead.

The mace still remained among our unused military weapons. We drew a huge mountain. Igor swung the mace and delivered a crushing blow on the mountain top. What power! The top of the mountain crumbled into tiny pebbles. Only a small hill was left in its place.

All we had to do now was test the last gift from heaven – the staff.

We drew a picture of a man. The staff sent out a beam of light toward the image, which landed on the crown of the man's head. The beam moved on as bright lightning into the tailbone, the central channel. The man came alive and looked back. He was given life and he now tried to understand what it meant.

We erased the curious man and drew a black bird instead. The beam hit it on the tail and the head – the bird became light in color.

Then we erased the bird and drew a rabbit. How could we revive it? We directed the beam toward its legs and its head, then touched the image with the tip of the staff and materialized it. It worked. Therefore, the sequence has been revealed: first, an idea, then energy and then matter.

That was intriguing. We cleaned up and descended to the first level.

We stood on the ground and saw names, formulas and geometric figures swirling around us. All together it resembled billions of threads. We intercepted one of them and lowered it into ourselves. It was now like a film strip. Planes, helicopters, naval ships, volcanic eruptions, disasters, typhoons – all this was now within us.

We intercepted another thread. Now we were under water, surrounded by fish and coral reefs. We could see what lived there, what developed and died.

Intercepting another thread we saw a city, cars, computers, network failures and ecology problems – all in all, a very stressful environment.

We replaced the film tape. Around were stars, the moon, satellites and spaceships. We received information about the danger of an asteroid on a collision course with the Earth. The powerful impact would cause the Earth to increase the speed of its rotation. This would be a terrible catastrophe.

The information was being processed very fast, in numerical form. We again heard the voice telling us that we were the second to get access to this information, which signified the beginning of the second stage in our lives. And if we could pass it and save the Earth from destruction, this would be the third and most important stage.

One of the information threads began to vibrate as a sign of anxiety. We intercepted it and saw a house with something like a self-made altar inside and a table. On it was an amulet, burning candles and my photo. There was a woman standing by the table. She was about fifty years old. She was full-figured and had a mole under her left eye. Her long black hair and eyelashes seemed to be glued on.

The woman was casting spells. The ritual was specifically directed against me. Its purpose –information coding.

Igor took an arrow and aimed it at the table. This seemed to cause an earthquake. Everything began to rock and fall. My photograph caught fire from one of the candles, and its corner was burned. The woman was in utter panic. Her mind filled with fear. She realized that she had encountered something more powerful than she was. She extinguished the candles frantically.

Hopefully, she will learn something from this lesson. Fare thee well, homegrown witch, adieu…

We ascended into the Bardo channel to complete our study of the levels.

The fifth level was on our left. There was darkness, hurricanes, vortexes and lightning. It was the state of man and nature. A huge bee flew past us: one of its sides was striped like a hornet's. This was hypnosis.

There was an opposite picture on the right – a blue sky, light clouds and spring storms. The sun was out and a gentle breeze was blowing in the birch grove. But this was also hypnosis.

Let's try to see how it works... We galloped to the site and drew two houses. There was a family living in each house. We revived the picture and galloped upward to collect two small bags of hypnotic visions. In one of them we gathered the wind, darkness and moisture. In the other – the caressing spring breeze and the landscape with the birch trees. We poured the contents of the first bag on the house. Something broke down there and went wrong. Everyone in the family began quarrelling and couldn't reach a compromise. We poured the contents of the second bag on the other house. Everyone in the family started smiling, beaming, laughing and working. The sixth level was on the left. It contained creativity but it was of a strange sort: mediocrity, scribomania and barren efforts. To the right were the great inspirations of geniuses. Here talented creators were given revelations to write their books and work on their paintings.

I felt good here, it was a pleasant place to be in and I didn't want to leave. But Igor was already tired. We had to go back.

* * *

Knowledge about the structure of control over the Earth triggered, in its turn, a cascade of new information. It appeared within me suddenly, as a given thing – out of nowhere and for no apparent reason. Somehow I knew that all the levels are formed because the Earth spins around its axis as the result of the electromagnetic separation process. Each planet of our solar system has a structural influence of its own in this planetary mechanism of control. It is worth mentioning that these levels spread like pyramids not only in an upward direction over the North Pole but also downwards toward the planetary nucleus. In effect, this process results in two pyramids, with their bases merging on the Earth's surface.

I made a pretty accurate drawing of this structure on a thick sheet of paper. I liked what I saw. A light silvery Bardo channel cut vertically through this structure. A similar channel cut perpendicularly across the first one. The cross was defined distinctly and undoubtedly. "And God divided the light from darkness." Divided by what? It appeared that the Bardo channel filled with mysterious silvery color was, in fact, the Divine divider. And its name was the Holy Spirit.

"And God made two great lights; the greater light to rule the day, and the lesser light to rule the night, he made the stars also." With "the greater light" the picture is more or less clear. The Sun is the solar system's star. As far as "the lesser light", it isn't clear at all: where is it? It isn't included among the stars since they are mentioned separately. Could it be the Moon? Its influence on events taking place on Earth is enormous. However, I was uncertain about it. I felt that I had to find the answer, especially since Lapshin had referred to a mysterious Sun-2 on several occasions, with which he connected the ambitious plans to ensure his own financial might. Provided that I no longer perceived his Napoleonic aspirations as proof of a seasonal spring attack of schizophrenia, it was imperative to get the proper answer and the sooner, the better.

Now it is time to enlighten some of my readers with limited knowledge in that area of one special feature of clairvoyance.

Let me start with a simple example. When somebody has heart problems he or she goes for an EKG test. Of course, the elaborate chart doesn't reflect all the details of the complicated activity of our "pump". However, it gives an idea of certain aspects of its functioning. The picture they get is essential for physicians, and sometimes they may not need anything else.

At this point in time we don't know what the subtle-matter essences the psychics deal with look like or what exactly they represent. But the essences themselves clearly want to interact with humans. That is why they present themselves to the psychic in terms and images of his culture and upbringing, using his native language and the figures of speech familiar to him since childhood.

So when someone comes to a psychic complaining of chest pains, the latter sees an imp blocking his aorta. It is not an EKG that he sees but an imp, the way we imagine him from pictures in books of fairytales. The psychic has the ability to talk to him, not out loud though but in his thoughts. Nevertheless, they understand each other. Incidentally, this little devil, the product of some as yet unidentified imagination, provides a considerably more accurate picture of the patient's health problem than the EKG diagram produced by a device.

I think that when the human brain's activity becomes upgraded, for instance, from its current average 3-4 percent to 50, it will develop the ability to imagine certain processes, phenomena, even abstract concepts as visualized essences. Otherwise, why do the notorious dragon or the little devil mentioned above, limit their activities to just one-two functions and have an obvious, quite primitive designation. Take somebody like multi-headed Cerberus: he doesn't drink or eat, has no time to chase after girls – his only function is to guard the Gates of the Underworld.

As for humans, they are multi-functional with a great number of degrees of freedom. It is the human mind that creates this world of ours as we have already discussed before. Thus, all these images, essences, or whatever else, are simply the way the right hemisphere of our brain instantly understands and assimilates those natural phenomena, which take the left hemisphere many years to explore.

Another simple example: about a hundred years ago, physicists opened the door into what used to be terra incognita – the micro world of the atom previously unknown to man. Since then the scientists have been studying this tiny indivisible particle very thoroughly and meticulously, collecting information on its purpose, its role in the world and also in the structure of matter and physical reality. The question, however, remains: were Max Plank and other scientists the first to see the atom at the core of the material world?

Those who studied ancient history must definitely be familiar with the name of Democritus, a Greek philosopher who spoke of atoms two and a half thousand years ago and left us his depiction of these tiny particles. It is strikingly interesting to see the similarity between the description provided by modern physics and the one left by Democritus from the ancient town of Abdera – the two are virtually identical. The only difference is that Max Plank, for instance, already had at his disposal theories and research work by other scientists accumulated throughout the centuries, and the fundamentals of a materialistic approach to reality, while Democritus had none of the above. And while one of them already had necessary equipment and experiments available to him, the other didn't have even the simplest microscopes, forget about molecular ones – none at all. Yet Democritus somehow managed to see, and, mind you, this happened two and a half thousand years before Max Plank, and what he saw was amazingly accurate. In other words, basically, his vision didn't contradict the modern understanding of the atom.

The only plausible explanation is that he obtained his knowledge somehow differently, through a sudden revelation, through intuition, or rather – we can now say this – through clairvoyance. Because today not just a select few but many people possess this tool or this ability at the practical level. They are able, by means of intervening in the processes inside the human body, inside a cell, inside chromosomes and even genes, to redirect negative events in a positive direction, resulting in recovery and, in many instances, even in a change within sequences of events.

How is it possible? Most likely, phenomena of this nature belong to a world which is basically outside the scope of what can be comprehended by the earthly mind, as the Russian religious philosopher Semen Frank rightfully pointed out. But let me remind you that we still don't quite understand the essence of electricity which doesn't prevent us from actively using it. Then why not to use for the benefit of man the images that are revealed to a psychic?

We imagine angels and saints the way they are depicted on icons; that is why we recognize them so easily. The canons of iconography help us distinguish them. The same is true of historical figures whose portraits were drawn by famous painters. Sometimes these portraits are not exact representations, so what?

Which brings us to yet another rule: the more educated the psychic, the more he can see. One can recognize Socrates in a painting only if one has heard of this philosopher's existence. No doubt, a psychic with the background of a mining engineer sees transcendental essences differently than someone who is a specialist in zootechnics. But if they work together they will engage their common cultural arsenal of visions.

I am sure there are many interesting angles to this problem. Regretfully, nobody has been involved in studying the history of clairvoyance, or engaged in a comparative analysis of our visions and how they are connected to the psychic's individual personality.

So, the transcendental world is interested our engagement and needs humans. I don't know the ultimate goal of such interaction. What I know for sure is that I will never give up my human dignity.

I don't claim to be the first person trying to understand the possibilities of the subtle world and its connection to physical reality. I have an advantage, though, since I am at the same time a researcher and participant in this process. Still, even in the former Soviet Union there were scientists who dared to express ideas totally heretical from the viewpoint of the dominant Marxist-Leninist ideology. Let me quote V.I. Siforov, Corresponding Member of the Soviet Academy of Sciences "The wider we expand the horizon of knowledge, the more aware we become of the limitations of cognitive and intellectual abilities of any one individual. Professional specialization and narrow specialization in science are proof that we accept this as a fact. Respectively, the way we see it today, our knowledge of the Universe remains a relative truth within the broader interpretation of knowledge about the Universe which is how Lenin viewed it. I am positive that we will encounter many surprises in the Cosmos, including some very 'weird' forms of matter. An in-depth study of space and time, applying to it the principle of discreteness, will open before us such new horizons in understanding the Universe, which we presently cannot even imagine and which, from the vantage point of the present, can be characterized only as 'crazy' and 'ridiculous'. Just as once the thought about the transfer of photon energy seemed 'ridiculous' to physicists. The degree to which an idea is unexpected and paradoxical may, in the long run, determine the degree of its activity. Niels Bohr was the one who formulated this paradox as follows: 'We are all agreed that your theory is crazy. The question that divides us is whether it is crazy enough to have a chance of being correct.'

Everything we have just discussed relates directly to the hypothesis of the 'intelligent Universe'. Perception of the Universe as a self-influence system, which is equipped with certain attributes and implements certain goals – such a perception goes beyond our present relative knowledge. Perhaps this is a situation where today's limited knowledge has to be aided by intuition."

Let us now return to the situation at my work in the "Khudlit" Publishing House. Precisely when it looked like we were finally getting out of the debt and showing a strong tendency for growth, Deputy Minister Grigoriev launched a restructuring of the industry, which smoothly flowed from the stage of industry scare into the phase of practical activities. We became witness to a horrific hysteria brought about by the new redistribution, the aim of which was becoming more and more obvious: to place his protégés into key positions, while dumping the rest into large mass graves of holdings, where they would eventually vanish on their own from the competitive market space. As a result, in addition to all the other enticing privileges, a substantial number of prestigious mansions were being vacated, and manipulations with distributing this coveted space promised not so much the state itself but its officials – servants of the double eagle – very good commissions. In other words, they embarked on a great gamble and showed no intention to play by the rules. Just as a few years earlier many top officials from the State Committee on the Press were kicked out of their offices, they now sacked the only people who saved their enterprises from final collapse in the same unconcerned, but methodical manner. The most tragic thing about the situation of these industry directors was that the state did not need them anymore. They continued to exist despite the terrible circumstances they found themselves in: the government refused to provide them with necessary working capital loans and would occasionally divert their money to its own coffers, withdrawing from their accounts everything they had earned. In the new market-imposed races where they had to compete with their private company rivals they had to stay on track without a drop of gasoline to keep their engines running... Because working capital is the fuel, without which no industrial project, whether private or state-run, can be implemented. While a company in the private sector could guarantee that it would repay the loans to the banks with their shares or real estate property, what could a government-run enterprise possibly suggest as collateral? The point is they didn't own anything they could call "theirs".

We witnessed prominent publishing houses being destroyed one by one – filled with great sympathy, we were helpless to do anything about it. The editor-in-chief of the "Knizhnoye Obozreniye" newspaper was fired while he was on sick leave. Yelena Nortsova, Director of "Detskaya Literatura," which was among the oldest publishing houses of Soviet times and quite a successful one, was thrown out of her office within two weeks. She sued, won the case in court, and yet could not make it back to the position she had held. The pressure was too much for her mother who suffered a heart attack. After she was hospitalized, she begged her daughter: "Lena! They will kill you! Don't you see what kind of people you are dealing with! Quit, if you want to keep me alive! I cannot live, knowing that your life is in constant danger."

This gives you an idea about the negative background – at work and in the industry as a whole – against which the further dramatic events unfolded. Despite these stressful psychological circumstances, Igor and I still found time to further explore the far-away kingdom we knew nothing about before.

On the seventh level to the right and left of us we found magic water –

alive and dead. We took just one step after entering the gates, and the fairy tale scenarios suddenly turned into reality. We knew that if we proceeded further along the path we had just discovered it might take several decades to see everything we could find there.

On the eighth level we saw a reviving cross and a cross bringing death.

On the ninth level we discovered the Biblical Paradise and Hell. All gates would open before us but so far we couldn't explore everything that was hidden there because we were afraid of getting lost.

Once we saw a large black raven in the Bardo channel. Since we were wearing protective shields, the ones Grigori Petrovich taught us how to use, the raven didn't notice us and flew right past us. We decided to check where he was going and galloped after him. We didn't really need to gallop anywhere… It took us just one large leap to catch up with him on the third level where he entered the gates of the Kingdom of the Dead. Those were gates to the left. Nobody stopped us when we rode into the gates following the raven.

The raven descended to the ground. Now he was half-bird and half-man. We knew who that was: it was Lapshin. So this is who he communicates with and where he takes his knowledge and strength! He is not human. From one side he looks like a bird, but from the back he is Satan, with a tail and hooves. He was greeted by a humongous dark figure. Its face was covered by a hood which made it impossible to tell whether it was a man or a woman. We saw a scythe on its shoulder. This was Death. They stood opposite each other, communicating by means of telepathy. We couldn't retrieve the information because they might have noticed us. What we saw was how a swirling flow of black energy was streaming from the chest of Death right into the chest, head and groin of this creature, this half-Satan and half-bird. So this is the place where he lives, where his house is and his kin. It was time to leave before they discovered our presence. I doubted that we were ready to fight against Death at this point. We retreated quietly, particularly since there was a scary crowd of zombies gathering in the distance.

In the evening we decided to pay a visit to Lapshin. He was clearly working against me lately. Many people who are close to me have been seeing hypnotic dreams with horrible scenes of rape. These night terrors weren't accidental. Especially for one who knew how the levels worked and who was capable of doing something similar. Yet there was a huge gap between what one "could do" and what one "actually did". It appeared that Lapshin had crossed the line. Well, it meant that he wasn't worthy of our consideration.

We tracked down our ex-guru in Moscow. He resided at the apartment of one of his supporters, where he was offered to stay for as long as he wished. He was reading a book and was doing fine! Well, all this was about to change. Without removing our defenses we entered his mind. We knew what to look for. Informational threads were like film footage. We looked through all the shots. Here they were, the zombies from the Kingdom of the Dead. He too came from there. His task is to collect the energy of those who trust him and deliver it through the egregore to the Kingdom of the Dead. He was fueling the dead with the energy he took from the living. Here we saw him creating thought-forms of horror and transmitting them onto other people. You'd never imagine the things he did for fun... Who would think that in our times – in an era of triumphant materialism – such mystical practices were not only possible but widely spread among the most ardent atheists? Indeed, God works in mysterious ways.

Lapshin sensed that he had been invaded, especially since our light energy was like holy water for his dark essence. It burned him like fire.

315

He stood up and activated the bio-computer (since it was his definition, let him call it whichever way he wants). He ascended to the levels trying to figure out the source of the impact.

But our defenses were impermeable for him. Lapshin's wife asked:

– What's the matter with you?

– Stay out of it. It looks like Petrov is invading me again, – the sorcerer snarled.

– You are obsessed with this Petrov guy, – Lusya retorted, releasing a geyser of indignation, and looked away.

Lapshin turned his face toward us. His scanning beam slid along our protective cube. The beam changed direction hitting its surface and then circumvented it from both sides. This way he won't be able to see anything. Igor and I moved to the left, while Lapshin looked to the right. Getting nervous, he dropped the book to the floor and startled himself.

We took the staff and encircle the book in red. Lapshin could see the bright circle around the book. His legs gave way under him and he collapsed into his armchair.

His wife asked him again:

– What's the matter with you?

– I am just tired, too much stress. My legs are wobbly. I feel lethargic.

He slowly fell asleep. The hypnosis we inflicted upon him worked.

– How about we show him a horror movie? – I asked Igor.

– Not a good idea, he loves them, – my companion in arms disagreed.

Lapshin's wife got up and poked him in the shoulder.

– Are you really asleep?

He reclined in his armchair and asked in a weak voice:

– Give me some water.

– Go to hell, – she replied, giving vent to her anger, and went out into the next room.

We entered his mind again to see what he was scheming lately. He had been working on his defenses. They weren't at all complicated. He was using various shapes created by man: pyramids, squares and spheres, which he interconnected like flying saucers. We entered deeper... Goodness gracious, he was so old inside! Believe it or not, he was several million years old!"

We recorded a message from us in his subconscious: "Repent! Think of God! Stop doing your dark deeds."

Now we can enjoy our fully deserved rest. We left this space and emerged in my office. Igor and I looked at each other and smiled. We were happy like children.

* * *

What we achieved in the virtual space suddenly received a concrete confirmation in materialistic terms. One of Lapshin's closest followers, who had been with him from the very early days, quite unexpectedly came to our Center. The woman was very anxious, even frightened. She told me that she was alarmed by the growing number of incidents of children developing mental disorders attributable to Lapshin's techniques. She finally mustered the courage to call Lapshin and not only shared with him her concerns but also objections.

One day later, a woman from Donetsk, who headed the local department of the Academy, showed up at the Center. The three groups of children, which she had trained, using Lapshin's techniques, were struck one after another by diseases similar to those that affected other kids who were subjected to energy training at the Academy. As was the case with the

317

children I had been training, they were tortured by nightmares and visions of graveyards.

Unfortunately, I didn't have a chance to talk to her in person. She had a conversation with our Center's manager who explained the situation to her in detail. I hope it will help her to sort out what was happening.

The next time Igor and I entered the non-material space we were already expected. An angel with large radiant wings appeared before us, summoning us to follow him to higher spheres. We immediately found ourselves somewhere above all the levels and stood together with him on a cloud, which felt like solid earth beneath our feet.

There were also clouds above our heads. They were swirling and blocking the light. Then a dazzling bright stream of light poured into the opening which appeared between the clouds. At first, we could see a geometric figure – a circle with a triangle inscribed inside it with golden threads. To one side, a lavishly jeweled icon with the image of Jesus materialized, gradually converging with the geometric figure. It smoothly entered the center of the triangle, solidified there, turning into a golden medallion, and suddenly started floating in our direction. A gold chain emerged from nowhere on the medallion, transferring itself to the neck of Pegasus. Then a man wearing the Monomakh's hat appeared out of the light, followed by saints and warriors. They formed a multitude. Passing by us they turned their heads and started at us sternly, attentively and vigilantly. The walls of an ancient city could be discerned in the place from where all they appear. The walls are tall and snow white.

A man in long white garments with wings on his back emerged from the light. He flew over the host of warriors and saints, smiling at us.

Hesitant, we tried to guess:

– Are you Archangel Michael?

318

– Yes! Don't you recognize me?

We saw more marching men who were carrying banners embroidered in gold and silver. More warriors came along in chain mail and helmets. Among them there were the saints of the Russian Orthodox Church and the priests. The opening between the clouds was getting wider. Suddenly a storm-filled sea emerged under them. The fierce waves were bouncing up and down an old ramshackle boat. The wind was tearing to shreds its rotten sail. But the people aboard weren't afraid of anything. The course of the ship was controlled by a beam from the skies.

The scene disappeared. Now we saw a huge man – a blacksmith. He was forging a giant sword with a large stone in a frame set at the crossing of the blade and the handle. The blacksmith handed over the sword to us. Igor took it and kissed the blade.

At once I stopped being Pegasus. I was standing in my academic mantle next to Igor.

Somebody from aside, wearing the garments of a priest, also a giant, sprinkled us with something from a yellow vessel. We were baptized by a huge cross, and we kissed the cross three times. The one doing the blessing placed his hand in turn on Igor's right shoulder and on mine.

– You have now received the true baptism! In the name of the Father, and of the Son, and of the Holy Spirit. Amen!

* * *

The next day, Igor and I went to see Grigory Petrovich. He met us, as always, with a smile and was already up to speed on what had happened in the nonmaterial space of events.

– Well, that happens. They betrayed us. The main thing is to draw the

319

correct conclusions from what happened. Victory is always achieved by the one who draws the correct conclusions. Think about how now to fight the hypnosis and holograms, how to discern the real enemy behind all these cartoons. And now let us begin working – he proposed. – Turn on your screens, and let's begin.

He concentrated.

– The experiment of sonverting space into the volume of one's soul. What do we do first? We limit the space around ourselves and draw it into ourselves.

Surprisingly, unlike the previous rising up the vertical Bardo channel – we instantly find ourselves above. Now we are like a genie who has broken loose from the bottle. The infinity of the Cosmos is around us. Everything is very clearly visible: the stars, the spiral branches of our galaxie, other galaxies in the distance. And below is our bottle containing the entire world. The second area on which we are standing is probably the cork from this vessel. We are now elevated, thanks to which we also have broken away to freedom. Here is what our space looks like if you look at it from the outside.

There is nothing here – no center channel, no left, no right. It is foolhardy to try to go upwards. This infinity suppresses, but we overcome the fear. This is possibly man's first venture into the outer Cosmos without a spacesuit, but not likely. There are some similar testimonies already, for example, in the Tibetan Book of the Dead. However, the authors of this book didn't have to go so high.

It leads us somewhere. And our path, totally unmarked, is hardly random. We are literally drawn by an invisible cosmic current into the depths of the universe. The Earth and the Solar System have long not been visible.

– Try to stop – we hear the voice of Grigory Petrovich.

We stop. Opposite us something like a large screen lights up, over which text is moving rapidly in large letters. It is something like a lecture. We read:

„Life is infinity, and infinity is life. But not every life has infinity. He who experiences this infinity, also experiences life.

Infinity is in each of you, in your soul. Turning this infinity around, you experience true life both on the Earth and in the Cosmos. Infinity cannot be interrupted, and life is also infinite, like the Cosmos.

Life changes, like the Cosmos. And it is the Cosmos that influences your life. Everything that you do, this is cosmic and inherent in the laws of the Cosmos on Earth.

The Cosmos gives Life both on the Earth and on other planets. It is erroneous to believe that someone created the Earth. Life created the Cosmos itself in the manifestation of the highest power of Reason.

Cosmic energy is in each of you. You should learn to use it, and then you will experience true life both on Earth and in the Cosmos.

This is the wealth which is given to each. And each who is trained can control this energy. Live in harmony both on Earth and in the Cosmos – and you will find everlasting life.

The Cosmos – this is the manifestation of you, and you – are the manifestation of the Cosmos. Take that which is due you. Plan life on Earth and in the Cosmos, since you have arrived to where you are now. Your only help is Faith.

Everthing cosmic is not alien to you. It is native for you, although it is not given to everyone. Only the chosen can utilize the energy from where you are now. The Cosmos gave you life, so don't reject it. Remember – you are living according to the laws of the Cosmos. That which you accomplish is also the Cosmos.

You discover nothing, but you read in the book of life that old which was written.

Hurry! Everything that occurring in the spiral is ending. But it is eternal, because it begins all over again.

The structure of life is not what you have become used to thinking alway and about which you have formed a specific world outlook. Life is the space, which is defined by the cosmic laws. Nothing can develop chaotically, spontaneously, by itself. Everything proceeds orderly in its development.

Life is structured according to the laws of the Cosmos, and it is erroneous to believe as if you are discovering or inventing something. All of this was before, and people are standing only on the first step of its development. And the stairway of knowledge goes far upwards. In order to correctly use unlimited knowledge, you must have complete harmony of the soul with the Cosmos. It is erroneous to believe that after death you dies or on some day discover something new. Life is infinite, and your discoveries are also infinite. They have already been accomplished both in the past and in the future.

Those who know their God through their soul, they will have access to the law of the Infinite Cosmos. They will be able to use the knowledge which will advance them so far that today's consciousness will not be able to imagine this and fit it in its reason. They will subsequently be saved from the heavenly punishment for an incorrect life.

The laws of life are very simple, but each who subsequently will read them in the Book of Knowledge must be ready to comprehend, to understand, and he also must know what responsibility will fall on him for controlling these laws."

This was something like an introduction. Then came the first section.

„Interaction of negative
and positive energies

Negative and positive energies are equivalent. But in some cases, negative energy can be more than positive energy, and vice versa. This occurs during the interaction of energy forces and the struggle of good forces with evil and evil forces with good.

There from where you came, there is almost constantly an equal sign between them, since events and life are described according to the law of the Cosmos. In order to change some situation and control your life, a third energy is needed, which you do not have where you are. In order to change events and the course of life, it is necessary to take energy from the source of life which is located higher, above you. It is namely above that place where you are working.

But you must evaluate the strength of the energy to be used, since you are changing not only the course of events and the standard of living, but you are changing the laws of Being and the laws of the Cosmos where they are in effect regardless of you or of the will of those living there. You must evaluate the scale of the energy being used, and also clearly understand the consequences of using this energy and understand from whom you are taking it.

Upon establishing the energy channel, judiciously use the force given to you, both in good as well as in other intentions. Be aware that the force being used by you is an order of magnitude higher than other forces of the world in which you are using it.

After testing, this force will be assigned to you. But know that this force is not the beginning, not the end, but just one of the forces which you will be allowed.

It will be rendered to you and for your affairs.

In the name of the Father, the Son and the Holy Spirit, amen!

The Advent of the Lord

Prepare for the Advent of the Lord, for God will go to that place from which you yourself came. And those who will not be devoted to the causes of the Lord and who will not have the power of God will inevitably perish.

The power of the Lord is in your soul, and find the faith of your soul. Then you will find peace and harmony in your life.

Know that each of you have access to use the powers of the Lord, which are much greater. And do not be afraid to take these powers, since you are granted them.

Know that these powers may change both the world in which you are located and the life, nature and everything around you.

Do not doubt the correctness of the decision, since your decision – this is also the wish from above. Act with faith and your soul in harmony, since they are prompting you. For you are the embodiment of the hand of the Lord which gives the both in the Cosmos and in the life from which you came. The fourth unearthly power is placed at your disposal. It is like a wall – without a beginning or an end. No one can overcome it or overpower it. You will need it where you must protect or confine.

Use this power for good, reasonable intentions and know that the power given to you will increase manyfold for assistance and concern about the place from where you came.

Using the power and abilities which have been given to you, know that always in using the power you are not alone. Our Lord stands behind you. And those forces which will oppose you are lost and trying to resist the anger of the Creator.

Let them see your greatness and they will be near you in service to you. This is how it foreordained both in the past, in the present and in the future. May God and all the heavenly power save you!"

That was all, the subtitles ended. The screen went blank and disappeared. We are alone in the in the endless Cosmos. Where to go?

Suddenly a chariot rushes about from afar, drawn by three white horses. It is glowing. It is driven by a huge bearded man. He is very similar to the one whose image is on icons. It is God the Father.

– What, are you lost?– a resounding, deafaening voice thunders over the entire Cosmos.

– Lord! Help us find Earth! – we plead.

He laughs. The chariot turns around.

– Hold on to the back!

Igor holds on to the wall of the golden chariot with his hand. It rushes through the infinity. We flew past the Sun.

– There is your Earth.

God the Father throws lightning in its direction.

– Thank you, Lord.

– They still call me Father, – he laughs loudly.

– Thank you, Father.

– Well, finally you guessed.

– May we touch You?

– You must not. You will burn up.

The chariot turns around and speeds away somewhere deep into the galaxie.

We enter the levels. That's it, we are again on Earth. Grigory Petrovich looks at us with surprised eyes.

– Do you know who that was?

Igor and I exchange glances.

– The Creator, – and sorrowfully adds: – Yes, lads, no one will become bored in your company. I personally saw this for the first time that the Creator Himself escorted someone around the Cosmos.

* * *

Things began to work out much better for Igor and me than before. We get to the levels more quickly, diagnose diseases better, and more quickly find solutions for eliminating pathologies in the organism more quickly – in ourselves and others. If we do not know something, we immediately turn to Grigori Grabovoi. He has his own place of residence on the second level on the left – a small palace with peacocks in the courtyard. Igor and I also begin to think about something similar. But for the time being we simply can't decide.

Things at the Center are working out pretty well. People are going. But it is basically the very poor, who cannot pay either for the training or for the treatment. Nevertheless, we don't turn them down. We need confidence in ourselves. And each complicated illness which we overcome with the help of the technologies given to us, this is a great celebration for us. People come with diabetes and receive the help expected. They come with cancer, and it turns out it is forced to leave.

Sometimes the presence of a foreign informational being in a person's aura is clearly visible. These are, as the people call them, demons. We can take them away, but we first sent the person to church, as a rule, to Father Herman at the Trinity Lavra of St. Sergius. Let the sinner understand that everything is not so simple in life, that the time will come to pay for everything. Father Herman will clean the brain. He is a stern priest, and we have special relations with him. When the army went, to whom we were introduced, we saw him among those giving blessings. If the Lord himself admits him into His world, into His Kingdom, that means he is someone you can believe. We went to listen to his service at the Church above the Gate and saw how energy-informational beings of the dark world were leaving the people – devils and demons. True, sometimes then and there they got into someone nearby. But basically they were drawn upwards, into the rising energy flow under dome of the cathedral, and they, writhing and suffering in the Holy Spirit, were deformed, dissolved, and faded from view in the sky.

We had a temptation to confide in Father Herman, but we overcame it. You see, his screen of inner vision was not working, and he himself might not have known that he was close to the Lord. He received his knowledge and ability to drive out the demons over the channel of intuition. So we remained kneeled before him, like the rest of the laymen, several hours and received the fatherly blessing. And we recommended that others do the same at any convenient opportunity.

Having returned one day after a tiring service with Father Herman, Igor and I recalled our beaten former adversary Lapshin.

It was in mid-May. The days were warm, sunny and long. We were again seated in the office under the tower with the dome, where our energy column, the same one as in the church with Father Herman, was formed. Thanks to it, we only had to wish – and we were already in the nonmaterial space, ready for work.

But is our friend Lapashin somewhere in Moscow? Aha! Here he is! He is walking around his office. There is a table behind the window. It came from Theodosia. We rewind the tape. What was he doing there? So,

327

he was walking through the cemetery. He brought flowers. There was a large grave, a small bench, and he was sitting. He was communicating with the third level. On the right was one of his relatives. It was his father. He is swearing at him. Lapshin does not hear him. On the left he is half-bird and has a tail in the rear. There are many dead people around him. He is like hope for them, like salvation, and there are thousands of them. They are giving him their energy. They say that he is invincible.

We dash over to him and sit next to him. Everything below us is black. The channel has opened. We flew over it. The first, second, and third levels. It is the gates! They open up. There are skeletons in long black robes. They are creating a dark-colored sphere. It is assembled in an instant. Lapshin drives it into his chest. He also has armor. A saber or sword for some reason is hanging on the right. There is also chain mail now. And the shield is now the same as we have. Only everything is dark. First a bird and then the devil alternately reveal themselves on the shield. There is a stone in the middle of the shield. There is a tall spear. He is our complete analogue, only black. True, only on the outside. His essence is different – a bird in order to escape, and a devil in order to fight. They are planning to use him to fight us. They have made a prototype of the Black Knight. This armament had just appeared. It expands his capabilities.

To the right of him is the father – short, thin, grey-haired. He says: stop him, all our family will suffer for him. The father has normal thought, the son – on the contrary. He is thinking how to take over the world.

Centers such as ours, other schools and academies interfering with him. We are dangerous for him, lone psychics do not bother him. Lapshin uses hypnosis. We put a mirror up to him. He looks into it and reflects himself. However, he knows about us and is ready for everything. In general, he has 100 percent confidence in himself.

Why is his system operating autonomously?

Lapshin doesn't seem to be exerting himself, and that is bad for the people! It is necessary to figure out where the thread goes from him. We see. There is a small black pyramid of spheres. From it the small beams draw towards those he wants to destroy. He operates in the automatic mode. What a clever deal. What if we try the same against him? The black pyramid crushes us, which means a light one will crush him.

We set up a pyramid of gold speres above the third level. We saturate it with the energy of St. George the Dragon Slayer. We aim at Vyacheslav the little demon. Aha! He prepared well! There is protection around him immediately in the form of a cube. How to get to him? We will hit him with a spear. Three birds fly away. Will that catch up or not? That time he has already deceived us in such a way. For the time being we fought with a hologram wolf, and he left for the third level. Now he can't leve. Even the birds don't fly there – the golden pyramid is interferring. The dead people on the left are becoming angry and are cursing. What is the sense of cursing?

We must remember how it happens in stories. There is a good reason why Lapshin has been reading tales lately. Waste shots on the vultures? Don't hold your breath! We release on them our native bird – the two-headed eagle.

We create it with a beam, and invigorate him. That's it, the holder is ready, and it flew. And it went past the birds. That means they are really not real! Again, our two-horned friend wanted to trick us. It is not good...

Our eagle flew down into Lapshin's office. And there some kind of strange, small cube formed in the middle of the room. Consequently, the devil here. We ask the two-headed bird to move and hit the small cube with all our might with a club, from which even big mountains could be flattened. The small cube cracked. Vyacheslav banged his head directly into the table. There is a vortex at the back of his head. The computer here indicates the input-output. We unscrew it counterclockwise. We press on a point, and a second later, it is restored as before. We repeat it and get the same result! We draw a line with the small brown beam and pull the stupid consciousness from the sick head. This is the kind of hole that ended up in the head!

But, as we know, nature abhors a vacuum. We stuff the previous spot with good intentions, mercy, and a willingness to help the sick and poor. Will it last long? His former friends and bosses, probably, will soon begin to suspect that something is wrong, and they will redesign the good person again into a diabolical good-for-nothing. Well, maybe he will survive another week without nasty remarks? And we will at least get some kind of respite.

The next day we are planning to lift the girl – the very one that ruined the whole show for Vyacheslav on the sabbath – to the top of the levels. Her internal vision screen is working well, but it comes from the lower levels, just as Lapshin set it up in the past. She is a talented girl, and we would really like to reorient her towards the path of light towards God. Moreover, it was she who had been able, a while ago, to undermine an important occult mystery of Lapshin. The only thing that frightens me is her overconfidence and arrogance. I think if she were to see someone from the divine hierarchy, that would help her to get oriented in life.

So the long-awaited moment has arrived. The young psychic puts a dark mask over her eyes and turns on the screen. We try to lift her to the tenth level. She is doing really well. No problems with the ascent. She is wearing a silvery suit with wide trousers, heavy boots with wings, like those of Hermes. She moves in space freely and very quickly. She is wearing a headband, like a Japanese ninja.

What a super-advanced child.

We are flying along the central Bardo channel. No problems. The girl feels in her element here. We move upwards.

There is a landing. Everything is covered in fog, no one meets us. Our charge is below, and she looks so small. We ask her how she sees us.

– You reach up to my chest, she says.

Something is wrong, but we can't seem to figure out what it is.

We are moving up the staircase. After a little while there are no more stairs. Just empty space. It was a very clear explanation that we need to go back. We did. We chose a different route. The teenager made a circle and returned to the same place.

We go up another stairway. There is a pyramid followed by a mountain. There are several old men, who are very tall.

We ask the superwoman: "Can you see them?"

„Yes, I can. They are very small," she says. „I am looking down at them."

The old men turn away. They are clearly demonstrating that they are not willing to communicate.

Why does the girl see herself as so large and that she looks down at everybody? In this space this seems to allegorically demonstrate some serious personal problems she has with her self-esteem. An exaggerated view of herself, her place in life... If she had not been a child, she might have been welcomed with more severity.

But the girl keeps her good spirits. She simply turns away from the divine elders and frivolously climbs up the mountain.

Two figures appear in her way – Life and Death. They look at her, she looks at them.

331

I think she just does not care about anything. She is simply thinking how to step over this unexpected obstacle. She is still thinking that she is big and they are small. Life and Death turn their backs to her, clearly demonstrating their attitude towards the reckless girl.

She wants to keep going. I protest. This is not a circus or a zoo. Everything is very serious. We need to leave. She is not welcome here.

It's also a lesson to us, her elder teachers. Of course, children are quicker than adults in opening up their internal vision screens; it's easier for them to feel the intricacies of the subtle plane However, their heads are also easily turned by success. It's so tempting to boast of their phenomenal gift in front of others, to show that they are the chosen ones! We have seen that later in some of our other students as well. So, we need to remind them more frequently to value their gift, to remember that this gift comes not from Igor and me, but from higher up. It is not vain arrogance that should reign in the heart, but pride in the forces that you represent.

* * *

There are becoming more and more people who have heard about our extraordinary healing capabilities. Almost every day they come asking for help. The complexity of the diseases is increasing as well. One woman with breast cancer came to us. Her name is Tatiana Vladimirovna. She teaches foreign language in a high school. An acquaintance of ours sent her to us.

What should we do? We have never worked with advanced cancer tumors. Moreover, her doctor demands that she undergo surgery immediately. The X-ray showed extensive metastases in the ducts of the mammary glands. Another complicating factor is that she both believes in and doubts our ability to help. She is just grasping at straws. This uncertainty of her consciousness is a very significant obstacle in our work.

Igor and I activate the internal vision. We look at the organism from the inside. It's a sad picture: there is blood poisoning in progress and the immune system is suppressed.

We filter the blood. The blood swirls as it enters the kidneys. There is a lot of hydrocortisone in the kidneys. We collected the filtered cells – they are as clear as glass. We dump them into the bladder. We filter once more, purify via the kidneys and bladder. We dump again.

A connection is present from the head to the tumor. We go to the cells from which the oncological process started. We work with the metastases. The liquid in the cell is cadaveric. It decomposes the organism at the site of the tumor. We reprogram the cell for positive function. We cut off the metastases at the information level and place them in a box of sorts – now they do not receive any nourishment, they are cut off. And the original cell starts to function as a healthy one. Its memory has been returned to it.

This is all for now; nothing more can be done during one session. We will work with the main tumor next time.

We finished working with her and wanted to deactivate the internal vision screen… Suddenly we found ourselves somewhere in the Cosmos. This is a sphere. We are inside it. It is twilight. The Sun is hanging. We allow it within us and play with it like children. Something is written on the walls. The letters are unknown. A voice within says that the writing pertains to the creation of man. It clarifies that it is the stairway of evolution. Animals are on the left, humans are on the right. It is all of their development, followed by man and technology.

There are inscriptions and a recess on the floor, with a five-pointed star within the recess. The same pattern is on the ceiling. This star is the formula of life. It can be activated – by the rays and by hand. We touch it: it is cold and slippery. But then a flow of energy rushes from it. A rainbow is formed. It rises from the floor to the star on the ceiling. If you touch it with your left hand, you feel warmth. If you touch it with your right hand, you feel something entrancing coming inside. We stand on the star. The ray passes through us. It does not create any special sensations, but it passes through. A portrait of the Mother of God appears before us. The sphere begins to rotate. The star rotates together with us. We must not move. We must show respect for the Mother of God.

But something happened. We are being rocked. In this geyser of energy a person with wings appeared and walks towards us. Everything changes instantaneously. The sun, a dove, and a small white window appeared. We are being shown an image: the sky, wheat and a field. The person with wings is standing in front of us. We come to our senses. There is a second sphere next to us. We need to enter it. Devils are running within it. But we are not afraid. Some woman appeared – young and beautiful, but immediately she turns into something horrible. The devils side by side are crawling, jumping and screaming.

The human lot is described in writing on the walls: greed, gluttony, drunkenness, adultery, envy, betrayal.

In front of this wall are sitting four huge demons – the monsters of people. They are the ones embodying greed, envy, fornication, betrayal.

– What are you doing to people? – we ask sternly.

They bare their teeth and laugh.

– We are doing what you are seeing.

– But why?

– So that there may be peace in the world.

– How can there be peace through this?

– And what do you think? Is it different?

– Do you serve the Creator?

They laugh:

– We all serve the Creator in our own way.

Demons around us are choking with anger. Small imps want to attack us, they crowd around. But there is illumination around us, and they cannot overcome it.

We leave.

Another sphere. It's the house of saints. We may enter. There is light there, and the smell is pleasant. On two sides there are figures similar to angels. They have wings. Saintly women and children are running around without clothes. It is similar to a room. Some are flying, some are walking, some are sitting on clouds. They are all smiling and looking at us. Some energy influence is going on. A saintly elder appears. We are shorter than they. Someone says:

– You must remember who you are.

We strain our memory. A vision appears – it is a horse and a rider. He has a white sphere on his head. In the middle of the nimbus there is white, a circle, a rainbow. And then Igor and I are again Pegasus and the prince.

Everything around us changes. It is nature: rivers, sea, mountains, forest.

We ask:

– Can you show us the structure of St. George the Dragon Slayer?

They show us faces with spheres. Jesus Christ is in the center. There is a drawing – six male energies and six female energies. The women are on the left, the men are on the right. There are signs of the zodiac.

Now the Cosmos is Christ, the horse is time, the guide to the Cosmos. The rider is the socium – the last part of the spiral, which, moving through space, receives liberation.

"Nature is the world surrounding you. But for you there is not just one world," – someone invisible clarifies. – „Very few have been given access to what you have been given access."

– What should we do on Earth?

– The task is to heal and protect the Fatherland, help people. You are gathering strength. You will preserve individuality, but will be united.

– Where is the place that keeps the power? – I ask.

– Search. Everything is in the power of God, in your power, – comes the ambiguous answer from the invisible interlocutor.

The TV set has disappeared, shut down.

We return to the levels.

We rise above the landing. We have decided to experiment. The color is gray. We draw a line in white, it turns black and disappears.

We draw a square. It is erased as well. It's useless to persist. We see an entrance and go in. It is a tunnel. There are six landings. There are doors again, made of iron, padded, very strong. There is another landing. We stand on it – it feels like fine matter. It is a film, like what greenhouses are made of. It holds us easily. There is something around, but we see it only in glimpses. We need to have some other kind of vision. We see sometimes an ear or a patch of dress. Those to whom they belong are huge.

We went even higher. There is a yellow color. Blue. We draw a yellow square on the blue. It becomes real. It turned to the left, tumbled to the right, hovers, still then flew. We erase it using the violet color.

We begin to move more slowly. We are pushed back, downward. But we stubbornly press upward. There is a landing. Igor uses one hand to catch on the edge which is thin as a blade, and pulls me by the saddle with the other. He could cut himself. They are pressing from above, not letting us in. Igor catches on with the shield and we barely climb up. We are being encircled by something white. In good time, too, or we would not have been able to stand the heat that surrounds us. We barely tolerate it and look around. Signs of the zodiac are around us. There are twelve of them. The view sometimes opens and then closes. It is very hard to see.

There is a red circle above. Using the ray we cut a hole in it. There is a black hole against the red, then it seals. We drew a green sphere – trees and animals began appearing from it.

We move higher still. The circle is near. There is a white color on the landing, again the signs of the zodiac. Everything there shines like gold. We climb up. We are blinded from above, as if by the Sun. There is pressure. We hang. We cannot climb onto the landing. There is golden ice. We need to leave, it seems like at this stage they do not want to let us in here.

We apologize for our insistence, that we were sneaking in uninvited.

– You were not sneaking in, you were led, – comes an answer from the Cosmos.

– But why was there resistance?

– But what did you expect? You decided to flex your muscles? So you did. And why did you not go through with it?

– We are afraid to be impolite to the hosts, - I feel embarrassed for the two of us.

– Yeah, yeah, we see how polite you are.

– We were training, - we try to explain.

– Yeah, yeah, – they say in agreement. – Go with God.

We found an exit, go down and flew. There is space, stars, we found the channel. The Milky Way is under the hooves of the horse. We see the Earth. We lower ourselves onto the landings. Below there are twenty-four elders waiting. We again apologize for our persistence.

– This is not persistence, this is will power, – they say in consolation. We descend to Earth.

Now we know: St. George the Dragon Slayer is the protector of the Russian Land. It is the system of the living God. The second coming of Christ.

So who are we in this system? Those who are acting or those through whom they act?

Questions, questions, questions.

Chapter 9

There is a new person working in the Center: – Tatyana Nikolayevna. She was recommended by Olga Ivanovna Koyokina from the Scientific Research Institute of Traditional Methods of Treatment. It is a weighty recommendation. Tatyana Nikolayevna herself also made a good impression – a little pudgy and smiling. She knows many ancient spells, particularly those involving water. We worked with her for a couple of weeks and activated her internal vision screen. She was literally overwhelmed when that happened.

Throughout her life Tatyana Nikolayevna had honed the ability to perceive the aura of a person, his biofields, through the sense of feeling. She has perfected the finesse of her perception and could, without particular strain, feel erosion and gaps in the biofield, and then, using the energy of her hands, sort of smooth over the appearing vortices. It is true that such treatment can help a person for a period of time. And all of a sudden the things she did by touch, blindly – she was able to see with the internal vision. People's auras and her influence on them. New, previously unknown possibilities of bioinformational effects overwhelmed her by the opening prospects.

She saw the latent world, levels, structures, databases, programs for influence and control. The internal vision screen turned out to be a door into the invisible Universe, which is always near us, is waiting for us, which harms or helps us.

We decided to raise her to the upper level of the Bardo channel for initiation. She was prepared. She has an attractive black mask with the silver sign of the healer. Well, if she has outfitted herself so, it indicates a desire to work together.

We turn on the internal vision screen. The ascent is remarkably easy. We pass the Earth level, enter the Bardo channel. We went upwards. In ten minutes we are on the landing. She can see everything very well and is happy. We lead her up the stairway to the divine elders. She carries herself with dignity.

The elders are sitting at the table – impassive, majestic, projecting the calm of eternity, a detachment from the earthly vanity. We explain to them whom we have brought and petition for her.

Tatyana Nikolayevna at first was rendered speechless. She cannot grasp whether this is real or just a trick of the mind. Had she been alone, she would not have believed this.

The elders are benevolent. They ask why she came and what she is seeking.

– I want to heal people with water, – Tatiana Nikolayevna replies, somewhat reticent but quite specific in her request. They give her a bowl of water. And warn her: "Don't spill it".

We fly back. Tatyana is holding the bowl carefully. She brought it back without spilling. On Earth we stop by a small lake.

– Now in this bowl you will be able to see everything you want, – a voice is heard from somewhere.

We have an opportunity to test it. We have visitors today.

We start seeing patients. And Tatyana Nikolayevna is working with us.

There is a male patient with glaucoma. We start working. We go to the third sublevel of the first earthly level. She is with us. We develop the information matrix. We can see the connection of this illness with the heart. This glaucoma is caused by very serious stress. We tell the man about it and he confirms. He explains that there was a serious breakdown at work, and he confronted his boss face to face. We work with the eye, and turn on the healing program. There is another stress, a very dangerous one, looming ahead for him – his wife cannot forgive him for something and is being very overbearing with him.

We worked with his wife. We lit up in her brain a program for attitude towards our patient. This should make her kinder.

The next patient is a woman, and she is very ill. Everything seems to be hurting within her. We see that her spleen, liver and blood are affected. It seems like a cancerous process is starting. Also, there is a major scar in her urethra. We ask her what that is. She explains that she underwent surgery. We go to the third sublevel. We create her skeleton, organs, tissue in the information space. Everything of hers is black. It is really impossible to work. The suddenly emerging black clouds are pressing from above. It is understandable. The patient is a client of the "furry fellows" from below. Something is brewing in her about which they are very worried. We raise our shield above our heads and protect ourselves.

At the same time, we keep working with the woman, even though it makes you feel like not doing anything – she is not one of us, not a person of light. Tatyana Nikolayevna is a real trooper. She works from below. She does everything very competently. Igor and I, in the image of St. George the Dragon Slayer, are protecting her work. But the pressure from above is becoming more and more intense. Why?

Suddenly, a black dragon escapes from the woman and grows in front of our eyes. It is not a very big one, but Tatyana Nikolayevna is shocked. She is seeing this for the first time. She is not morally prepared. It very quickly climbs onto the horse, that is, me, and hides under Igor's shield. We fight the dragon. It escapes the lance somehow very easily. But finally we get it right in the mouth. It fades and disappears. You can say it's her first baptism by fire in our special field of implementation.

The pressure from above dissipates momentarily. We continue to work with the woman. We illuminate her. For how long will this work? This is what obsession is. There is a dragon in one person, a devil in another, and something unknown in the third. And even I have something weird feeding in the protective square. How it will show itself in the future – God knows. However, so far it seems to be a peaceful dragon, it does no harm, but actually helps. Does it mean we will coexist?

* * *

So here we are, the love of our dear Ministry has finally rolled around to reach us. This love is called the restructuring of the sector. It sounds beautiful: to combine all the state-run publishing houses by field of specialization into large holdings. But this is just the showcase, and what is behind it?

If the publishing houses were to be merged without working capital, without the ability to finance their publishing programs through loans from the state-owned funds (and where are these funds?), they will only be able to do one thing – lay people off. Thus, the new holdings without the conditions necessary for them to develop (and these conditions are what is not provided) turn into the peculiar stagnant swamps of the state-run domestic book publisher or large mass graves.

Behind all these ideas are clearly visible the ambitions and prospects of the commercial publishers, first and foremost "Vagrius". An industrious donkey (the logo for this publishing house) decided, within its sector, to pile up with its silage everything that has not yet been stomped and crushed by earlier reforms. The prospect is quite clear – peaceful green grazing grounds for just a single head of cattle. And that head of cattle could be quite easily seen behind all the announced reforms.

So here it is, the earthly embodiment of the astral projections. Something very important is beginning. First, they show you what is forthcoming in the form of an allegory, like a film. And now you have to lift, in real life, your cross and pull it up the hill, keep the promise you gave at his coffin to your friend Boris Mozhaev: „I will save "Khudlit". You have to answer for your words. Now pull your cross, keep pulling.

A staff meeting is held regarding the upcoming restructuring. Everyone showed up, even the ones out on sick leave. Everyone knows not to expect anything good from the ideas of the new management in the Ministry. The people are well-known. The press is overflowing with their administrative and criminal escapades – searches, arrests, millions of dollars confiscated from the apartments. The regal instruction from Yeltsin to stop all prosecution of the friends of the Family; new appointments are made in the government, but the journalists continue their investigation. Convincing and verifiable versions are created showing that the ministerial management is involved in more and more large-scale crimes.

The "Khudlit" employees are afraid of those reformers and unanimously vote against joining any holdings. They don't want to lose their right to exist that they won through hard battles. The resolution, supported unanimously, has another line which is quite pleasant for me: „The publishing house must be run by the same people who saved it from bankruptcy." That means my team and me. This is an important sign indicating that our course is approved. It was quite logical, however. We have started steadily and quite noticeably improving the profitability indicators.

These days in the May issue of the journal „Birzha Avtorskih Prav" [Copyright Exchange], journalist Olga Peskova presented a detailed analysis of the situation at "Khudlit". I would like to share a quote from there:

„Kniga Encyclopedia" notes that in 1996 the publishing house published 38 books. However, there is a situation that was not mentioned, even though it cannot be called insignificant. The debt of the publishing house at the end of 1996 reached 4.5 billion non-denominated rubles. However, already in 1997 it reached a break-even point, and in 1998 it showed a profit of 50,000 rubles (now denominated). In 1999, this figure reached 300,000. Expected profit for this year (2000) is 6,000,000 rubles. Such are the numbers. They tell us, in particular, about the crisis that hit the publishing house in the mid-90s. Actually, it happened even earlier. This we can also see from the numbers. Thus, in 1991, the publishing house published 277 books with a total number printed of nearly 38 million copies. In 1994 – 58 books with a total of 2 million copies, and in 1995 no books were published at all. In 1996 – 38 books with the number barely reaching 0.5 million. So that was the declining curve. We already know what the financial situation of the publishing house was and what it is today.

„Given the dynamics, it would be easy to forecast what was to follow: books would no longer be published and the publishing house would go bankrupt. In 1997, the situation was following this very scenario: only 25 books were published with a total of 235,000 copies. The publishing house was dying. But, as I already mentioned, this year the debts of the publishing house were paid off.

„In three years the publishing house climbed out of the debt hole and set up a normal production process, resuming multi-volume publications of classic Russian and foreign literature. First of all, it published the scheduled volumes by Andreyev, Kuprin, Graham Greene, Maugham, Hoffman, Hamsun, which had long been expected by the audience. After all, "Khudlit" has always specialized in publishing complete works of authors.

344

Those sets involved work by the greatest Russian and foreign specialists: philologists, historians, archive researchers, bibliographers, translators, textologists, artists, literary and art figures. This is what the publishing house was famous for. Many of the books published and now in print by other publishing houses are variations on the work of "Khudlit" from the earlier years."

And just as we have on our own clawed our way back from the brink of the abyss, we are again facing the threat of destruction. Someone was not very happy to see the "Khudlit" that rose from its knees and was gaining strength. A dangerous competitor must disappear. It was not without a reason that the former director of "Khudlit", Georgi Andzhaparidze, now working at "Vagrius", has acknowledged among his new associates that he is proud of the role he played in destroying the publishing monster "Khudlit". It seems that some people enjoy any kind of fame, even if it is that of Herostratus.

But now I know how powerful is the influence of the informational plane, of the informational field of the Earth on current events. I know, but I am still not very capable of using the new knowledge. So, I must learn. Now when we visit the levels there are three of us. Tatyana Nikolayevna is with us. She is already accustomed to the virtual plane of existence of the lower levels. We decided to give her a closer look at the areas with which we are already familiar. We start the tour from the palace belonging to Grigori Petrovich on the second level.

We enter the Bardo channel. Second level. We turn left. We quickly find Grabovoi's palace. It is surrounded by a wall. It has tall gates. A guard protects them. He is wearing a cloak and armor. We are wearing armor, too, more accurately, Igor is. Tatyana is sitting on the saddlebow, which means on top of me. I am already used to function as a horse, and I am not

345

at all embarrassed by that role. I know that Pegasus is the favorite horse of the Father of the Gods. Therefore, it is a great honor to be given such an image.

The guard is not hostile, nor is he surprised by our appearance, and routinely asks the purpose of our visit.

– We would like to visit our teacher Grigori Petrovich Grabovoi.

The guard steps aside and lets us pass:

– He is expecting you.

We cross the yard and a beautiful garden in which peacocks are walking. We go up the stairs and enter the palace. There are spacious halls, a lot of paintings, and antique furniture. It looks more like a royal palace than a dwelling of a Russian scientist.

We pass through several rooms. At the end of the suite of halls there is a large well-lit room. A man is sitting with his back to us at a desk adorned with elegant inlays.

– Grigori Petrovich, forgive us for coming uninvited, but we wanted so much to see it all from the inside. I suggest to Igor the words he ought to say. He carefully repeats them.

Grigori Petrovich turns around:

– If you were uninvited, you probably would not have come inside. What, did I not welcome you well? Was someone trying to prevent you from coming inside?

– We also come to you with our hearts wide open...

Grigori Petrovich suddenly emits a ray of light from his forehead and an image of a fawn appears next to us.

– Your lady is like a fawn, he says.

I would not have necessarily called her a fawn. Actually, Tatyana is rather on the heavy side, even though rather attractive. She obviously

346

melts from the compliments. Another two or three such passages– and she will leave our team for the palace with the peacocks. It's not a baseless concern. Tatyana's actions speak louder than any words. She has already left the saddle and come almost right up to the master of the magical world.

I whisper to Igor what he should say. He repeats:

– We would like to spend a day with you on Earth sometime so that we could discuss everything together and get to know each other better.

– I will call you, – promises Grabovoi.

– And your dream will come true – you will have a hut on chicken legs, – he is talking to Tatyana now.

He points at a tree. It is a very tall oak.

– Your house is up on it.

Just in case, we put Tatyana onto the saddle again. Grigori Petrovich laughs.

– That's right, take good care of your treasure. Since you are heroes, sooner or later you will have to rescue the princess.

We say our good-byes and leave the palace.

We rode to the right. It's the information level. At the crossroads we see an owl. It's very large, with huge eyes. We keep going. It is an enchanted forest, and we need to get out. But somehow we know the way. We do not meander at all. We simply keep walking and then come out. There is a sacred tree. Under it there is a road. We are given a huge chariot straight from space. We get in it. It rushes upwards. There is a light tunnel and a crescent moon.

Someone is chasing us. It's a wolf. That is someone we have known for a long time. The space turns silvery white. Igor continues on horseback. We leave the gray tracker behind. There is some kind of landing, surroun-

347

ded by rocks. We are being shown ancient signs. The color is green. We zoom in. Here is the sign of Sagittarius – this is Igor, Ingvar, which is the same thing. Now there is Capricorn. He is wearing a bell. Now the images turn into something scary. There is a snake. It has wings. It's alive. We remove it. We bring closer the next image. Some person bars the way, not letting us through. He has a feather on his head.

The next sign. Two people – and they are sort of barring the way as well. They look like American Indians with bows. Half-naked. Now a Lion appears. He is very beautiful. His fur is glossy. He wants to be petted and rubs up against us. We stroke him. He enjoys it.

Next is the Cow, or, actually, a Bull. Now there is a Jug, water is pouring from it. It is a zodiac sign. It is made of marble. But the water is real. It makes you want to drink some of that water. Above the sign there is a bird, and it is wearing a crown. It is a Phoenix. „If you drink, you will fall asleep" – someone's words appear in the mind like a light breeze. So, we shall not drink. Now a man with a shovel appears. He says:

– Dig down! There is a treasure, and a dragon guards the treasure.

– Some other time, perhaps at leisure if we have the time, of course, - we elaborately decline the treasure.

Now there is the last sign: a live Scorpion. He is wearing a green mask. He is covering something up with his wings. We part with him as well. Quickly, we enter the tunnel. Third level. To the left. Chill creeps about, it is damp. Some kind of moat, skulls, bones. Dead bodies are around. Tatyana is frightened, and we reassure her, saying that no one can see us. We should not have: some yellow stain is watching us. Ancient hieroglyphs appear. We zoom in. Besides hieroglyphs, bolts of lightning – crisscrossed, and there is a skull above them. Nearby there are huge beds like in a hospital. People are piled up on them. They are all heavily ban-

348

daged. So, this is the historic birthplace of Lapshin, this is his floor. We go back. We move over to the right side and enter. Birds are flying. The sky is blue, and the clouds are light. There is joy around. Building, cars. All the cars are convertibles. There is a column in the shape of a man supporting a balcony, bunches of grapes are hanging down from the side, and there are children in holiday attire with wreaths on their heads. It looks like a modern city. This is also the Realm of the Dead, but here the good people are gathered, who are being prepared for a new incarnation. They study the mistakes they made in their previous incarnations on Earth, along the way towards Godly humanity. When they work through their karma, they will come into the era of immortality. This is already close, very close.

Level four. On the left. There are entities– white flying ones. There is a streetlight. It is alive. It looks at us through the glass. It is in a friendly mood. A cow with shining eyes is looking at us as well. There is no threat. People are dressed in something strange – some are standing, some are lying down. There seems to be a temple nearby. Oh, those are not people. There are clothes, but there is nothing inside. Non-embodied souls of people. Further on there some frescos. They depict a horse and rider, who is slaying a dragon. The frescoes are hanging in limbo. They look like folds of gas, not fully materialized.

We move to the right. There is also a temple. The style is very interesting. Everything is helical – pillars, arches, friezes. We enter a room, there is a throne in there – it looks like a shell with someone sitting on it.

We proffer a greeting. The person answers us, but it is hard to distinguish whether it is a man or a woman. In its hair the person has a crescent moon. Some kind of golden animal skin floats towards us. It is a present for us. We take it. Oh my God! It is the Golden Fleece! Igor places the present on me and thanks the giver. The latter is also glad that we accepted

349

the present. We ask if we can be of any help.

– You are already helping by the fact that you exist!

The giver blesses us. Invites to come again if we need help. Presents us with another gift: a scepter floats on the air towards Igor's hand. The master advises that it needs to be held firmly.

– Save it for yourselves – he repeats. Once again, he warns us: You must hold the scepter firmly.

Level five. On the left there is a tempest and thunderstorms. The weather is the state of the humanity and nature. Then followed hypnosis: something is flying like a bee but not quite. It has stripes on one side like a bumble-bee, and its buzz also seems split in two. Rocks are falling from the cliffs. Igor and I have visited this place before. Tatyana has had enough for the first time.

On the right there are woods – birches, the sky is light, it is warm, and there is wheat in the field. There are little bags sitting on the ground, one could collect medicinal herbs in them. There is moss – it is always useful when you travel. A bag is proffered made of air: please gather. Then they say: you need to place it in water and reconstitute it. It is good for healing wounds.

Level six. On the right there are cliffs, sea, and the ocean. We walk towards the water. Tatyana sees the water flowing from the mountains. This is the flow of talents. We wash our hands. Water is dripping from our fingers. The light washes us from above, we feel very well. We water the horse. That means me. This is the way knights do it. The knight's best friend is his horse. We were given so much light. It was a generous and friendly deed! Thanks.

Level six on the left is the symbol of the lack of talent. Everything is topsy-turvy, things don't work. Projects that were started and then abandoned. Territory for losers.

Level seven on the left – there is dead water. People are mucking about in muddy wet earth. The soil is very sticky. It's clay. There are small dippers on strings and a pit with swamp water. Something is written on the dipper. It is broken and has a crack. On the side there is a picture of a person in a wheelchair. That's clear: if you want to become an invalid, drink some water from the swamp.

On the right, there is the water of life. People are dressed warmly. There is ice. Snow. Ice holes. The dipper is made in the shape of a duck.

Level eight on the right. There is the Life-Giving Cross. The grass next to it starts growing lushly. People have beards. Very long beards, they reach the ground. This is a hint that they were given a long life because they live believing in God. The Cross is very beautiful. On the top it is shaped like a bow. Rays come up from it in a cone. The clouds are drifting. Ahead there are mountains; they are lit up by the cross, which is taller than they. It lights everything up: Egyptian pyramids, Russian temples, Catholic churches and oriental minarets.

On the left there is the Death-Giving Cross. Everything is burnt and dry around. In the distance there is a sphinx. His mane is large like a wave. There is stone around. Everything alive in that area dies or dries up. We leave.

Level nine is heaven and hell. We will not go there today, but the next time. There is a landing above the ninth level. The elders are there, St. George the Dragon Slayer, Life and Death. One cannot come there just out of curiosity – it may end badly. Under the best of circumstances, no one will welcome you, under the worst – there will be a new client for Ward No. 6*. This had happened before. This is not a game or a cartoon, this is the Path.

* In Russian hospitals, Ward No. 6 is the mental ward.

The Path with a capital P that leads either to disgrace or to immortality.

Igor dismounts the horse and helps Tatyana. He takes her hand. Around the landing everything keeps rotating. Tatyana, wearing the helmet and the mail, looks very striking. We come up. There are stone boulders and the elders on top of them. They look and wait for what we have to say.

Tanya [diminutive for Tatyana] thanks them again for the gift, for her bowl.

One of the elders reminds Tatyana, that it is not a simple bowl and that she will need it. He says that soon there will be a meeting with a knight near a big lake. Some kind of riddle of life. Oh well, Tatyana will solve it.

We go to another staircase. The entrance is semicircular. Inside there are two birds. On each side of the door there is an angel. We go there. The light is mild and not blinding. It illuminates the road and us. There is water ahead and a shining emanates from it. We walk on the water like Christ. We passed across the water, it is now behind us. The light intensifies. It is hard to see, and we squint. Tatyana leads the horse. From on high, gold flakes descend on us like golden light. This means we were granted some kind of protection. A large bearded head appears above. We know who that is – it's the Father of the Gods. He looks affable. We greet him.

He asks Igor:

– Who is that with you? Do you come in peace?

– Of course, in peace.

He stretches his powerful hand from above. We need to give him a present. The Fleece? Tatyana hesitates. She is feeling stingy. Igor and I have no doubt that in our mission gold is not the key. We can do without. We pass on the golden fleece. Immediately our eyes are not blinded any more. This is a sacrifice. Gold should not bind us, and we should not be bound to gold. We are free to go on. The horse looks golden now, and the

352

rider is golden too. Now we are given freedom to act.

We know that had we kept the golden fleece, in the physical plane the golden calf would have become favorable to us. But we made a different decision and we do not regret it. The Father of the Gods asks what we would like for ourselves.

– We want to accomplish our mission on Earth.

– Fine – the Father of the Gods agrees. – And in addition I will give you freedom. So that your soul would expand. Your soul will become very, very large.

We thank him. We go back. We have become taller than we were before. And we have become filled with something on the inside.

Another staircase. On it there is St. George the Dragon Slayer. He is enormous – his head is surrounded by mists and clouds – a very beautiful sight. St. George the Dragon Slayer takes Tanya up onto his hand. He shows her the finger with a ring: read this. But she cannot read the inscription. The divine warrior feels that she is a little frightened. St. George the Dragon Slayer explains:

– It says on the ring: „Honor and Dignity". – He lowers Tatyana. – Now you may go. This is hard for me.

We go down.

Again we walk down the stairs. There is a tunnel on the right. We enter. There are human remains. We shall not go there. We go into another tunnel. There are large teeth, it's a mouth. We are in a jaw.

Tanya is dragging me somewhere. I follow her. She is led by female curiosity and not intuition, like she says. She brings me to water. The river is flowing from above to our feet. There is a Mesozoic fern. The water is very cold. We take some water. Create a flask, tighten the lid. Fill another flask to put in the saddlebag. There is an inscription on the flask: „To victory".

Tanya again leads us somewhere. We go around the circle of the landing. There is a field. But is not a simple field. It is a battlefield. We gather nuts from the ground. What should we do with them? Crack and eat them. We crack them. We sat down and ate, following them with water. That restores our strength. That means soon there will be a battle.

* * *

Unusual events on the informational plane astonished Tatyana Nikolayevna to such an extent that she decided to bring her best friend to help us. The delicacy of the situation was such that for the first time we were asked to help not with health problems but in a specific family situation, a complicated relationship between a husband and wife. We were also interested to see how the information field of the Earth would react to a quite a private conflict in everyday life.

The friend was named Olya. She worked in the Supreme Court. And the fact that already officials of such rank are ready to submit to the higher judgment of the noospheric intelligence makes one feel better about the future of the country.

Olga arrived on time, as we arranged with her in advance. Besides Tatyana, another apprentice of mine, Yura, a sixteen-year-old kid, is participating in the experiment. His internal vision screen is working perfectly, and he was supposed to sort of follow along with the process as an independent observer.

We activate the internal vision screens. We ascend to the information level. We start the analysis. The planetary mind decides to maintain a dialogue in the form of images this time as usual. There is a crown above

Olga's head, but it is weighing her down. She would not give it away, either, since there are no candidates, and the family would be wrecked, too. Her lifeline greatly depends on external circumstances. What are they? We see a person – he is frantically clutching onto his chair. This is her husband. He is the director of a large plant. Is he tying to hold onto his job?

We zoom in. What is this: he is tied to a chair? His hands are pulled together behind his back with a rope, and one end of that rope is tied to the bar of the back of a chair. Behind the chair there are two figures: a man and a woman. The woman is putting some hood or bag over his head from behind. She is very determined – she has a good figure, long hair – she is beautiful. We ask Olga who that is, and describe her appearance.

Olga explains: this is her husband's mistress. She is a lawyer and helps him to win court cases.

The image expands. Now it is shown to us that from the side a train is rushing towards the man tied to the chair. A few moments and he will be overcome and crushed. Man and woman leave. What should we do? We stop the train. We need to figure this one out.

Yura suggests:

– Let's untie him.

Tanya objects:

– We must understand what is going on.

We are shown a cow, and the man, sitting on the chair, sees his double next to it. The cow has been milked and there is a pail of milk. The cow is a situation with which a lot of work has been done. The milk represents money, and there is a lot of it. The man must decide what to do with it. His life depends on his decision. Literally in the next few days.

No – he does not want the money, he refuses it. And immediately he gains strength. He snaps the rope that was holding him to the chair and stands up. He is very determined and kicks away the chair. This means he has refused the deal with the bank, which wanted, for a bribe of four hundred thousand dollars, to buy out his plant. And which had lured to its side his mistress, the lawyer. She needs the money. She had chosen the money, and set up her boss and lover to die.

The man is standing with great determination. He will not sell out the plant and his team of employees. He has a lot of good and bad features in his character, but he will not do such a thing. This is firm and final. But his hands are still tied. He cannot completely free himself. What is the matter?

A house appears. That is his home. He is not sure where to go and hesitates. He stands still for a minute or two, thinking. Finally the decision is made: he walks towards the house. This is the correct decision because he is returning to his family. Tatyana unties his hands from behind. Igor erases the train. For now the situation is resolved, but the threatening factors still remain. Now everything will depend on his behavior. We now know: things occurring in the informational plane are mirrored on the physical plane. Olga is amazed. This allegorical story is fully in line with her specific life situation. She does not want to leave. She stays with us to have some tea. What occurred is a shock for her. No one close to the man knew about his relationship with the bank, including Tatyana.

Kirill has arrived. He is a spy from Lapshin. He says that the Moscow Department of the Academy wants to leave Vyacheslav's patronage. They come to ask for help. Because he is feared.

He is telling lies. We can see that by clairvoyance. But why? What does he want? What is he trying to achieve?

* * *

Igor left Moscow for a week. The three of us are working – Tatyana,

Yura and myself. We decided to sort out the databases of the large planetary computer. We are interested in the programs for magic. I have access to all the databases, so I am certain that we will be able to pursue this field and get results.

We enter the program. All the books pertaining to magic are recorded there. We look through them. There is the first, second, third... The Ninth books catches our attention for some reason.

It has a shield and a sword on the cover. There is the image of St. George the Dragon Slayer, slaying the dragon. The cover is made of metal. We open it.

We see a field. Some events are happening there. It is a scene of sending troops off to battle. A woman hands a double-headed eagle to us. It is alive. Close to us on the left there is a lion. The trumpets are sounding, calling. They are long trumpets. Tanya mounts the horse, and Yura is behind her. St. George the Dragon Slayer sends us on. He gives us a weapon –his huge sword. How Tanya is going to wield it is not clear. We hear something knocking. A troop is gathering. A large troop arranged in a line. They all wear helmets and have spears and shields.

There is music. The troops start marching. The lion runs along to the left of the horse. That is me. Tanya and Yura have suddenly become giants.

There is a city ahead, with a lot of buildings. It is a baleful city. On the right there are rocks and cliffs. The landscape is very forbidding. It is dark and cloudy. A bolt of lightning pierces the darkness ahead. The clouds become thicker. Someone is standing ahead in a loose dark red garment. There is a thunderstorm coming – a storm. The cloaks stream in the wind, slap into our eyes. The city is locked, everyone seems to be trapped there. We must free them. Our opponents are gathering – they are of normal height or even a little shorter. They are calm and are advancing towards us.

Our troops turn, line up like a wall. But at the same time the ones opposing us are not ordinary people. I am worried: something has gone awry. And I don't perceive these events as being like a cartoon any more. Igor should be participating in this battle. We have set in motion something very dangerous. Our enemies are non-humans from the Realm of the Dead. So that's what the energies of Lapshin's students were used for.

They send some kind of bird towards us. Yura shoots a white arrow and hits it. It falls down and dissolves in the thunderstorm. Now some kind of device rolls out from the castle. It is like a helicopter with a large rotor. The rotor is used to bring about more clouds; they get thicker and thicker. The things happening around us are oppressive. What have we started? We need to stop the events. I tell Tatyana and Yura to come out of the book and close it. Delicate silk cloth, red in color, billows from above. It is a veil. It falls over us from above. It is guided by a woman's hand. Tanya says: this is motherly protection from the Mother of God.

Our accidental battle with the monsters from the Realm of the Dead has, already in the next few days, turned into quite real trouble for everyone involved in the events. All of a sudden we all fell ill – our health problems descended on us like an avalanche. Tatyana was coughing, her eyes were red, her handkerchief was continuously at her nose. Yura also had symptoms of acute respiratory disease. My situation was even worse. All at once it affected my throat, liver, and kidneys. I had a splitting headache. I had not felt so awful in many years. And there was no one to help. The internal vision screens of all of our team have gone dull. They barely work, and even so – only in the emergency mode. And Dina, Nina Andreyevna, Svetlana Nikolayevna and others from our team – all of a sudden everyone is out of shape, following our example.

One fateful mistake – and the whole thing goes to the dogs. Some working with magic that was! We had been warned that magic would not agree with us. It is the enemy's weapon. God Himself lends strength to us, and still we venture where we shouldn't. To be precise, I do. There is no fault on the others. They followed me as I was leading them. And so I led them astray – now everyone is sick and miserable. I wish Igor would return soon.

I went to visit Grigori Petrovich for advice. He has already been informed about the events. He looks at me with sympathy.

– Had some fighting, didn't you?

– I just wanted to see what our opponents' capabilities were, to do some fighting reconnaissance. I try to justify myself.

– I understand, –Grabovoi shrugs his shoulders. – But think for yourself: what will happen if a horse without a rider leads the troops into battle? At least you had the sense to stop the battle. It could have happened that from that battle you would have proceeded straight to the next world. When will all of you understand the meaning of the word „responsibility"? What happens there inevitably is implemented here.

– What should I do? – I ask in despair.

– Eliminate the violent stage of the confrontation. Turn the events back, before they manifest themselves into reality. Roll everything up into the point before the active fighting started. Bring it back through the database, by counting the time backwards.

Fortunately, Igor returned the next evening. Everything was okay with his clairvoyance! It makes work possible. We sit down together. Find the magic program, extract book nine. It opens on the page where events had been stopped. The troops are at a standstill, the non-humans are ushering in the clouds with their rotor. We activate the backward counting of time. That's it, those bastards turn their harmful contraption back into the city.

For an instance the Black Knight riding the black horse flashes among their troops. How could I have not noticed him the last time?

Now their troops are retreating back into the gate. And then we leave from under the city walls. The farewells, St. George – everything is rewinding up to the first page. The book closes. We return it to the databases. At our exit from the Bardo channel next to my name others' names have been written. As if the mountain-climbers had inscribed their names on the peaks they conquered: Chumak, Kashpirovskiy, someone named Mirzoyeva... The largest signatures are Juna's* and mine, almost a kilometer tall.

– Let's remove it, – I suggest to Igor.

– Why? – he asks.

– To eliminate the arrogance, – I explain. He understands and agrees. We remove my immodest announcement. Igor is right in saying: „One has to be simpler, humbler!"

We study the levels. What do we see? Nine levels, each of them has three sections. So there it is, this unknown distant land, unknown distant kingdom! The tenth landing is like the cork from a bottle that holds the punished genie. Those who get accepted here – have passed the initiation. And not everyone is accepted, as we have already found out. And those who have passed the initiation do not need the cork in the bottle.

The levels on the left represent the past. The ones on the right represent the future. And in the center, where the past meets the future, that is, in the Bardo channel, – there is true time, the past-future. The levels go down underneath the ground as well. Straight to the planetary core, which is the second Sun of our Earth. Was it about that that Lapshin had talked: Sun-2, Sun-2? And hinged grand personal plans on spe-

* All four names – Chumak, Kashpirovskiy, Mirzoyeva and Juna – are names of Russian psychic healers.

cial relations with this underground celestial body. Dark levels below are also filled with information, power, and knowledge. But it is somewhat different – through temptation, greed, lies, thievery, envy, and fall from grace. I would have to think this through thoroughly. And also it is necessary to understand how the levels and the landing interact. In principle it is already sufficiently clear that each level is connected to such global components of the Cosmos and Man, as informational essence, karma, fate, spirituality, existence, space, time, connection between heaven and earth, etc. The will of man leads him through complicated labyrinths of life towards himself. But will he find himself in the invisible matrix of existence, which is full of dangerous stumbling blocks and unpredictable tests, in order to ascend the steps of complete liberation? God knows! I know of only one such person. His name was Christ. He found the way in the labyrinth of His fate, conscience and desires.

They say that His second coming is expected. And perhaps He is already on Earth? Who knows? And those levels are like the genie's bottle. And who is the genie? Is it Man? All that is needed is to wipe clean the glass, which has gotten dusty from time, and remove the cork. The one enclosed in the bottle would find it quite difficult to do so. And the cork is not so simple – twenty-four of the elders are guarding the way out of the bottle. They cannot be deceived. They can read minds; instead of granting an expected gift, they can reject and punish the applicant. Little children should not venture to go to Africa!

One girl did go, and what happened? They did not give her permission and turned away. At least they did not punish her. I say to Igor:

– Let's take a look at her. There may be attacks against her. Maybe she needs help. She is a member of our team after all, we are responsible for her.

361

We enter the information flows. Quickly we locate the right line. By now we can do it almost automatically. We look at her consciousness and ask for a view of the general situation. They show us: a sphere, divided into two parts. Both halves present the image of an ocean, differing only by color of the water. On the left it is black, on the right it is white, and a mirror divides them in the middle. Waves come from the different sides and hit the mirror. This is a battle occurring in her consciousness. She does not understand yet the meaning of the process of life, rushes into extremes: now she does good deeds, now she thinks about her superpowers and how to use them for her personal ends. There is a never-ending storm in her consciousness.

* * *

Every day we learn how to work with the levels of the planetary computer. And strictly in line with the results, more and more new patients come to us. Almost at the same time, a boy named Misha – he is autistic and unable to speak at all, – and a girl, or actually a young woman – Dasha. Dasha is deaf. My deputy at the publishing house, Sergey Kolesnikov, asked for her. She has been seen both by doctors and sorcerers without any result.

– If you can restore her hearing, I will be the first to testify to anyone who asks that you are capable of performing miracles – Sergey said with his usual flourish. Dasha was seen by the best audiologist in Moscow. He said that her condition is not treatable. His opinion is like a sentence. Try to refute it.

Over recent years Sergey had slowly drifted from total denial of the possibility of healing using fine plane influences via the consciousness to a partial acknowledgment that such things may be possible. The words did not have much of a convincing effect on him, but once, more like an experiment, he asked us to take a look at his knee. An old sports injury over the years had led to pain in his knee that would not abate for weeks at a time. Sergey suffered, could barely bend his knee, but soldiered on, since the doctors promised him no miracles and recommended that he get used to it. Sergey asked us for help. Naturally, he received it. He was then immensely surprised when a few days later at a friend's summer cottage he calmly assumed the lotus position at someone's request and, lifting himself up on his hands, performed a few elaborate yoga exercises. With belated horror he thought: „The pain is going to be blinding now". But there was no pain. None at all! It did not come back either that day or any other day – not a week nor a month later, as if it had forever forgotten about him. This resulted in a certain change of heart, and Sergey decided to continue the experiment, knowing Dasha's situation.

Misha and Dasha came to us on the same day. A mute patient and a deaf patient. And we started working with them on the same day.

Misha is a normal healthy boy. But between the right and the left hemisphere there seems to be a thin dark film. This is a wall. And breaching it will not be so simple. We had never had any cases like this.

We look into the causes. So, it relates to the inheritance. Very large sums of money. We are shown houses, gardens and Catholic churches. It looks like Poland. A stern old man. Great wealth is in his hands. But it does not belong to him, it has come to him as a dowry. The woman to whom the wealth belonged has not been living with him for a long time. She wants him to return what was hers. She has taken him to court. And it seems she is very close to reaching her goal. He is afraid; he wants to leave everything to his son. And he hates the unknown boy in Russia, who will receive everything in accordance with the ruling of the court. The woman in question is Misha's grandmother, and she wants to leave everything to her grandson.

We relay this to Misha's mother, and she freezes in shock in front of our eyes: the situation is exactly the way we saw it. We can't make a decision right away and ask for a time out.

Dasha's situation is not so simple either. Physically, there is no cause for the deafness. But she has two informational plugs in her ears. We need to figure out why. And again the information flow takes us back to the old times. Her grandmother, quite a religious person, at some point had an abortion. The soul of the aborted child was unable to return to the Realm of the Dead and was hanging in limbo between the levels. It was calling for help to her niece, who was able to hear her due to a particular sensitivity in the right hemisphere of her brain. The information plugs were put in place so that Dasha would not lose her mind. We look at the forecasting phase: in the beginning of 2001, Dasha would regain her hearing. The plugs need to be removed carefully. The neurons in the brain are not prepared to hear sounds. It will result in shock and stopper of the entire system that controls the organism. At first we will take down 0.3 – 0.5 percent per week. We set that in motion. The process is activated! We are shown that Dasha is sitting at a concert and listening to music.

– Dasha! You will hear music, – I say slowly. The girl reads my lips and nods. She understood.

* * *

Since the time we stopped the unsanctioned magical battle that we almost unleashed, everything is calm. The battle participants are not sick any more, and the events around "Khudlit" are sort of frozen. All around there were screams and moans of colleagues from other publishing houses regarding the heavy pressure from the ministry, threats, redistribution of property which gets taken away by the new bold guys who managed to insinuate themselves into power. And on our front everything is strangely quiet, as if someone on high is guarding and protecting us. We can guess who that is! We talked to them, we saw them, we know now that there is a God!

Of course, some atheistic habits persist. But there is already a cross hanging around my neck. And another one is burning in my soul. During my entire life prior to this I had not attended church so much as in these recent years. Even though, my attitude towards the church is uneven. There are too many unenlightened, reactionary, ignorant people in it. Some of them are fit to serve not to Christ, but His antipode. And was it not the priests that two thousand years ago rejected His coming to Earth? Of course, the current ones would say – it was not us, it was it was the other ones. But those who sent God to die in torment on the cross did not consider themselves different. They thought **He** was different. History could repeat itself, since the second coming of Christ is going to be announced at any moment. We know that, we see that.

In the religious teachings, the Church is represented as something supernatural, as the "mystical body of Jesus Christ". Alas, besides the Church with the capital C, there are many churches scattered throughout the world where the "c" is decidedly small. Simple, mortal people – priests – act there as intermediaries between God and the flock. And they are far from always blessed with sanctity.

Here is a small town on the outskirts of Moscow, with a small wooden church in the center. But already a large brick temple is being built nearby.

Several devoted worshippers with art education paint icons, which are then sold for the benefit of the future temple. It has been several years that they have been working for free, denying themselves normal secular joys and comforts. There are always some lay sisters easily susceptible to persuasion. Meanwhile, the rector of the temple, (it's just so tempting to call him the boss) during these years bought himself a two-story apartment in a prestigious brick house and hired a housekeeper, even though his wife is not working…

Is this the way of Christ? Or maybe it's the way of Lapshin, who asked bitingly: "So why don't you ask for money from God then?

My son Nikolay came with a request. His friend was injured in a car accident. His backbone was broken, his tailbone shattered. There is practically no hope that he will not become an invalid.

A day later, we received a recent photograph of him that was taken right in the hospital. The lad is quite a horrible sight. We enter his consciousness. There is one thought beating in his head like a wounded bird: he wants to keep living and for this situation to come to an end. He himself did nothing bad. He is grabbing at life, but he lacks strength. Life and Death are next to him. Doves are flying above him. We read the information. He is both alive and not alive.

There is a hematoma in his neck. The silvery color goes up his head, the green color into the hematoma. It disappears, but a tinge of yellow appears. Without an energy information matrix we won't be able to do it. Igor activates it and spreads the hologram. The correction is aligned along the spine. We lift him and turn him so that we are looking at his back. We remove another hematoma. The Mother of God comes from above to us. She watches us work.

More silvery color. We assemble the vertebra, fix it, strengthen the

366

norm. The energy starts flowing. Now we place the norm over the tailbone and the vertebrae. The green, white, silvery colors are working. The vertebrae set into place! The muscles are torn near the tailbone. We have assembled the tailbone correctly. That seems to be all. We send a command to the pituitary gland:

– Remove the hematomas and restore the blood vessels!

We strengthen the control from the head. We look at the nerve endings and the nerves themselves – the connection with the head is restored. He is in pain, he screams. It is clear why – the nerves have started sending signals to the consciousness.

The left kidney– the color is lilac. We overlay the norm.

The right kidney – the color is red. We surround it with a square and remove the hematoma. There is a table of restorative processes. The kidney vibrates. It starts functioning. It assumes the normal shape.

There is a spot underneath the heart. It is black. We supply the white color. The norm is over the heart. The head – the color is silvery. We increase its flow throughout the body. We create a pillar of energy.

Through the internal vision screen we request the forecast phase. It shows the patient on crutches. The right leg has not resumed its functions. A red arrow is showing the reason. It is clear: a nerve is pinched.

We activate the norm again and overlay it on the problem area. We increase the energy flow directed towards him. He needs energy now. Energy is life. If the doctors could see and know what we see and know now! But they are firmly clutching their scalpels, devices and pills. It looks like they themselves need some treatment. And it seems as though they are starting to guess that.

We look at the forecast phase again. The guy is sitting on a bench smoking. Everything is fine with him. The doctors will be happy with their work. No one was able to accomplish that before: shattered tailbone and broken spine, yet the guy is in fine shape.

We wanted to leave that space, but didn't quite make it. Below appeared the Black Knight with his warriors. He prances so that we can see him, obviously trying to attract our attention. We descend towards him to the central crossing of the Bardo channel. Our troops appear at once. Where did they come from? But there is no time to be surprised.

– So, what do you want? – we ask.

– I want to do battle! – he answers merrily, without malice.

– There will be time to fight; let's talk. How long have we been fighting, do you know?

– From day one, – the Black Knight replies.

– And what have we achieved?

He laughs, and prances in front of us:

– I am capable of everything, but you are still learning.

– And what else do you want to achieve?

He replies that if he wins he will grow and receive the force that is within us and whose strength has no bounds. The puppies need to be drowned while they are still small, – he hints.

– Maybe we can achieve that by cooperating rather than fighting?

– People have never come up with that idea. – And adds that we are no match for him. We look closer – this is not Lapshin. This is someone else.

We activate the fourth power. Surround him. It does not work. He falls through the ground and then reappears slightly to the side. He also possesses a strength that is unknown to us. It has been granted to him and he is walking on our ground with impunity.

– I can ride out here, – he yells, egging us on, – but will you go a down there, below, where the Realm of Darkness is?

– I am not afraid, – Igor responds.

He laughs:

– I know. You are brave, but careful – what a combination! Even the fact that I come up here is a victory for me. Because you don't visit me down there.

– You want so much to fight, just fight – and that's all?

– No, I don't, – he turns serious, – but that is the only way I can find out what is happening on the face of the Earth. I have knowledge that has been there forever, and you have recent information.

– May be we can trade knowledge for information? – I suggest to Igor.

The Black Knight is thoughtful, stopped riding around on his horse.

– I would be all for it, but you cannot make such a decision independently, – he says.

– That's true, so we need time.

He turns around, and his troops leave after him.

The Bardo pillar lowers itself down into the ground. The levels are visible there, similar to ours.

We need to go up and ask what we should do. Small children with wings are flying around us. They are little angels. There are a lot of them. Our troops are not leaving yet. They are waiting. We go up and into the central flow. An updraft lifts us within the Bardo channel, it's like an elevator. The Earth levels and the golden landing. Igor dismounts the horse. The angels flutter around.

The Creator is in front of us. Igor kneels, takes off his helmet and prays.

– Rise, My son, – says God.

– I am human.

– You were human, but now you are My son.

369

He instructs us to be very careful. The dark forces are treacherous.. What the Black knight said is true. They want negotiations. But is it possible to believe those who have cheated many times before?

– Be careful, – he warns us once again.

– Do we need to learn to negotiate? –asks Igor.

– Yes, – the Creator agrees. – You may descend down and nothing will happen to you. But it will be horrible there. Here there is no place where you can see things like that.

St. George the Dragon Slayer is next to us. He is enormous. They talk with the Creator about us, but for some reason we cannot hear. On the right there are a lot of saints. They must decide on something. They are talking about a major horror– it is a very major horror, tears, change to the man.

St. George talks to them as well. The priests and the saints are standing. The Creator is sitting. One of the saints asks Igor:

– Are you ready? Do you know what will happen to you?

– We do not know what will happen to us, but we gave an oath to serve The Lord.

Christ stands next to the Creator. He tries to offer support:

– Do not be worried; prepare yourself. You have received God's gift, the power. But use it for good.

– May we go down?

– It is not prohibited, but you have to realize and know what will be waiting for you. You have been told everything that is allowed.

We are blessed, and a prayer is read for battle, for eternal life, for glory in heaven. All those around cross themselves. Some shell has appeared and it glows. There is reverent silence. We are being purified. George shakes hands with us. The Creator thumps his staff, and we find ourselves down below.

– The troops are with you, – the voice roars from the sky. – They will appear immediately at your summons.

The children lift Igor onto the horse. He is completely exhausted. He is almost unconscious. Drops of sweat are rolling down his forehead and cheeks.

* * *

And already the next day Kirill again appeared in our Center. This strange boy, who in terms of intellect and knowledge could outperform any professor, came to seek employment with us. I knew that his internal vision screen operates excellently, he is well-versed in the technique of bio-informational impact, but it was his strange relationship with Lapshin that was disconcerting. Within the entourage of the magician from Theosia he took a special position. I noticed that Lapshin, who could be very rude to any of this staff, for some reason never quarreled with or yelled at him. Even though there were plenty of reasons for doing it: Kirill simply never worked. At any time during the day he would be drinking tea or coffee, chatting up the girls and blatantly ignoring whatever job responsibilities. When Lapshin caught him idling, anyone would catch hell, except for the actual culprit.

And so Kirill came and said strange words:

– Well, you wanted to exchange knowledge.

– You are here for the exchange – Igor guessed.

– Yes, – Kirill confirmed the situation only we understood. – Besides, Nina Andreyevna has been inviting me to come and transfer to you for a long time. So I have arrived. – And he put a smile on his face stretching from ear to ear.

– Whom should we send to you as an exchange? – asks Igor.

– That's up to you, – Kirill responds, again quite on the topic. It feels like he is completely aware of all the otherworldly events.

We started working together with Kirill. It is a completely new technique. No less effective, but completely unfamiliar to us. There are very grave doubts as to whether it is beneficial for us to use it at all. But we are bound by a treaty: he shows us his capabilities and we show him ours. However, sometimes Kirill takes it too far. All of a sudden Tatyana Nikolayevna fell into the habit of endlessly squabbling with everybody. Soon she stopped it, even though on the face if it the pretext she used was extremely minor. It seems like she herself understood that it was not for no reason that she was inclined to quarrel with everyone. Later, when we retraced the events, Kirill's influence was clearly visible. He deftly arranged quarrels among the employees of the Center. It turned out the boy was carrying quite a big stick even though he was hiding this hitting instrument very professionally.

We did not yet arrange the paperwork for official employment of Kirill. He was considered to be on a trial period. So we decided to hold off with the employment, to take a closer look at this present from the Black Knight. Or else with such eager help we risk losing all the staff completely.

Meanwhile, innovations were occurring constantly. Igor and I do not need the internal vision screens anymore. We can see everything clearly without it. We come out into the space we need and observe continents and oceans from our enormously tall height. We can see planes, rockets and satellites. Sometimes they fly right through us without adverse effects to either party. Every day there was something new. And most importantly – everything became more and more interesting.

We exchange telepathic messages with Grigori Petrovich Grabovoi almost every day. We consult with him constantly – and it seems we wore him down quite a bit by our questions. Sometimes he just says openly:

– Guys, you are capable of doing everything yourselves. I really have to work now.

We offer our apologies and go to other levels. They are very strange: sometimes you can cover them in several minutes, and sometimes it seems that ten years would not be enough to study just a single sector. However, soon our explorations came to an end.

In the morning, just as we entered the other space, we were met by messengers. These were two angels. Having seen us, they announce Armageddon and call us to the battlefield.

Igor and I feel as though we are frozen from the inside. At that moment we feel the burden of responsibility not only for ourselves, but for the whole Earth as well. And we also know: if we lose this battle, our death will not be an illusion but a very real one. And most likely instantaneous. It's just that in my office, where we are sitting, two strange crumpled bodies would be found and taken to the nearest hospital in order to understand why two healthy guys kicked the bucket all of a sudden. They would all wonder and inquire.

But we knew what we would be facing when we asked the Creator for the honor of saving the Earth from the sad fate foretold to it. We were granted this right and must prove that we had been asking for it from the true calling of heart and soul.

The angels bring us to the Bardo channel, where at the crossing of two worlds, at the very border of the upper and lower levels, the Black Knight and his troops were already waiting for us. It must be that he has tired of the truce. He must have decided that since we were asking for cooperation, we have not reached our full strength and are just stalling for time. "The puppies need to be drowned while they are still small." And quite a few of the famous entities have gathered to watch this procedure.

Beyond the ranks of the dark warriors there are three thrones. The largest of them is for the King of Darkness, next to it – two for his supporters. High presence of low entities. Behind the thrones there is an eloquent structure: two black crosses on special stands. This is an element of psychological pressure. It is easy to guess for whom those are intended.

Oh well, if it has to be a fight, we shall fight. We have gotten ourselves into it. With a mental effort we turn over the crosses on our chests. We know that the inscription "Save and Protect" will protect us in the battle. We are not alone either. Behind us there is the seventeenth legion of Power which belongs to the Lord. He Himself is also above us together with the Mother of God. They have settled in the spheres, surrounded by angels and saints. Blessing us for battle. They say its outcome will determine what is going to happen to the Earth for the next thousand years.

Igor and I are in armor and fully armed. He is the rider and I am the horse, Pegasus as usual. A double-headed eagle alights on Igor's shoulder, and a lion appears down at my side.

Two great forces, whose struggle pushes mankind along the spiral of evolution, have met in a deadly fight for the Earth.

Above the rows of the dark forces a huge raven soars up. Our eagle flies up to meet him. They meet at the very center of the Bardo channel, and their chests sent sparks flying from the impact, as if both birds were made of metal. The battle for the skies did not start very well for the eagle. He started losing strength and spiraling down. Igor sends some force and energy of his own. The snow-white bird revives and throws itself back into battle, started beating the enemy with its beaks (it's a two-headed bird!) and its wings. The raven and the eagle fight for a long time, until the light bird gathers its strength. Finding an advantageous angle the eagle hits the raven so that the latter tumbles down wings over heels. Black Knight watches the fall with dismay, but does not lend his assistant even a spark of personal force. He considers that his fight is the only one that will determine the outcome and does not want to waste his power on a secondary fight. Meanwhile, as the raven comes to the center of the cross, it crashes and burns.

And so the skies were held by the Lord.

Now a wolf rushes forward from the dark troops: it is the gatekeeper of the Gates of Hell. The powerful lion rushes to meet it in great strides. They clash, and the lion flies from the center of the cross. The wolf crowds it, pushing with its chest and tearing at it with its fangs. And following the wolf, step by step the ranks of the Dark Forces advance.

Igor decided again to support the lion with some of his energy. The animals are fighting, roaring in rage, and the situation gradually changes. Now the lion is crowding the wolf. The gray one runs off and hides among the nonhumans. The lion jumps after him in the heat of battle.

A moment later he returns victoriously. But there is something alarming in his powerful leaps. Just a moment ago he was tired and starting to weaken. Literally just a few meters before our ranks, Igor lowers the wall of the fourth unearthly force in front of him. The lion turns into a wolf as he hits it. Immediately the real lion breaks free from the ranks of the enemy and rushes towards his adversary. He is enraged by the deceptive, non-knight-like behavior of the enemy and bites the hellish monster stunned by its encounter with unknown force right at the throat. He tears hell's gatekeeper, throws him around on the ground and drags him, barely alive, to the dark ranks. Gathering his strength he tosses the defeated enemy up and throws him towards the three black thrones.

The outcome of the fight is decided. It is not allowed to finish off the wolf – it would upset the balance of the primary forces. Now everything that lives under the ground will be the wolf's domain, and everything that is above it will follow the lion.

And no matter how important the first two victories have been, the main battle is to take place now. Igor has already twice given some of his strength and energy to help out the eagle and the lion. I know that doing so was correct. We could not leave our comrades without help. But would we now have enough strength to overcome the powerful and experienced Black Knight?

So we set out towards each other. The black horse and I circle around the cross, and with our hooves we shape the even circumference of the tournament landing.

On the planet only a few suspect that this battle is taking place. While Armageddon is playing out in the heavens, the unsuspecting people keep at their small affairs of going to work and running about their business in general. Only a few know how in the information field of the Earth the main flows of future events are being reshaped.

The Black Knight hits Igor, and his magical sword strikes sparks out of the armor. The protection holds, but Igor sways and nearly faints. The black horse, shaped out of a murder of crows with black magic, redoubles its efforts. It is pushing, trying to force me out of the circle. I become enraged. I push back. It seems as though Igor has regained his senses; he flares up his spirit by the force of will and directs a barrage of heavy blows at his opponent. The swords clang, raining blows on the armor and the shields. Already the sword plunges into the black body of the horse, and stays in it, so that the open wound would not let out the crows, which would then reassemble into the monster that devours space and time. The horse falls over as its rider jumps off.

Then the Black Knight turns into a dragon. The old legend again comes alive, and the spiral way that was shown to men by Christ is again barred by the poisonous maw of the Primal Serpent. In the circle, where in the center of the cross the whirlwinds of Heaven and Earth have come together in four dimensions of space, the events of the ancient mystery are underway. Igor hits the dragon with the spear. But it is very difficult to penetrate its armor. Igor is pushing with the last of his strength. Just the fury and fighting fervor keep him going. He stands up in the stirrups, and the weight of his body drives the spear into the defeated monster. The blow of the spear, armed with divine lightning instead of steel, the path of the initial creation was opened, returning Earth to Heaven. "And the dying serpent bit the white horse, then exhaled its hellish fire and crashed into the bottomless pit, where it was torn apart by its own kin, who devoured its power and immortality". Nicely said, isn't it? Just in the spirit of the ancient Russian traditions. However, the white horse is me. And for some reason I am not feeling any pain from the poisonous bite. But this is not the most important thing. Right now I am overflowing with joy and jubilation. With the toppled dragon an important stage of human evolution has been completed; the day of the second coming of Christ has come closer!

The rest was easy to foresee. When the two armies engaged, barely a third of the nonhumans were left, and they fled into the underground levels.

The seventeenth legion of the Power, angels, saints– everyone is jubilant. Helmets are thrown into the air. The warriors yell: "Glory!" And The Lord Himself wipes a tear from his cheek from excitement. Armageddon, on the outcome of which vents for the next thousand years depended, is completed, with the full and unequivocal victory of the forces of Light.

A golden light shines from above on Igor and me. Something is happening. The Lord himself stood up and is waiting for something. We stand next to the center of the circle where we fought. The main pillar of light shines down on the center of the cross. Something appears there. Along the perimeter where the black horse and I marked the tournament circumference with our hooves, the signs of the Zodiac line up. The first one is the sign of Sagittarius. There is a ray of energy stretching from it to Igor. Igor dismounts Pegasus. He is drawn towards Sagittarius. I lose the appearance of the horse and once again become a human wearing an academic cloak.

There is a ray of energy extending from me to the center. It extends from me, not towards me. It appears in the center of my chest and stretches to the center of the cross, where in the flow of the shining coming down from above a powerful double-headed human being appears – an Androgyne. He has the torso of an ancient God; one of the heads is male and the other is female. This being represents the harmony of the two great original forces of the universe and the beginning of the Golden Age that had been purported to be lost; for which humanity has been waiting to return for a long time. Next to him the ominous figures 666 are blazing with fire. For an instant they burned clearly and firmly, but suddenly they were turned upside down, signifying the new meaning of events. Now three nines are burning in the center of the circle strongly confidently and magnificently – 999. For the first time the two opposites of the world are harmoniously combined in one archetypal symbol, determining the development of subsequent events on Earth.

The Androgyne stands up and all the levels suddenly reverse. The dark ones come on top and the light ones move down. Another rotation, and what was on the right turns to the left, and vise versa. What was dark is immediately lightened by the Holy Spirit.

Everyone around is jubilant again, throwing whatever they have to throw into the air.

The new Human-God looks in our direction, and Igor and I exchange glances. It seems that our height is too pompous, we look like giants. The Androgyne addresses us:

– You have accomplished the mission that was entrusted to you by God the Father, the Son and the Holy Spirit. You have achieved everything honestly, in the way of knights, without tricks or deception. For that, you are granted divine power, and there is no doubt that you will use it to save the Earth and for the benefit of people.

His voice rumbles like thunder and rolls far across space.

– We are now connected by an unbreakable bond, and at any time you may call on me for help. You are worthy of this honor and this glory. There is much work ahead of you, and you will have to learn a lot. I believe that you will not be intimidated by future dangers. I bless you in your endeavors.

Again everyone rejoices and shouts: "Glory!" Something sweeps us up from above and starts pulling towards itself. We are flying, surrounded by angels. The Creator Himself is standing in a cloud. The ray that had come down on us from above was coming from His hand. We kneel in front of the Lord. He sits down on the throne.

Angels bring a gold bowl with water and golden towel. We carefully wash the feet of the Creator with holy water and dry them with the golden towel. He smiles and regards Igor and me as if we were His sons. He does not look at all like the images we used to see in church icons. Certainly over thousands of years the artists – both the icon painters and secular

379

ones, of varying talent and professional level – have depicted the Almighty in different ways. But here He is in front of us, and we are aware that in every previous depiction of Him there is His true Likeness.

The Creator stretches His hand out to us, and we take turns kissing his ring, whose stone is gleaming with multitude of colors.

– You may now stand to the right of Me, – directs the Creator.

We stand where we are told and, despite all our height, we barely reach the knees of all those who are standing there already. We are still little. This word "little" is spoken with gentle sympathy by those standing next to God, and it reverberates in our consciousness. We understand that in this world the height is determined by real actions and deeds. When will we grow tall?

The Creator is benevolent:

– From now on, this place will be like your own home to you. And you can be on Earth.

Igor answers for both of us:

– We must fulfill what we promised.

The Creator is satisfied by the answer.

– Bring truth to the people, – he instructs us. – Have no doubt in anything.

We kiss the hand, the cross. The Creator Himself crosses us three times.

We proffer our thanks and return to the levels. Someone suggests that I need to be washed with the dead and living water to counteract the effects of the venomous bite.

We go to level seven. We request permission to bathe in the dead water. Permission is granted. Igor pours the dead water over my thigh where the dragon bit me. Six black beads roll out of the wound and dissolve in the dead water. That's it, I am free, free from the ominous six, the six heads of the dragon, of my ambiguous role in the game of patience of the dark forces. I defeated my dragon in the center of the labyrinth at the border between the words. No one can have any claim on me other than myself. And only my heart, my soul and my consciousness from now on define my actions and deeds. And still – the lofty word "Responsibility". My actions ought to be equal to the power that has been granted to me. In this respect, it is easier for Igor – he had not had the six black poisonous beads in him to start with. He had not grown six dragon heads on his body.

But it is easier only in this respect. With respect to everything else, by the will of God the Father, the Son and the Holy Spirit, we have the same lot, the same fate, and the same responsibility. Neither he nor I are afraid of it. We know that God the Father, the Son and the Holy Spirit are now always with us, and we are with Them. Amen!

* * *

Now it was possible to reflect on what has happened. The events we saw and took part in corresponded to an ancient prophecy that it would befall Russia to become the field of the battle of the Gods in the year following the End of Times. The End of Times was in 1999, the end of the cosmic cycle. And the eclipse that occurred announced this to the creation and everyone who was made knowledgeable of the essence of the ancient prophesies. The end of the world was in 2000, the year of the millennium, the year of change that has been viewed by many as a direct physical process could have easily occurred if events had taken a different turn. The outcome of Armageddon determined everything.

For hundreds of years the dark and light forces had been preparing for this decisive battle. On Earth people were carefully selected, in whom, through a series of sequential incarnations, specific character traits were developed. Those were the people who entered the annals of history and left quite a noticeable mark. Their names are known to everyone: monarchs, military commanders, outstanding religious leaders, scientists, writers. Once the average number of incarnations of the people currently alive reached the number of 13, and when the ominous figure 666 was stamped on the foreheads of men, the duration of the redemption of Christ and the Earth, bought back by His suffering, blood and life was a no man's land once again.

The dark forces had been insolent and arrogant after the previous Armageddon, which ended in their complete victory, and they had no doubt that this time they would have the upper hand in the battle again. At their disposal were the knowledge and all the advances of civilization; black magic and the energy of the people whom they had molested by filling them with material values without spiritual development.

Russia, which entered in the beginning of the XX century an extremely important incarnation for this purpose, and which successfully completed the painful act of birth in the bloody events of the revolution, had become the place where the new God-person was predicted to appear. This is where the prophesies of Vladimir Solovyov, Evgeniy Trubetskoy and other seekers of the truth had come true.

It was specifically to bring it about that the Holy Trinity had in advance created a special spiritual structure which was included into the state symbol of Russia – St. George the Dragon Slayer.

And so the prophecy has come true. The slogan written on the ring of St. George the Dragon Slayer, „Honor and Dignity", is shining over Russia. It was Russia's regal bird (the two-headed eagle) that fought next to

God's warrior. It was in Russia's Bardo channel of fine material space that the great victory was won. It was due to Russia's sons that the ominous number 666 was turned around and signified a new code for humanity: 999.

Evil's power is now limited, but dangerous years are still ahead. The tentacles of evil have penetrated the souls of the people too deeply, but it is not so simple to cut them off. Because free will is still given to man, and he is the only one who can decide whether to follow the winners via the difficult road of the ascension or to stay with those who so vigorously encouraged all the human weaknesses – lust, drunkenness, envy, greed, betrayal and professed betrayal, arrogance, etc. – and instigated the people to break their promises and find self-justification in all cases.

The last of the above-mentioned temptations is probably the most treacherous! We so loathe criticism, instructions, even the slightest comments! „Who is he to tell me what to do? How can he understand my soul, my sufferings, my desires?" – this excuse is the mildest one. Even the person with the most deceitful soul and the weakest spirit considers that in reality, potentially, he could easily be the „chairman of the whole globe". It's just that luck was too fickle and too many conniving enemies were around. Besides, the times are not so good for real men, it is various crooks who insinuate themselves into power. It's quite a consolatory position! But the treacherous part is that outward humility proves to be simply the other side of the same coin, the same sin of arrogance. Our ancestors knew that and coined the precise description: humility more than pride.

A truly distinguished personality knows his place in life and his value. Mikhail Lomonosov wrote to his patron Shuvalov (letter is dated 19 January 1761): „Not only do I not play the fool at the table of eminent nobility, nor any rulers on Earth, but even for the Lord God Himself, Who granted me my mind, lest He take it away from me". What is this – pride, blasphemy? No, it's the dignity of a working man chosen by the fates, proud of his mission, before his destiny. Without such an attitude towards life, great achievements are impossible. It is for good reason it is believed that another Russian genius, Pushkin, knew this letter of Lomonosov by heart.

Therefore, I regard the fine material events that have been revealed to Igor Arepyev and me via clairvoyance as a kind of learning process, with the help of which we gained access to secret knowledge. It seems impossible to gain it any other way – only through the test of the mirror-lined sphere of one's own consciousness.

But I would like to say again that as long as a person is inside the sphere, as long as he lacks the capacity to leave the limits of three-dimensional space – he will never be able to cope with this on his own without having any help nor specialized knowledge. Only after exiting the limits of the sphere of the three-dimensional material world it is possible to regard your consciousness sort of from the outside, looking at that mirror ball. Find out what is filling it, what problems are there, what mice are running in that head. What about you – can you see what mice are running in your head? Well, not in the literal sense, of course. You understand that there is some allegory behind this statement. The mice running around in one's head – it means I have a disease, I have this, that or something else, or a predisposition to it – tophus, for example. This conviction of a person is received by some sort of consciousness reflector, which creates a problem and immediately superimposes it on itself, multiplies the symptoms at the level of the body. And in reality on the skin of some woman some spots break out like a rash, the protective functions of the skin are disrupted, streptococci enter the body, etc. The same occurs at the planetary level. The noosphere – what is happening to it? This is where the consciousnesses of everything that exists and of everything that possesses consciousness are arranged – which includes minerals, animals, plants and, of course, humans. Actually, humans – first and foremost. Some levels form and acquire a rather stable form of existence. In general, as I said, – these are the levels of consciousness. But the material structure of their manifestation is supported by energy-informational toroids that appear due to the elementary particles spinning around their axes. Those toroids are globally initiated by water, snow, ice and mineral crystals – including sand.

So the first level is everyday functioning consciousness. The next level you may conditionally classify as a „magical country".

„The magical country" reflects a certain path that humanity has traveled, sort of its level of the world outlook, when each brook, each tree, each event – everything was associated with some unknown spiritual forces and was personified in the form of gods, in myths, in whatever. So here, at these levels, you can find the same thing – whatever. If you get here using your consciousness, you are certainly in for some encounters. Well, to put is as precisely as possible, likes attract here. For example, if you have a pugnacious character, and you want to have a wrestling match with someone to test your respective strengths – you will find all these adventures here. And if you like Greek mythology, you run a chance of encountering a Cyclops or some kind of a similar monster. If you prefer Russian fairy tales, there is Baba Yaga and Gorynych the Dragon. I want to give you a proper orientation with that – don't think that this is some virtual arrangement that has nothing to do with reality. Why? Because as soon as you touch a phantom with your consciousness – and this is indeed, up to a certain moment, a phantom and nothing else, but when you touch it with your consciousness, it stops being simply a phantom, it becomes a character equal to yourself in the training program in which you are now

385

involved. In principle, this is also a training program, like the Earth and what happens there. All this is a training program for humanity.

But you must perceive the events not superficially, at the level of the pattern of external events. Let's look, for example, at the new character in our story: the Androgyne. Why did it appear? For what purpose? To what events is he the key as an archetypal image?

There is an ancient legend about the Androgyne. That this allegorical character is a being that combines the male and female origin. It is stated, that the Androgyne was harmonious, whole, that it had outstanding powers and capabilities. But once upon a time, the Father of the Gods, Zeus, took up his sword and cut the Androgyne into pieces. Thus men and women appeared, and the wholeness of the humans was lost.

How should we perceive this legend – as a pretty made-up story or as a cosmogony that has quite real meaning and sense? Personally, I perceive it as the latter. I see in this legend quite a definite methodology for creating the world and humans. Let me tell you how I see this.

Human life starts with two reproductive cells: the ovum and the sperm. By uniting they become a single organism. In ancient wisdom, this embryonic cell is usually shown as a circle divided in two. One half of this circle is dark and the other is light. But this is at the micro-level. At the micro-level – this is the first of the generations. Also this is the abyss when the path is created. At that, the dark half of the circle does not mean that it is bad. This is female energy. That area accumulates stable features and attributes, important to future development, in order to pass them on to the offspring organism.

In ancient times, there was the concept that the embryonic cells already have the prototypes of the future child, which, in turn, enclose within them their future children.

Nikolay Kuzanskiy, one of the most astute medieval philosophers, in his work „On Scholarly Ignorance" (M., 1979, vol. 1, pp. 50-95), investigating the concept of trinity in unity, also pointed out this strange circumstance: „The Father is not before the Son, and the Son is not after the Father; the Father precedes the Son only in such a way that the Son comes no later than Him. If the Father is the first person, the Son is the second but not after him, but in the same way the Father is the first person without preceding, the Son is the second person without following; and in the same way the third person is the Holy Spirit".

How should this be applied to our research?

It is known that the program of life is inherited. Genes are the carriers. Genes, being discrete units, never mix with each other. This is a very important quality, and it explains a lot. From the original starter cell the organism starts to build. But first in that cell itself the DNA spiral needs to be built where all genetic information necessary to support and continue the life of the organism is encoded. It is that moment of prototype cell DNA building that the legend about the Androgyne reflects – a single body from which from which two threads of deoxyribonucleic acid molecule appear. In the course of differential dyeing, cross-striping appears on the chromosomes, so-called disks or bands which carry their specific information. They are similar to beads on the DNA threads. The threads are connected between themselves by four types of nitrogen-containing compounds which are called bases, which form sort of an endless ladder, the ladder of our life. Maybe that's what Nikolay Kuzanskiy wrote about in the above-mentioned work, meaning both the microcosm of a man and the microcosm of the Universe: „Whenever I say „Unity is the maximum", that I already express the trinity. Because when I say „unity" I name the beginning that has no beginning; by saying „maximum" I name

387

the original origin; connecting and tying the two by the bond „is" I name something that emanates from both. The maximum is whole because the minimum, the maximum and the connection are one, therefore the unity itself is minimal, maximal, and unifying…".

And further on he wisely suggested: „The visible is indeed the image of the invisible… You can see the Creator in the creation as if in the mirror and the likeness". Because „any image is obviously striving to repeat its prototype".

How many centuries did it take so that symbols and signs behind the myths, legends and allegories would become visible, leading to the truth? And the labyrinth of yet another myth, the one about the Minotaur – is it not the reflection of our endless search for ourselves in the spirals of the DNA? We most thoroughly research the endless Jacob's ladder – we probe, measure and weigh its elements, not understanding that the minimum and maximum are infinite, and are united besides. And that the knowledge obtained in such a manner would be valid only in the land of the blind. Meanwhile this land is drifting into the past already now, today. You need to hurry in order to understand and see.

What else can be added to that – perhaps just a wish: „Wake up, sleepers of the Land of Shadows! The prophecy has come true. And now everyone can decide for himself what he wants to be – a person or a shadow of the person imagining it is God-man. Now, the way to becoming a true God-man is now open, but it is the way of service, creativity and spirituality. The state of being a true God-man has to be deserved!"

* * *

The next day my internal vision screen flatly refused to activate. That was strange, for one could have counted on exactly the opposite. Igor and I decided to call my student Tamara so that she would help us figure this out. I sat downcast next to them and tried to guess what my transgressions were.

Something odd is happening at the levels. Sometimes odd spheres pass floating by, or a frog hops around wearing a crown. Igor and Tamara are telling me what they see. Their internal vision screens show that I am with them. I am wearing a black robe and an academic hat. As for myself I cannot see anything, so Igor holds me by the hand, and Tamara follows us at a short distance as a backup.

Suddenly, a clock hand started rotating around me, as if I were the center of a clock. There are hints all around: the time is passing by, and what are you thinking about? A black bird appears from somewhere. Rivers of mud flow from the levels. That is not surprising, for only yesterday evil spirits were ruling here. The mudslide carries Igor and myself into a pit. We struggle, but what should we do to get out? Igor is holding me – he will not abandon me.

Someone else is stretching a hand towards me. Igor warns me: don't touch it, it has claws, it's something evil. Tamara from above confirms:

– It's some kind of a devil.

Igor manages to strike the clawed hand, and the demon jerks it away with a scream. Tamara above fashions a rope with the power of thought and lowers it to us into the pit. Then she pulls us up to the surface. We are covered in mud leaking off of us. We need to go to the dead and live water to cleanse ourselves. As we walk, crowds of imps and devils move towards us. We are covered in mud and they are paying no attention to us Some of them ask:

– Have you seen the Seeing One? We need to find the Seeing One.

Everything can still be changed.

I am still blind. Igor is dragging me along by the hand. What Seeing One are they looking for? Could it be me? But I am blind. And why am I blind today?

– So that they would not find you, – Igor explains.

– They are looking for me? Am I the Seeing One?

– It wouldn't be me, would it, – Igor grumbles good-naturedly. – Why do you think I am acting with such certainty – because I can read this information off you. I don't know why, but you take to this space like fish to water. You know everything, as if you were born here.

We are passing again through throngs of evil spirits, who are leaving to go down to their new levels.

– The Seeing One, where is the Seeing One? – they cry to each other.

We keep silent and grunt, push, go against the flow and Tamara is flying above us as a guardian angel. Finally we get to Bardo channel. Immediately it becomes easier. We rise to level seven. Ask permission to use the water. Wash ourselves. Tamara looks at us and says that we have become small again. This satanic dirt turned out to be very harmful to us. We need to go through purification at the Earth level as well.

That same day, the three of us went to the Holy Trinity-St. Sergius Lavra. We went to the temple of St. Sergius of Radonezh and placed candles there. Then we went to the source of holy water across from the Ascension Cathedral. The visit to the gate church, to Father Superior Herman, where we spend several hours kneeling completes our trip.

When we were leaving the temple and kissing the cross, we wanted to tell Father Herman about Armageddon. But the crowds were pushing from every side. And how would we explain our joy in passing? Would he believe us, would he understand? Even though we saw him among the priests sending the troops off to battle and blessing Igor and me with holy water, it was possible that he had no idea he was among the chosen. He has no internal vision screen. He just heard the voice within and trusted it. And was he told about us? It could all turn out rather silly. So we left a good person without saying a word.

The next day, we decided to figure out the situation with the levels. Kirill joined us. He already knows about the events and demonstrates his loyalty strenuously.

– Lapshin is an idiot. It was all in his hands, but he wanted it for himself alone, he wanted to get ahead just by himself, – Kirill accused his former boss.

– You are not afraid to scold him? – I ask the boy, who is at least five million years old.

– I have more authority than he does, – lashes back Kirill. – I come from the Beginning of the Beginnings, from the Spirit.

He makes a meaningful face, trying to increase his importance.

– From what Spirit? Would that be from the Holy One? – I clarify.

He is silent, snapping his eyes about. We decided still to take him along to the levels. It's hostile territory. We don't want to get muddy all over again. Let him look out for himself, and we will see through his internal vision screen.

So, we start. Six of my students follow Kirill, observing him via the internal vision screen. So that he wouldn't think up any tricks. Kirill goes into his former element and reports:

– The levels' configuration is completely different now. Two pyramids are joined at the base at the Earth level. Along one diagonal in the shape of a figure 8, there are nine levels above and nine below. Along the other diagonal of the sign of infinity there are six levels above and below. In the center, they are connected with a cross.

He winces slightly at saying the word „cross", but controls himself.

– With what shall we start our study?

– Let's start with the new, six-level structures, – I reply. – We are already familiar with the nine-level ones.

Kirill obediently goes via Bardo channel to the six-level structures. The first level up is an informational one. There are twelve gates. All are sealed with the Seal of the Creator.

– I am not going there, –Kirill states, trying his best to demonstrate his loyalty to the legitimate powers of the Cosmos.

– Nobody is asking you to, – I dispel his doubts.

– The second level, – he continues the tour, – has the male and female energies. There are four doors there. One pair of energies is light, and the other pair is dark. There is no interaction so far. The gates are sealed up.

Since the gates are sealed up, everything is clear. We shall not go there.

– On level three, there are 12 small gates; they connect with each other by images, like an hour-glass. These are the gates of the signs of the Zodiac.

– Go higher, – I urge the tamed demon.

– Level four has three doors on each side, right and left. They are sealed up as well. There are dark and light energies there.

– Higher.

– Level five has three gates. One is white, one is black, the third one is silver. These are the three colors of the Creator, as on His staff, and the seals on the gates are His seals as well. There are holy symbols here as well, and a rainbow.

How does he know about the Creator's staff?

– Level six – this one is like the start-up generator. It sits above everything in the shape of a bulb. If it is activated– the levels will start functioning. And it is activated by the ray. But who has that ray? – Kirill asks spitefully.

We come out to the landing. A gigantic screen appears and shows information. On the right there are Satan, the Antichrist and a wolf. The wolf is Lapshin. His human face sometimes appears through the wolfish snarl and then fades again. The Antichrist is supposed to appear on Earth, but now it is difficult for him to reach the earthly plane. The previously planned path is destroyed. He will appear secretly, and it will only possible to discover him through personal communication.

The map of Russia appears. At its center there is a star and within it the numbers of the new code of humanity that are so pleasing to us – 999. In Moscow there are already several thousand people with this sign. And there are hundreds of thousands throughout Russia. Nowhere else in the world are there such multitudes of people with the new code of the new Man. They will save humanity.

The Antichrist must create obstacles to their activities. The calculation is that everyday life problems may dampen the main purpose of attaining the state of God-man, and that will make those people weaken. A lot depends on who is to lead them. Everyone is waiting for a general, a warrior whom people would follow. There are seven forces in the world, each of which has an Initiate heading it. Which of those will lead mankind?

Kirill conscientiously and in detail tells us everything he sees, without deception.

– There will be three in the lead, representing three forces – suddenly his voice begins to tremble. – I knew that. Lapshin is a bastard. I told him... He was thinking only about himself.

He is swearing, and those who followed him through the internal vision screen say that the big screen is showing images of Igor and me. It is not yet apparent who the third one is. The invectives spouted by the demon indicate better than any other words how serious his problems are.

– One of the two of you should become the top leader. Also there is the Antichrist. He still has not given up on the struggle. So it's too early to call it the end. What if you start fighting for power?

In the way he said that was so much hidden hope for just such an outcome that Igor and I felt pity towards him. Why did he decide that the third one will be the Antichrist? Perhaps it will be Christ? That would be somewhat more logical, at least for us. And why are we the leaders? What made him decide that? Might he be trying to lead us astray again?

The tour is finished. We ask the others to leave us alone in the room and thank them for their help. We need to think over the information and discuss it.

Once everybody leaves, Igor suddenly, instead of discussion, goes into clairvoyance mode again.

– We are being called, – he explains briefly.

– There is a circle there – he is telling me what he sees. – Within the circle there are three nines and a sign that looks like a T. You are with me again, wearing your robe and hat.

He says that I am next to him, but I still cannot see anything. I cannot get the clairvoyance ability to work.

– You need to enter into the center of the circle. The Androgyne is there. I am leading you by the hand.

– Lead on, – I say in agreement.

He brings me into the circle, right into the center.

– What is going on?

– You are joined with the Androgyne. The signs of the Zodiac are

394

around. I have entered the sign of Sagittarius. They are all rotating around you.

Down below are the levels. Information and energy have appeared there. They are filling everything up. There is also some kind of tree there. We enter it. We are carried up inside the trunk. Now we are among the branches. We are moving along the outline of a figure in a somewhat circular pattern. It feels like it could be a figure eight. This apple tree is the symbol of the division of the world into darkness and light, into the three dimensions of space – the Father, Son and Holy Spirit.

Now concerning time – the events are developing so quickly there that Igor barely manages to relay them.

– Now we have our own apple in this tree.

We are on the landing again. Someone is coming, he is enormous. Behind him on a string like two balloons – the Sun and the Moon. The familiar ring shines on his hand. This is the Creator. Igor says that He made the sign of the cross to us. We fall to our knees.

– Have we done everything correctly? – I ask.

– Yes, that was correct, – God the Father responds, the Father of the Gods. – You already possess that Holy Spirit, which helped you in your quest. For the victory you deserve a reward. You may choose between power and knowledge. What do you choose?

– Knowledge, – I say to Igor. And he agrees with me.

– From now on, you have been granted the Holy Spirit and the knowledge. Those will be with you until the third event occurs. Measure the strength given to you and the responsibility, that you have taken for the people and Earth as a whole, – solemnly says the Creator, as if the proceedings have some global significance which is yet unclear to us, which He wants to underscore with the intonation in advance.

– You are granted knowledge and abilities which are unusual for the people of the earth. By the power of your thought you will be able to heal others from the gravest illnesses, know future events in advance and see where good is and where evil is. Go forth and tell people the truth, as I have revealed it to you. And may the strength not leave you, and your mind be clear. Learn everything that is there in My Kingdom. From now on all doors are open to you. I bless you, go.

He turned around. Igor cries out after Him:

– Father, may we come with You?

The Creator stopped, turned around, and bent down to us from his unthinkable height.:

– You are always walking with Me, My children, and I with you. Don't fear anything. My protection is always with you. You need to work, study, gain knowledge. Go on. Both Christ and the Holy Spirit are protecting you as well.

Igor comes out from the different world.

– We need to have some tea, – he says. His face is pale and fatigued.

Kirill is stalking us in the hallway already:

– I want to talk to you, this is very important.

We go into a different room while the women are preparing the tea and setting the table.

– So, what cosmic problems have sprung up? – I ask.

Kirill is sitting in front of us, his face is serious.

– You probably think that I am from the dark side?

– And are you from the light side? – I deride him.

– You have seen, I travel around Bardo freely.

– Let's cut out this childish nonsense, – I ask. – You are five million years old. It is time to grow up.

– Five and a half, – corrects Kirill.

– All the more so, – Igor notes with a serious expression.

– Fine, – agrees Kirill. – There are two of you now. The rules of the game require that there be a third one. I propose myself.

– And the reasons are?

– You have everything now except one thing. You do not know where to go. You are alpha and omega. There is infinity between you. Which one of you knows how to go through it?

Igor and I exchange glances. He is an interesting boy, very interesting, but he is right: we do not know. We do not know yet. But do we need a third one like him?

– You want to jump on the bandwagon at the right time?

– Exactly, – he confirms. – And there is another problem you don't know about.

– So?

– The Confederation.

– What is that?

– Have you seen Star Wars on TV?

– Yes, as it happens.

– Very similar. There is a space fleet, laser weapons. I have the red button to call up the fleet. They are ready to interfere. They are unhappy with the course of events. I could push it at any moment.

– Look what a cute child we have here, –I say to Igor. – In his little baby vest pocket he has the little red button that would destroy the Earth. And he seriously threatens to push it if we don't give him a ride on our wagon. Imagine a sixteen-year-old kid sitting there threatening an academician to blow up the Earth. One shouldn't frighten an old weak man in such a way

– You call yourself old and weak? –Kirill moves on the offensive. – For you there is no difference now, whether it is one hundred years or one hundred billion! And your arms are stronger than steel now. Weak? – he repeats again. – And who toppled the Black knight?

– Not I, – I raise my hand in protest even though the sweet ecstasy of the remembrance of our victory is already spilling within me. – That was Igor. He is so… wild...

But still, what is this strange boy talking about? What billions of years?

– Well, so everything has changed now: the control system, the levels. They still need to be activated. The Earth cannot exist in disequilibrium. At any time nuclear war could break out or some other global problem. Do you know how to activate them? And where to stand for control - on the right, on the left, on the top, on the bottom?

– We already activated them, –I cannot help boasting. – And for some reason the Center is missing from your list. It's right between the top and the bottom.

Kirill pales, and immediately activates his clairvoyance. He checks the information concerning the levels.

– Yes, the process is underway, – he agrees reluctantly.

There is a knock at the door. Nina Andreyevna stands in the doorway.

– That's enough talking, boys. The tea is getting cold.

What interesting dialogues are coming up. Events are obviously making someone nervous, some confederation. What kind of a zit on the body of creation is that? May it be some evil galactic civilization? I have a feeling we will hear about it again, and more than once.

398

Chapter 10

Just as the Creator promised, all gates were open before us. And at each gate we were greeted by a holy man. There are many gates. Today we choose the one with the Sun depicted on it. The gate is large and made of iron. There is an elder with a staff at the gate, waiting. I am wearing the academic robe again. Igor is wearing a loose white shirt.

We greet him. We kneel, and he blesses us.

– Why have you come? – he asks.

– For knowledge, – we reply.

The elder says that we are allowed to enter the Kingdom of God, because the Creator himself let us in here. We enter the gate. There is a garden within. We stop at the wall.

– We need knowledge of medicine, – we specify.

– To you the gift of God is given, and you are acting directly from the power of God, – he reminds us.

– We are interested in cancer diseases. How to neutralize the tumors once metastases have already appeared? – we ask, understanding too late that our question belittles our capabilities, about which we would be told without constraint. But the holy man is not arguing, even though it is obvious that he is upset by our lack of understanding.

– Look at the wall, – he says. A screen appears on the wall. – The cancer is similar to a foreign body, a tick that is lodged within the organism. This tick needs to be removed – its body and every limb. Then it needs to be neutralized. Then every cell needs to be healed, – the elder explains, and images appear on the wall illustrating the healing process.

– Here is the throat, there is the tick. The tumor is like jelly. What is on the right is normal. What is on the left is affected by disease. We make this tick transparent. It breaks down the small cells first, then the large ones. At the informational level it really is a tick. Here it squirts its poison into the nucleus. And that makes the cell uncontrollable.

Your task is to take the divine silver color and discolor the cancerous tumor. Have you discolored it? Now we can see a fine spider web, a nucleus, a liquid. Fill it with energy now, fill it again.

Tie the leg with a thread and pull it towards yourself so that it would not dig itself into another cell. Do the same with the other legs, too. Pull the tick out at the cellular, informational, and energy levels. Is it out? Tie the silver thread around it and destroy it. Treat each of the damaged cells with a silver ray. Spot by spot. Illuminate the red areas that have not been treated yet with the norm. Treat them. Check the norm – there are red cells again. Repeat the treatment, don't be lazy. Overimpose the norm again. The red is still not completely gone. Repeat the treatment.

Use the norm one more time. There is no margin for error. Enhance the norm. Look, the cells are now identical to the healthy ones. Set the time for healing, say, one month, and after that apply the enhanced norm again.

– How much time does the cure take?

– Usually about two to three weeks. If you superimpose the enhanced norm again, you will destroy the remaining cancer cells. Sometimes they hide very skillfully. That's why you need to control.

– And how do we accomplish organ regeneration?

– Look, – the elder continues the lecture. – Let's take, for example, a kidney. The first task would be to restore the interaction of the kidney with the urogenital system and the adrenal glands. Take the enhanced norm and overlay it. Take the silver thread and affect the kidneys directly. On top install the program for health enhancement and healing. Then, using the silver color, we shatter the stones and remove them along the canal to the bladder.

Now comes the main part... Using the silver thread, we restore the cells in the kidney so that new young cells will appear. The old cells die off, the new ones are created. We create them anew, you see? We take the enhanced norm and overlay it on the pathological area. We see in the right kidney that cells are dying. We restore the cells, apply the enhanced norm. Now we take the silver thread and start the process of energy cleaning.

We follow up a week later. There are still problems. Again we take the enhanced norm. We apply the program for health enhancement and healing. We work a little using the silver thread. That's all. Any questions?

– And can we hear about the gallbladder?

– About the gallbladder which you do not have, – the elder notes, pointing his staff at me. – The gallbladder on the right has been removed. We take the enhanced norm and apply the silver thread. We activate the program for health enhancement and healing via the pituitary body. Now we have to create the external form – this is a hologram. And now the internal. The process of cell division needs to be activated so that the new cells fill out the new form. I repeat: with the right hand we take the silver thread and create the external shell; this is now complete. We take the norm. There is a gap on the bottom. We repair it. Take the enhanced norm.

With the beam we create the internal structure. We overlay the norm, check. We restore the bile. Overlay the norm, there is not enough bile. Take the norm. Apply. Check. This is all. The program for health enhancement and healing via the pituitary gland. The timeframe is fifteen days. Take the enhanced norm, apply. There are gaps. We repair. We enhance the silver thread. We apply the norm. Interaction is under way. The program is complete.

Another elder appears nearby. We look at his hand – there is the familiar ring. We fall to our knees. He lifts us up. And sort of continues the lecture. He says how we should relate to money, power, and health. He advises that we need to have our own opinion on any issue and that any situation needs to be assessed and resolved without doubting our own actions.

– You must not be proud, – He instructs. – Don't let your future blind you. Everything always needs to be evaluated from three sides– from the left, from the right, and from the middle. Then you make the decision – that's the fourth action.

We kiss His hand. He makes the sign of the cross at us and disappears. We agree with what He said.

It's a strange type of learning, unusual. Just to think who is teaching us! Any medical professional would read these pages and say: this is drivel. Meanwhile, Igor and I are seeing the patients twice a week with just those diseases that are taught to us in the celestial academy. And the strange thing is that they really do recover.

Neither I nor Igor ever studied even the basics of medicine. And can this really be considered treatment? We do not touch the body – we do not cut, do not disturb, do not prescribe pills. We just look and see how another person's organism functions, issue commands to an organ, and the organ obeys us. People get healed – even if they are blind and deaf. Later they stay in our Center as if it were their own home and try to help in any way they can. The relatives of the cured and the patients themselves every day bring us pies, fruit, other gifts. They know: we returned life to them, which medical science had denied them, helplessly throwing up its hands.

So many people die in the hospitals – and the physicians are not held responsible for anything! And here we see completely the diagnoses that do not offer any hope – and a fast cure. It is not even possible to accuse us

402

of anything, since the final official sentences had been issued to all these people. The only thing possible to do is to pretend not to notice us, which is what the representatives of conventional medicine do. Here is one of the typical cases from our practice. Anastasia Kvakova is an 18-year-old girl from St. Petersburg. Rapid deterioration of her health forced her to seek medical help from doctors. A medical examination discovered a brain tumor, which made the physicians bring up the question of urgent surgery. The horror of the need to have her head opened pushed Anastasia away from giving consent, which she was being pressured to give. She was being coerced, but time after time the girl refused to make the final decision.

Meanwhile, the disease kept progressing: Anastasia's vision was weakening, her field of vision became narrow due to growths on her eyeballs. After that followed problems with her gastrointestinal tract. And new diagnoses: a duodenal ulcer, a stomach ulcer. Some time after that, unbearable pains in the heart appeared, accompanied by regular fainting spells. The last consolation the physicians delivered to Anastasia was their sentence of sterility.

The girl had a very hard time coping with this slew of illnesses affecting her and admits she was on the verge of losing her mind.

It is hard to say how the events would have progressed had it not been for a chance conversation with a friend, who had read an article in a newspaper about our Center.

And so Anastasia, all but against the wishes of her relatives, came to Moscow, to our Center. Three months later, her brain tumor disappeared. Both ulcers, in the stomach and in the intestines, vanished without a trace. The heart function returned to normal; normal vision returned as well. It is hard to believe, but some pages of this book were typed on the com-

403

puter by the very same Anastasiaя Kvakova, whose eyes were no longer covered by the horrible growths.

As it turns out, it is possible to cure the brain from a tumor without sawing the skull apart and to heal the ulcers without slashing the body with a scalpel. Everything is possible if you do not hinder but help those who are capable of doing it in accordance with the will of Providence.

Now Anastasia is studying in the first year of the Law School of the Engineering and Economics University of St. Petersburg. And who would be able to say, looking at this merry, sociable, pretty girl, that just a year ago her life was with a certainty turning towards disability, an unbearable existence and perhaps even death.

But the physicians who were pushing her to undergo surgery do not even know that, contrary to their professional convictions, Anastasia Kvakova regained her health without scalpels and medications. It is Anastasia's health that now separates her as an insurmountable wall from those who still believe that it is only possible to cure a person by cutting off his organs or poisoning his body with kilograms of medications. It feels as if within the same space two parallel universes coexist, and things possible in one are utterly not permissible in the other.

We started working with the autistic child, Misha. Now we seem to have the necessary knowledge. And it is working. The mother is noting more and more positive changes in her son. But this work is very difficult, at the level of human consciousness.

Our deaf girl Dasha can already hear. And she speaks much better, too. She has begun studying at a medical college. Another piece of good news is that her internal vision screen has been activated. Now she can see for herself everything that we are doing with her and is learning to work in the fine plane. Soon a fine specialist will appear at the Center.

However, not always are we capable of helping people so successfully. Sometimes we are flatly advised against doing so. As a rule, the bans extend to people who have committed a lot of bad, horrible deeds in their lives.

But there are other reasons as well. Once a woman came to the Center. She did not come alone but brought her husband. Both were scientists. They were tense in the extreme. They conversed in a very strict manner, as if they were auditors.

– What is this strange methodology of treatment? Why have we never heard about anything similar before? – This is what she asks. It gives you the impression that she is trying to be intimidating with her unsmiling, accusing facial expression. – Prove to me that you are capable of this. I do not believe it! This is not clear to me!

For a whole hour I was delivering to them a lecture on how we work. Something thawed within them, but not very much.

I apologize for not being able to deal with their education alone at the moment, that I have a lot of things to do. A rebuke follows immediately.

– If you want us to undergo treatment with you, you should prove that you can perform your work better than others.

The situation is becoming downright absurd. It is interesting, if this couple were to go to a church and demand from the priest: „Prove to us that there is a God, and then we will put up a candle for Him and give you some small change for the needs of the temple", – would the priest agree to a deal like that? Most likely he would show them the door and explain that one ought to come to the temple when the soul calls you.

But we still invite the woman to a diagnostic session. When we look, we see small ulcerations in the stomach and some problem with one eye. Nothing serious that would require urgent intervention into her organism.

– No, you are not seeing it! I have cancer. I have already had surgery and am supposed to have another one. That's why I came to you – the biddy is „exposing" us.

We look again and again – but there is nothing to see. Finally, a black square floats out from behind her back and fully shields her from our attempts to diagnose the tumor. This is her consciousness. She came to us for help, but she does not believe that clairvoyance exists, that we can help her. She considers us to be quacks. This is her position of principle, and she is convinced of it.

As with any person, she has the right to her opinion and the right to follow it in life. Since for her clairvoyance does not exist – it means that a black wall appears between her consciousness and us.

We cannot help her. She must leave together with her principles, suspicions, ill-will, and... the cancerous tumor. She should go to an ordinary hospital – there they will cut off what they can and sew up whatever she wants. We can only feel pity on this woman from the parallel world. She already has no present. Perhaps she already has no future either. But who is to blame that she is so tightly limited both by a one-sided perception of reality? How can those whom she does not believe help her?

And we are still attending the celestial academy. We are taught how to work with vision, the heart, stomach, liver, prostate and spine. Once we are called up straight from the class to the landing that tops off the levels.

Something extraordinary is happening. Again all the high-ranking entities from above and from below are gathered. The Black Knight is standing with lowered head.

– This is the judgment, – we are told.

We kneel in front of the Holy Trinity. There is some sort of energy cloud above us. This is the Cosmic Mind. It is the entity that will now

406

announce the final verdict in connection with Armageddon. The decision is already made. This is just the announcement of the verdict.

The voice sounds from above. Everybody hears it differently, but everyone understands him in the same way.

The voice speaks about the Black Knight. About the fact that he lost the battle, he repeatedly violated the Great Laws of the Cosmos and therefore he will be imprisoned in the center of the Earth for three hundred years. The place where he will be located is to be sealed with a special cover with the seal of the Creator. And no one has the right to remove it. And as to who is going to be present on Earth from the side of the Dark Forces as a liaison to interact with the Light Forces has not yet been determined.

We did not consider the verdict unjust. Our victory was acknowledged. We were granted the right to safeguard the Earth, and we were allowed to always use what we had.

The Dark Knight disappeared. The rest followed suit. We remained alone on the landing. We did not even get a chance to thank anybody, we were so overwhelmed by the events.

Had I been there alone, I would have thought that I had lost my mind! But, first of all, I am not alone– dozens of people already are actively involved in developments. And what is done there is quite accurately reflected here. We really can help people in the most hopeless situations. Actually – and that is very strange – we can help others better than ourselves. On the other hand, we practically don't work on ourselves.

Kirill became very nervous. He demanded negotiations again and received them. Listen to what this sixteen-year-old boy said. I recorded his words practically verbatim. He already knew about the sentencing and began speaking at once.

– You call this the plan of God. And we call it cosmic idiocy.

407

Kirill is very handsome, intelligent and witty. But there is something demonic about him. He speaks in such a way that it is impossible to catch onto a thought unless you are familiar with the events. But we understand.

– This is happening for the fourth time already, – he enlightens us. – The Black Knight got ahead of himself, and started the battle without permission, at his own initiative. He wanted to win everything. And he lost everything. And so what have you won? The Earth? And what are you going to do with it? Who cares about it? You have now two buttons in your hands. Number one is for emergency destruction, and number two is for indefinitely long assistance. Who is there to be helped? There is nothing worthwhile left here. Look at those freaks, idiots, drug-addicts. That's why none of the serious cosmic beings wanted to meddle with this. One has to pay for everything – for millions of bucks, and for saving mankind. What do you need salvation for? May it be that the millions are better?

– And how are we going to pay you?

– Are you offering your souls to me? – His face expresses irony and an expectant smile at the same time. What a cute boy! But it seems he is not taking this situation seriously. He is just joking.

– Shall we sign a bond with blood? – I ask sarcastically.

He instantly senses that there is no use in pressing this topic further, and instantly changes the direction of the dialogue.

– There are two powerful cosmic corporations. One of them manufactures this and the other one manufactures that. Let's exchange this for that. Let's be more practical. Enough of sitting in a pompous position.

– So what has happened, after all, that the negotiations are necessary? – I press on.

– The year of the millennium – the change of authority. The one who has authority gets to feed on energy. That's the foundation on which the

408

supersystems are built.

– But the Black Knight lost? So, you are left without food then – I tease him habitually.

– This planet had a destiny. They wanted to build sort of a kindergarten here for future Creators. One hundred and forty-four thousand new Creators; at the End of Days they were supposed to transition to other spaces and unfurl new Universes. Earth is the master class. However, it turned from bad to worse. Three times everything was obliterated. Everything was taken to the point of madness. People found out about the Apocalypse. Why should people know that? How does it concern them? The dimensions of space, from zero to infinity. Life on all the levels. What's the point of crossing swords? What is Earth? Particularly now! Who would ever covet it? Come over, dear guests – there is no food left. Right?

– What about the destiny that you talked about?

Kirill looks us searchingly in the eye.

– Devoted servants of the Lord... The servants betrayed by the Lord, – he says clearly. – So, you will do everything as you planned, and what's next? There are two roads again: if you go to the right... if you go to the left... it's a figure eight, infinity. You are going to just keep going in circles along this rut?

– And we are doing everything correctly? – I inquire.

– Correctly, yes, – confirms Kirill, – but will what you do be correct? To the right, to the left... If the Soul joins the Ego, an Archon appears. Since he is an Archon it means he did not sell his soul to anyone, light or dark. That's also an option. The rays may be different – dark or light ones– but they are all reaching towards the same Sun at the Center of the Universe.

– How do you know?

– Because I am nobody. I am the air, the wind– catch me. As I said, I am a spirit! – the boy is mocking, openly mocking. He is laughing, but he is actually frightened.

– Why should we catch you, air?

– You want to breathe, don't you?

– What should we do?

– Learn how to behave adequately. Everyone was just doing whatever they wanted here. And now they have remembered about destiny. The entities far on high have gotten down to work, the Creator himself, too. And others as well...

– Are you trying to imply that it is we, the entities far on high?

– You were there purely by accident. Your places in the queue to become manifestations of St. George the Dragon Slayer were one thousand two hundred and five and one thousand two hundred and six. At the very bottom. It's just that you happened to be at the very right time at the right place together. And of course, you are also lucky that you did not lose the battle.

– And so what now?

– Now you have the power, but you don't know what to do with it. Meanwhile, I have knowledge, but do not have the power. I can show you the way. Do you want to see purgatory – the energy flows are gigantic there and not claimed by anyone yet. Why do you need to bother gathering one hundred and forty-four thousand? It's better to have fewer but of higher quality, don't you agree?

– The three of us, everyone gets a half? – Igor asks.

– A half! – Kirill confirms.

– It is not possible for three to divide it by half.

– Well, you will then decide who will be the second, – Kirill kindly

410

agrees.

– Together we are one whole entity, – I remind him. – And besides, what about conscience? Abandon everything and make it good for ourselves? And what about others?

– I am so fed up with that conscience of yours, – the boy roars. – There is still the Last Judgment ahead, – he is attempting to intimidate us. – They will whip you from alpha to omega and it is not clear how the whole thing will end. And now you have a ticket to any point in the Universe – it would be stupid not to use it. And you have the seventeenth legion of Power. And you know who has the eighteenth – Lucifer does! There are two roads – the dark one goes forward, but will take you backward, and the light one – back to the future where you came from. Why do you need to go there again? There are only two doors, and only two ways. God's position is to leave this system. If you don't leave then from the small figure eight you transition to the big one. And so ad infinitum. And so what?

– There is also the Creator's position.

– At this time you have absolute power in your hands. If you wish, a Mercedes will be waiting for you at the door and the president of the globe himself will be opening the door for you. Do you understand?

– What do you gain?

– But do you need a third party?

– In order to share universes? – I want to know.

– In order to ride the Mercedes, – Kirill corrects, tired of our lack of understanding. He is like a chicken from an incubator, without mother and father, without kin or family. Incubus – that is how they referred to male demons in the medieval times.

– And we are going to take the commuter train now, aren't we, Igor? – I ask my friend.

411

– Yes, the commuter train would be calmer. – And, already talking to Kirill, he adds:– As for you, young man, you must be more modest. More modest. That is the same mania between you and Lapshin to rule creation. Simply some kind of epidemic in your academy.

* * *

Igor and I usually tried to work with the internal vision screen early in the morning. This was very convenient. This schedule allowed us time both to learn and to work with patients. Sometimes there was also time left to discuss some problems.

Frequently we were called upon. Sometimes we initiated important events ourselves and went into the fine material world.

This time we wished to meet the warriors of the seventeenth legion of Power. They were the ones going to battle together with us, risking their immortal souls. We could see them only as lines of warriors. But those lines consist of individuals. So who went to battle on our side in those lines, whom did the Lord gather into His troops over a thousand years? And are there any of our compatriots, Russian people, among them?

Together with Igor we enter the different space. Barely had we stepped into the other world when our structure turns into the image of St. George the Dragon Slayer, to which we are no longer so used lately. We rise through the Bardo channel. Here is the landing where we fought with the Black Knight, the cross. Suddenly our legion appears. Igor dismounts the horse, that is, me. I immediately turn into a civilian ass: black robe of an academic, four-pointed hat with a tassel.

Igor goes down on one knee. I am next to him. And the entire legion goes down on one knee after us.

We thank the glorious warriors for having, with no fear and no regrets, followed us into battle, for never doubting us. We thank our Creator for having blessed, strengthened and granted us the Spirit. We thank the Russian Land for producing such warriors.

We also ask Our Lord to bless us and give us strength, and to preserve us from the evil one who walks around us.

– In the name of the Father, Son and Holy Spirit, Amen!!

Suddenly the saints and the Lord Himself appear on the landing. We thank Him personally and ask Him to bless His sons, to protect us from the evil eye, hex spells and other misfortunes.

– Our Father in Heaven, hallowed be Thy Name, Thy kingdom come! – the troops proclaim.

The Lord makes the sign of the cross at each of us and all of us together. He thanks us for our faith. He proclaims that He will never leave us, as we did not leave Him. May none of us doubt the honor and dignity of each one in our army. From now on we and the troops will be inseparable and protected from adversity, evil-doers, the evil eye, and devilry.

All the saints make the sign of the cross at us and bless us for battle with the dark forces. Now we are a single unit and shoulder to shoulder with each warrior in the legion of Power. Our strength shall increase by as many times as there are warriors in our troops.

We are given a ring as an award, with the inscription „For honor and glory". The ring has nine colors and a passage from one world to another, from gate to gate. No one can resist that ring. Because this is the Ring of the Lord! It is impossible to buy or sell it. It is the same size as we are, the same mind, intelligence and essence. It does not have a name, a title nor a definition. It is impossible to measure it or touch it, divide it or combine it with something else. It does not obey any powers and does not belong to any powers, but only to us and to our army. Its power is limitless.

– And if the evil one tries to tempt you, – the Lord raises His voice, – this ring will punish each and all who doubt the power of God. Because this is the fire of God! It effects God's Judgment!

We are touched by this magnanimity and the fact that the Lord Himself cares for us so much.

Priests are passing by, and again among them we see Father Herman from the Holy Trinity-St. Sergius Lavra. They sprinkle and bless us. From now on we shall be of a single spirit and a single faith with our troops. We are granted the strategic power and knowledge of each warrior. We also receive the connection with all our prior lives in all the worlds past and present.

We offer thanks. The Lord and His entourage disappear. Igor and I rise from our kneeling position and walk along the line of warriors. There are many people not from our times, and from different countries. But many are impossible not to recognize. There are Kievan princes, saints, Dmitriy Donskoy, Alexander Nevskiy.

Each row shows great warriors whose faith was steadfast and very strong. There stands the famous reformer of Russia, Stolypin. And next to him there is Nicholas the Second – the last tsar of the Romanov dynasty.

Igor and I look in his face, and a voice comes from an unknown source:

„Starting from 1901, Nicholas the Second knew what feat of martyrdom he would be facing. Because on the day of the hundredth anniversary of the murder of his ancestor, Emperor Paul, he learned prophesies of the clairvoyant cenobite Abel".

I have heard about Abel. Peasant Vasiliy Vasilyev (1757 – 1841) took monastic vows under the name of Abel. He foretold the fate of Catherine the Great, Paul and Alexander. All those rulers imprisoned him, and he died in prison. In total Abel spent 21 years in prisons.

Paul in his conversation with the clairvoyant asked him not only about his rule but also about the fate of the House of Romanovs and Russia in general. Abel's prophesy was written down and placed in a special box with the instruction to be opened by the ruling descendant one hundred years later. The box was kept at the Gatchinskiy Palace. Learning about its contents radically changed the way of thinking and behavior of the emperor; since then he repeatedly mentioned 1918 as the fateful year both for the dynasty, and for him personally.

The prophesies of Abel were confirmed by other clairvoyants. In the summer of 1903, in Diveyevo, a letter was handed to the tsar written by Reverend Seraphim Sarovskiy (1759 – 1833) shortly before his demise. Warning Nicholas of the tribulations to come, the priest exhorted him to strengthen his faith. Other legends regarding these events are also known.

The voice continues:

Nicholas II was aware of his fate, and consciously sacrificed himself for the sake of this country. He could have pusillanimously looked for another way out, and there were plenty of well-wishers willing to help him and his family to live long and happy lives. But the tsar accepted his death consciously, believing in God. Thus he earned honor and glory and the title of a martyr saint.

What was foretold for him came true. Many later regretted what they had wrought. And the people, ungrateful and forgetful of their responsibilities, have come to understand that it shifted the burden of its responsibility to the tsar alone for their sinfulness and lawlessness. The tsar accepted the burden of other people's sins, and carried them valiantly".

Following the voice, we see the courtyard of the Ipatyevskiy House in Yekaterinburg, a cart. There is a pile of stones on which the emperor is sitting. Nearby there is a stack of firewood – dark and wet. There is a large gate with an overhang. Two soldiers with rifles are standing guard.

A girl and a boy are running around in the yard. The boy is very sick. He coughs, and blood mars the handkerchief. His lungs hurt. Nicholas hears the children laughing. He knows that they will all be killed soon, and he is considering the possibility of poisoning his family so that they die in their sleep and do not see the horrors that are in store for them. He does not want them to be shot and killed, like rabbits during a hunt.

He knows what honor and dignity are. We can see today that by his death as a martyr he preserved over Russia the channel of the Holy Spirit which could have otherwise closed because of the blood of the innocents spilled during the Civil War and because of the subsequent horrendous experiments of the Bolsheviks.

* * *

There is some bustling around "Khudlit" again. In the ministry, restructuring papers are drawn and initialed again. In the newspapers there are articles by Grigoryev regarding structural reorganization and the need to concentrate financial resources in the newly established holding. At the same time, where the holdings are established, there are complaints precisely due to the lack of promised government financing of the projects. And the salaries of the staff did not increase by a single ruble. There are no new dazzling effects in the book field. Now it is particularly clear what was hiding behind the catchy pretty facade. Commercial publishing houses, via their appointees, are clearing the future marketplace. In addition, where government investments are expected, their own trusted treasurers are immediately appointed.

How shortsighted that is! Government-run publishing houses provide scientific and editorial preparation of works of literature prior to publication, they have a professional approach to the process of publishing a book. The professional interests of commercial publishing houses are mainly limited by raking in a hefty profit, and without compunction they simply reprint books that we have already prepared. Without our profound school they are doomed to degradation. All the book markets are filled with adventures of the „Daredevil" – an interminable project of "Vagrius", and the rumor goes that each book in it is written in a month or two by a team of literary old farts. It is good hackwork! But the reader does not have to use his brain. A book like that will always be in demand. Because by association it is connected with an interminable action TV series and it continues the same destructive work in people's souls.

As for demand – how can this serve as a justification? There is demand for vodka as well. And for drugs. Actually, such books are not any better than drugs. Because in one fell swoop they can undermine in the souls of the new generation all the achievements of civilization and thrust millions of human fates into the abyss of spiritless development.

Here are some "Khudlit's" and such getting underfoot, publishing the classics! If it were only possible to crush "Khudlit" under their own influence, make it into a Cinderella subordinate to "Vagrius"'s" donkey! But here difficulties of which the reader is already aware came about. The director is against it, the employees are against it, public opinion is against it, and the only one in favor is the donkey. Seems a little thin on votes though.

Again, smart kids in glasses, eager to receive green dead presidents [dollars] from the donkey, sat down to create devilish schemes and design

417

posters. And so there are photos plastered across every newspaper, with suggestive captions „Grigoryev knows!", „ Grigoryev has the skills!", „If it were only given to Grigoryev!". And what can he be given when he is a deputy minister already anyway? It sounds like a saying teenagers like to use: Vova is grown now, Vova knows it all, leave Vova alone.

Over a year and a half Grigoryev never bothered even to meet with the directors of the largest publishing houses. And for the ones with whom he did meet, it was only to inform them that they were fired. Oh well, so they are fired – no one can keep the same job forever. But who is to replace them? So that's some situation, all in the name of increasing productivity!

As I am writing these words, I am hearing in my head a line from Vysotsky's song „Everyone is eager to punish the Mages". Do you remember what comes next? Oh well, whatever. God willing, things will turn out all right.

Things at the Center are going better and better. Now Igor and I need just two or three minutes to see a person's problems, and a few more minutes in order to help him. This is the result of our new initiations. We have already noticed that whenever we meet with the Creator, our capabilities increase dramatically.

But there are not only pleasant surprises in store for those who are allowed to visit the unmanifested world. Once Igor and I were being sucked into a huge energy funnel. We understood this was not an imagined danger but a real one – and there was almost no time to make a decision. After all, the Lord said that from now on we are a single entity?

Igor sent a telepathic call, and the legion immediately appeared. At the very last moment, when the center of the energy whirlwind had almost sucked us in, the warriors of the legion formed a human chain holding each other firmly by the hands, and the last warrior connected his hand to

Igor's. So we had a living chain made of people. And no matter how the abyss roared and tried to pull the friends' hands apart – it did not succeed. We were thrown and lunged around, but the human chain was stronger.

High energies, mystical deeds, but the results depend on simple mutual assistance – like in a good old Russian village. On whether someone lends you a helping hand – or not.

A little while later our teacher, Grigori Petrovich, appeared next to us. He looks at Igor and me with surprise and delight. Then he laughed: „Good work!" Later he seriously clarified:

– The energy of this abyss does not obey anyone. In the tunnel there, one can see dents on the walls. These were due to the magi or the Initiated, who were sucked into the funnel and crashed against the walls there. These are the marks of their deaths. No one has ever come back from there – you are the first.

We were the first because the great warriors of the legion did not leave us in adversity. The abyss could have sucked in all of us. But they were not thinking of themselves, they were thinking of us. This is a lesson that needs to be contemplated.

Thank You, Lord, for the lesson!

We decide to explore the lower levels. We create ten mirror spheres and three scanner balls. We lower the mirrors through Bardo. Then the scanner balls. Thus we have a mirror trail leading to our computer. It will gather and analyze the information, then bring it up on the screen.

The first level. In the Bardo channel, in addition to the gates, there are some strange side openings. It seems like they could be back door passages. From here „the mohair ones" come to Earth, when they don't want to attract attention to themselves. So, that's useful knowledge. It looks like

419

in addition to those whom they are supposed to let out on Earth to do work in accordance with the agreement, they also use the back doors and let out whomever they want above the limit.

Igor suddenly exclaims in surprise:

– Look, they have paradise and hell, too.

They sure do! But they are reversed compared to the similar places on the top side. On the top they are located correctly, but in the lower realm they are reversed. This is how they create protection for themselves.

We send a scanner ball to the paradise of the dark ones. The tunnel goes in. There is a hall; in it there is a pedestal and books are sitting on the pedestal. The one in the center is open. There is a bookmark in the pages. It has a picture of a snake wearing a crown. On the tail of the snake there is a ball. The sharp end of the tail sticks out from the ball just a little. Presumably, that is how they imagine the globe: sitting on the snake's tail.

So, what are those books? We magnify the image. The one on the left says „White Magic", on the right „Black Magic", and in the center „True Magic". So here's an answer for you as to whom the white and black magicians are serving. No matter what color you call them, they all have one master. That very one, with the horns and the tail.

Our scanner ball suddenly shatters with a bang. It could not withstand the low-frequency vibrations and high temperatures. We launch the second one.

The room on the left is full of weaponry: swords, bow, arrows, incantations, talismans. Also there are necklaces, earrings – just about everything. Interesting means to boost success in business, love and politics. Quite a large-scale market. Anyone could receive whatever they wish. But how are they going to pay for it?

Igor is looking at a bead necklace. The necklace is made of small stone

420

beads with a dark stripe.

– Look, – he says. – The same one that Kirill has. So that's where the little imp got his equipment!

Another scanner ball shatters to smithereens. Right, this way we can torture ourselves till the end of time. This is not a very efficient technology. We need to think of something else. Particularly since we, as usual, do not have much time. And now we have to leave everything we started. Time to go to work.

It is a difficult day today: an international book fair at All-Union Exhibition of Economic Achievements is approaching, and the books are late coming from the publisher. Besides, soon it's going to be the 70th anniversary of the founding of "Khudlit". It would be nice to come up with something that would get noticed. Igor is going to the Center. He is already good at doing those things, even when he is alone. I have my own things to do.

By lunch we have sorted things out with my deputy for financial affairs, Mr. Kolesnikov, to see what we can afford. There was an idea to order ten „Golden Pegasus" medals and present them to the oldest employees at the publishing house. This would serve as an equivalent to awards that were almost prepared for the anniversary by the previous management of the government committee – five orders and seven medals. But restructuring of the sector and transformation of the government committee into the Ministry caused the need to redraft the documents for awards. Naturally the future award ceremony aroused no enthusiasm from the new deputy minister. Instead of the orders there was again red tape with the contract, even though with the right to operate as the acting director until the special decision is made. As months went by, the special decision was not forthcoming. The profitability indicators of the publishing house were climbing steadily, and in the ministry no one, except, perhaps, Grigoryev, was inclined to crush our publishing house.

After lunch, I got a phone call from the chief book publishing government department. The loud commanding voice of Irina Yakovlevna Kaynarskaya was ringing at me from the receiver:

– So, what shall I tell you, Arkadiy? I have nothing good to say, but nothing bad either. The middle path was accepted for "Khudlit" – a merger. Do you understand? Not a holding company, as everyone around was blabbing about, but a merger.

– How would that work?

– We'll attach you to two or three other publishing houses – merge them as your editorial departments. And you will have to sort it out with them yourselves. And don't count much on financial assistance.

Kaynarskaya was certainly correct: this was not the worst outcome, even though it was bound to make our lives complicated. The wage fund will grow, and the working capital that we were accumulating so painstakingly over the recent years would be reduced.

Quickly I gather the directorate. We discuss and analyze the possibilities.

Inara Stepanova, our chief accountant and brilliant financial specialist, prepared a quick outline on the computer showing how the main indicators are likely to change. It looks like if we manage to preserve the same rate and trend of growth for several months – and at this time we have already been confidently showing quarterly profits of 300,000-400,000 rubles – then we could, even though with difficulty, survive the middle path.

The main negotiations on this topic Kaynarskaya scheduled for the days of the All-Union Exhibition of Economic Achievements Book Fair. We decided to prepare counter-proposals.

In the evening, Igor and I went to visit Grigori Petrovich. Grabovoi's reception area was full of people. A slender, well-dressed woman was standing by the wall. I don't know why, but she drew our attention. As it turned out later, that happened for a reason.

Rather quickly we were called into Grigori Petrovich's office. He greets us at the door, shakes hands with us, and smiles.

– So, I can congratulate you on receiving the ring of the Lord, – Grabovoi immediately, before the conversation even begins, shows an amazing degree of knowledge about the event on which we have not yet shared information with him.. But Igor and I have long since stopped wondering about his abilities. Moreover, we also discover in ourselves more and more qualities that are weird and outlandish for a normal consciousness.

– And it is not very efficient to explore the lower levels with your scanners. But at least it is safe, – Grigori Petrovich comments.

– Well, at this time that is what our skills allow, – I weakly attempt to deflect the criticism.

– I want to ask you for help, – says Grabovoi.

That is an unusual turn of events. Normally we ask Grigori Petrovich for help. This is apt to swell our heads.

– I have prepared a book, – Grigori Petrovich continues. – Its title is very specific: „Resurrecting People and Eternal Life – Our New Reality".

Igor and I are exuberant inside. May it be that we have gone to this level: we shall be allowed not only to regenerate the organs, but also bring dead people back to life? In essence, it seems as though we are getting clearance for this program right now.

– This book deals not with mythical capabilities, but with a quite real practice that I perform already. But people are not ready to perceive the word „resurrection" in the literal meaning, the way it should be perceived

423

in reality. Even though the facts of bringing dead people back to life that I have performed are confirmed by official documents, are verified by notaries and filmed on videotape, – the consciousness of modern man is not at this time capable of perceiving such events as a reality, as something that can happen to him personally.

– Is the book already written? – I want to clarify.

– Basically, yes, – Grigori Petrovich confirms. – And I will give it to you today. The only thing missing from it is chapter four. I will need a month or two to complete it. You are a publisher. I believe that together we will be able to explain to people how to enter the age of immortality.

– We would be glad to help.

– By the way, you noticed the woman at the reception, – Grigori Petrovich was stating the fact rather than asking. – So, she is one of those I resurrected. She had committed suicide – cut her veins. Then her body was lying in a bathtub for nine hours. The body was found and taken to the morgue. Then her relatives came to me. They had read somewhere that I practice those kinds of things. It took several days to prepare the documents. And so there she is standing now, quite alive... You, by the way, may also start working using this book. You already have the preliminary knowledge.

As we were leaving Grabovoi's office, we looked again with attention at the woman standing by the wall. Scars from a razor were showing very clearly on her wrists.

The next day, as it was a Saturday, Igor and I settled cozily in my office and started working on Grabovoi's manuscript. We were reading very quickly, inasmuch as the topic of the book was mostly familiar and understandable to us in view of our own explorations of the unmanifested world. We felt that even though Grigori Petrovich had been working with extrasensory perception for a long time and had been using the internal vision screen almost since the age of three, we have come very close to matching his abilities, and, as the saying goes, are stepping on his heels. We were at it with a passion even though the person we were chasing was at the same time our teacher and did everything possible to help us achieve the fulfillment of our most heartfelt wishes. Grabovoi really was not afraid that we would be able to do what he is capable of doing. Moreover, he wanted it. We were reading with fascination the written experience of this unique man, to whom there are no equals perhaps in the whole world. In this book he was expressing his thoughts simply and clearly. It was quite different from his previous works filled with most complicated mathematical and physics formulas and definitions of the physical constants of the universe. I cannot resist the temptation to quote him, particularly because due to the absence of chapter four the publication of his work may be delayed. People must know that the great discovery is just around the corner.

„ Clairvoyance is the universal method for accessing information. With what can this way of obtaining information be compared? Actually, there is already something similar in our modern life. This is the Internet, a global network. Using this network one can obtain any available information from any point on Earth. So, as it happens, there is something similar to a cosmic Internet, where the data on absolutely everything is contained. A man can be compared to an operator in this case. Then clairvoyance is the method for the operator to enter the cosmic network with a query. And its speed of operation is so high that the answer comes instantly.

This brings about an interesting question: how are discoveries made? Discoveries, and sometimes outstanding ones, are made in different areas of life. First of all, this can be observed in the instance of science, but in other areas they are naturally present as well – for example, some changes made to a technical process in a plant or in society. New knowledge and skills are generally one of the phenomena in our life, even though the most visible examples of discoveries are observed in science, I would say.

That raises the next question: what can we say from the standpoint in question about discoveries made by people who are not clairvoyants?

When a brilliant thought occurs to a man and he makes a discovery, that thought, the answer to his search, of course, originates from the same database of the cosmic network. And in a sense this answer does not come to him randomly, in the sense that frequently that answer would be received as a result of many years of searching and determined hard work. But it is never possible to say when an answer is going to come or if it is going to come at all. So one has to admit that such a breakthrough into the database, unfortunately, is still an accident, since it cannot be managed or controlled.

The following comparison is possible. For example, there are two men who need water. One of them folds his palms together, stretches his hands forward and stands, waiting for it to rain so as to gather a little water. The other man is aware of the existence of a piped water supply network. Moreover, he knows how to use it. So when he needs water, he simply comes up to the faucet and opens it. He draws a glass of water, a bucket or a whole barrel, depending on how much he needs.

Therefore, one needs to be able to use a standard procedure for accessing the information. The point is that there are very many questions and too few random accidental breakthrough answers.

There is an important comment to the statement made above. For clarity of illustration, I compared using clairvoyance to entering the cosmic Internet network, in which one can find an answer to any question of in-

terest to one. This comparison reflects more of the external appearance of this phenomenon; it does not convey its true depth and multiple possibilities, so it requires a few clarifications.

It is of course possible, as was mentioned, to enter the cosmic network with a query in order to obtain information. But it is possible to act differently. Information can be obtained directly from the place where the sensor is located that broadcasts that information. Moreover, and this is important, the information exists already within the being of the asker, that is, in the form of direct knowledge, when it is not yet deciphered and the man is not aware of it, but it has already determined his behavior. In order for that information to be understood and immediately used by the man to select the path down which he needs to go - it requires a high level of development of the consciousnessя, and this is precisely the goal which I have already mentioned.

In chapter four, we shall talk about the new medicine, the medicine of the future and already of the present. At the foundation of this medicine lies the practice of resurrecting the dead. It is precisely the resurrection practice that defines the principles of the new medicine, and, first and foremost, the principle of the complete re-creation of matter. This new medicine has already begun resolving its main task. This task is – to make sure that the living do not die."

Unlike Igor and me, Grigori Petrovich is a specialist precisely in the areas of knowledge that are directly related to the subject of clairvoyance: he is a doctor of physics, mathematics and biological science. As if it were not enough for him to have this sublime gift, he kept studying throughout his life. God helps those who help themselves!

The fact that it was this man, well-versed in the system of traditional

427

world outlook, who achieved astonishing and widely recognized results in the areas of esotericism and extrasensory perception, by inevitably demonstrating: the materialistic outlook in the vulgar understanding that is common in the modern scientific and philosophical concept of the perception of the world is already undergoing a deep and insurmountable crisis. This is perhaps a slow process but a sure one. One hundred fifty years ago, Engels criticized the vulgar materialists Focht and Moleschott. Today a new reappraisal of values is looming.

That same Engels in his day warned that philosophy was supposed to change with every major scientific discovery. Today, we need to think through very many discoveries and build a new „dialectics of nature". The main question of philosophy – what is primary, the material or the ideal – has disappeared by itself. Will there be something to replace it? And is the replacement needed? Then, what is life? Is it just the „way of existence of protein-based bodies", or can it take other forms? When they say, for example, that some idea is „at the end of its lifespan", is it just a commonplace metaphor or another indication of the eternal struggle between Life and Death? And so on.

In recent centuries, science has been too categorically dismissing „ghostly otherworldly fields". The reasons are understandable. The issues of Light and Darkness, Good and Evil, God and Satan have been monopolized by world religions, whose clergy vehemently persecuted everyone who dared to undertake independent investigation of spiritual issues so as to say a new word in this area. The „dissidents" seeking unorthodox knowledge therefore preferred secrecy, they encrypted their text into such metaphors that no Dante would be able to figure it out. The works of the alchemists, astrologists, Rosicrucians and other masons are quite curious from the historical standpoint. But to find in them that grain of truth which

428

would help people in their trouble radically rather than offer a consolation is the same as looking for a pearl in the ocean. Purposeful closeness, secrecy, the hermetical proclivities of these fields, schools and teachings. It is possible that on a certain level some of these works could contain the secret of Being. It is too early to say so. Or maybe it is already too late. Because the new knowledge arrives. One thing is clear: in the exploration of man, nature, past and future the esoterics we know did not step outside the circle of understanding of contemporary science.

We don't need to descend into the gloom of history. Here is an example from the late XIX century: theosophy, claiming to offer an all-encompassing knowledge of God, to develop a universal concept to tie science and religion. The names that are known to the entire world: Blavatsky, Steiner, Krishnamurti. The selection of teachings from which „all the best" elements seemingly were taken – Hinduism, Brahmanism, Buddhism... I want to clarify – I am not against theosophy. Moreover, via the mechanism of clairvoyance one can see how much the theosophists understood and guessed correctly. But unfortunately, today the knowledge they brought does not have any practical value, as the public consciousness is not ready to perceive it, and it is interesting only to the most hyper-excited personalities. That was why during the peak of the popularity of theosophy, the Russian philosopher Gustav Shpet wrote: „A theosophist is a voyager through all religions, sciences and „wisdoms". He rides in any carriage that belongs to religion, mysticism, natural sciences, philosophy, the occult, or telepathy. There is as little essential connection there as between any rider and a hired carriage."

It's the connection that is the crux of the matter. There is no need to search for truth – it has been known for a long time. One needs to live according to the truth. Do you remember the biblical story about Jacob's ladder? Everyone must create his own ladder to God. Or find one that has already been built by someone else and use it. There are many ladders leading towards God. But it is not possible to climb several at once. Life is not a stunt in a circus, and its purpose is not to make the audience clap.

Any scientific theory, any religious teaching is valuable to the extent to which it helps a man to find his Jacob's ladder and get closer to the Creator by using it. It was precisely from this standpoint that we were reading the book by Grabovoi.

We were reading Grabovoi's manuscript and realized that it is not just a book, but sort of a guide for the magical country that we had not known before. Every letter and every word offered a key to the new knowledge that had not been available earlier. But it needs to be read not with the eyes only but rather using the internal vision screen. We decided to start this wonderful experiment immediately.

We would first read aloud some section of the book, then activate the internal vision screen and look at what happened. Here, for example, Grigori Petrovich describes how birds fly:

„Since childhood we have observed how birds flutter from branch to branch, from tree to tree. We are delighted by the ease and casualness with which they do it. Or, how they soar high in the sky.

However, there are a lot of unexpected points in the flight of birds. For example, at this time science does not yet know that birds fly only partially due to the beats of their wings. In their flight a significant role is played by the anti-gravity that they create. For example, the gravity in a pigeon's head is ten times less than at the tip of its tail; that means it knows how to distribute gravity, which results in the specific flight dynamics. For different birds the changes in gravity and its distribution throughout the body

430

occur differently. Even the flight itself may be based on a different princip-
le: for example, for the flight of an owl, which is a night bird, the principle
of flight is different than it is for birds that fly during the day.

The most interesting is the case of the eagle. It also has the capability
to create antigravity, but in addition it also has the ability to demateri-
alize. If you observe an eagle as it attacks, it seems like a small round
lump flying. One would think that it became so small because it drew itself
up into a ball. You have to take into account, however, that an eagle can
change the volume of its body by several times. So it is not really just the
tightening of the muscles, even though this is present as well. But mainly
the volume is reduced because of the dematerialization of some parts of
the body. In addition, the eagle can change the shape of its body depen-
ding on the task at hand. The only bird that can, at least to some extent, do
something close to what an eagle is capable of is the falcon.

Eagles have other amazing capabilities as well... It is no accident that
primeval peoples throughout the world have connected the image of the
eagle with the Creator. It is also for a reason that the image of an eagle
can be seen in the coats of arms of a number of nations. We can see an ea-
gle in the coat of arms of Russia, too. In that case it's a double-headed ea-
gle. An eagle with two heads is a sign of a stable and prosperous future ".

So now we'll take a look. Igor goes into that space, creates an image
of a flying eagle and externalizes himself into it. He becomes as one with
the bird's body, thoughts and desires.

– What does it want, where is it flying? – I ask.

– It wants to find a gopher, – Igor responds. – Very interesting. In
its feathers it has informational channels, and all these channels are connected to the brain. The feathers can transmit and receive waves. This is

radar! But this radar operates not in space but in time. You see, it can feel time. It does not just see it, but it scans it. On the right – no gopher. On the left – no gopher. And now there is something. The wings and the head transmit rays, that's it – the gopher is in focus. It is five minutes away. The eagle gets closer. It sees the prey. It plummets down and close to the ground it teleports itself. It takes some time to manage the correlation of time. It simply dives into a different space at the moment and thus arrives straight at the target. This is also necessary so that the prey would not see him. Impressive. Now it's understandable why it is the king of all birds. It can teleport itself and see the future.

There is another topic that arises as we study Grabovoi's book. But first here is a short quote to explain the ideology of the process. So as to make clear to everyone why this is needed globally, in the philosophical sense:

„In subsequent books, we shall look also into such phenomena as levitation, materialization and dematerialization, telepathy, telekinesis, teleportation and others. For a long time these phenomena were mysteries. Now the time has come to provide the answers.

Mankind generally has approached a qualitatively new stage in its development: we see on the agenda the non-dying of the living and the resurrection of those who have gone. And this is not a theoretical but already a practical issue. This is finally become a living reality. Living reality for actual salvation for everyone.

It is important to note that instances of factual resurrection prove that it is possible to restore matter, and that in turns points out the non-feasibility and absence of logic in any destruction.

In our time of accumulating weapons of mass destruction, the practice

432

of resurrection would offer a method of saving humanity. It points to an alternative means of developing civilization.

Developing mechanisms of regeneration, the mechanisms of recreation would enable us to work on the tasks of creation without destruction. The principle of restoration can easily be spread to all spheres of human activities. It can also serve as a basis for the development of constructive thinking of future generations.

Any so-called aggressive medium can, using this approach, be transformed and after transformation act as a non-aggressive element of the primary environment. As a result it is possible to develop an effective strategy of behavior that would make it possible to avoid environmental disaster and ensure further development without destroying the environment. Because it is necessary to bear in mind that resurrection is actual control of all the external space.

The highest level of harmony with the environment can be ensured by creating, for example, materials that would not be subject to wear, or cars that would not require significant additional resources to run. And all of this is completely realistic. The same as resurrection. And this is all within our hands.

One must always remember one very simple truth: a man is born for joy, happiness and a full endless life ".

So there is the philosophy – the philosophy of salvation, the philosophy of the Savior. It does not contradict any scientific or religious conventions because it will result in saving both man, and the nature that surrounds him. So, how does resurrection occur?

And here are some quotes again. The texts of the statements quoted here are taken from the book: Grigori Grabovoi, „Practice of Control, the

Way of Salvation „‟ Vol. 3, pp. 756 – 757. The book was published in Moscow in 1998 by the publishing house „Soprichastnost‟.

Statement by Emiliya Aleksandrovna Rusanova, dated May 27, 1996:
„On September 25, 1995, during a personal meeting with Grigori Petrovich Grabovoi, I requested of him the complete restoration of my son, A.E. Rusanov, who was born on August 22, 1950 and died on 16 June 16, 1995. My son was born in Moscow and died in Moscow as well. Before coming to G.P. Grabovoi, I was in complete despair and suffered a heart attack. After my request to G.P. Grabovoi some time in early October 1995, I regained hope for my son's return - I started feeling his (spiritual) presence in the house. I went to the cemetery, and, having approached my son's grave, I saw that there was a deep fissure along the entire grave, and in the middle there was sort of a concavity that looked as if some soil had been ejected from beneath.

Somewhere around midnight, I could see very clearly (even though my eyes were closed) that from my chest two white cords stretched out towards my son's grave, toward the concavity I saw on it; then I sort of pulled those cords towards myself, and this felt heavy. All of this lasted for a few seconds. My son was buried at Vostryakovsky Cemetery, and my vision of his grave occurred at the level of my apartment window, which is on the 7th floor.

When I came with the request to G.P. Grabovoi to bring back my son, A.E. Rusanov, I shared this information with my son's ex-wife, Tatyana Ivanovna Kozlova, with whom we continued to be friendly after their divorce. She had attended my son's funeral. Subsequently, during our conversations from October to February, T.I. Kozlova has told me several times that frequently she saw on the streets of Kaliningrad and Moscow people

434

who looked like my son, A.E. Rusanov. In early February 1996, she was traveling by the train named „Amber" from Moscow to Kaliningrad in the Baltics, and in the train compartment with her there was a male traveler who looked very much like my son, A.E. Rusanov. He had a likeness in appearance, manner, behavior, gestures and glance, but he appeared distant and lost. He was traveling with a man, who sort of accompanied him, and controlled him, but throughout the trip never called him by name. T.I. Kozlova was surprised when my son, A.E. Rusanov, upon seeing some money (one thousand rubles of the new design) clearly expressed that he was not familiar with this bank note design."

Statement by Tatyana Ivanovna Kozlova, dated May 27, 1996.

„I was married to A.E. Rusanov from December 1975 until October 1982. After the divorce from A.E. Rusanov, I continued to maintain a friendly relationship with his mother, Emiliya Aleksandrovna Rusanova. When I saw her on September 26, 1995, she informed me that she had asked Grigori Petrovich Grabovoi to revive her son, A.E. Rusanov, (A.E. Rusanov, according to the death certificate, died on June 16, 1995, in Moscow). After that, knowing that Grigori Petrovich Grabovoi was working on resurrecting A.E. Rusanov, I noticed during the period of October 1995 to February 1996 people on the streets who looked in appearance like A.E. Rusanov. During my trip to the city of Kaliningrad in Kaliningrad Region, as I was traveling by train, there was a man sharing the train compartment with me. Looking at that person gave me the impression that he was dragged out from some other world. This man who entered the compartment looked like A.E. Rusanov in the following ways: hair color, eye color, overall appearance and facial shape.

The manner of behavior of the man who entered the compartment was exactly the same as that of A.E. Rusanov, including his character. He ex-

hibited the same habits (silent, propensity to read: throughout most of the time he was reading a newspaper). The man who accompanied him was a man of medium height, who throughout the trip never called his companion by name. And when that man brought out some money, the man who looked like Rusanov was surprised at seeing the new design 1,000 ruble note; the accompanying man explained to him that this was the new style of money. It gave the impression that that person (who was accompanied by that other man) had spent some time in seclusion outside of real life. Even though it seems as though he retained his professional skills, because the man who accompanied him said that they transported cars.

The meeting described above took place on February 2, 1996, during my trip from Moscow to Kaliningrad on the train „Amber".

Here is the description of this occurrence as provided by the actual participants. Those descriptions reflect a number of important points, which we shall consider in more detail. We shall start our review from the statement by Emiliya Aleksandrovna, the mother of the deceased.

Actually, in the very beginning of the statement, Emiliya Aleksandrovna says that after I started my work on resurrecting her son, she began to feel his spiritual presence in the house.

The thing is that even when a man suffers biological death and he is buried and located in a specific grave, his consciousness still retains all the knowledge he acquired, and he is aware of his connection with the body, which no longer possesses life or what is normally called life. In view of this, the body, even though it may not have vital processes going on in the organism – in this case, the body of the son – in case of a fixation of the mother's consciousness on it, it reacts adequately to the external consciousness touch, to the information contained in an impulse from the external consciousness, and therefore provides an adequate response. This

436

indicates that when you imagine the body in front of you, you can send to the soul knowledge concerning resurrection.

Subsequently, already after the resurrection, when questions were posed to one of the resurrected, it turned out that at the time of the query sent to him by an external consciousness he realistically perceived all this and correlated his physical body with his own „I", even though that physical body was in the grave and was, naturally, limited in terms of many of its capabilities. Moreover, the revived person mentioned, and this is a well-known fact, that his presence at the general information level indicated that his physical body continued to exist and possesses all the possible and necessary qualities in order to continue to be a part of the general socium, part of the society. It is important to mention that this knowledge contained both earlier information, correlating to the former functions of this particular physical body, and new information, which already correlates to its biological death.

We keep reading the statement. When Emiliya Aleksandrovna came to the cemetery and approached her son's grave, she saw that there was a deep fissure along the entire grave and in the middle there was sort of a concavity that looked as if some soil had been ejected from beneath.

The explanation for this is as follows. The ejection of the soil from beneath needs to be regarded as the primary materialization of the consciousness, the very consciousness that inhabited the physical body. After initiation of my work of resurrection, there is primary materialization of that consciousness in the spherical form and bringing it into the informational channel of the planet. This is followed by the stage of creating the material structure around the soul, the structure, which we normally see when we look at people. One can say that both from the theoretical and practical standpoints a man can be viewed as a structure of conscious-

ness, which possesses a specific bodily shell.

There is another comment to the statement. I have mentioned primary materialization of that consciousness in the spherical form. So, after this sphere passes the informational channel of the planet it may be projected either into the next embryo (and then a baby will be born), or its projection may be sent to the structure of resurrection. That is, the same body and the same person would be re-created. So here the same thing was done as accomplished by Jesus Christ, when He revived Lazarus. Only in this case not several days but several months had passed from the time of biological death.

Further, Emiliya Aleksandrovna writes that one night, around midnight, she saw clearly, even though her eyes were closed, that from her chest two white cords stretched out towards her son's grave, toward the concavity that formed on it; and that she sort of pulled those cords towards herself, and this felt heavy. All of this lasted for several seconds. From the further description, it follows that Rusanova's son was buried at Vostryakovsky Cemetery, while the vision of his grave occurred at the level of the mother's apartment window, which is located on the 7th floor.

The two cords that are mentioned characterize the transitional stage. The first cord was created when the mother gave birth to her child, it is the structure of the birth of her son. The second cord is the structure of possible prolongation, extension of his consciousness or his essence. I have already said that after the biological death of the man two options are possible: either to be born as another child, and, therefore, to undergo reincarnation, or resurrection, and, therefore, recreation if the same body, which includes not only restoration of the formerly existing matter, but also all the consciousness structures. In this case it was the resurrection option that was implemented through the use of external control.

438

Appearance of the two connecting cords and perception of the son's grave at the same level with the apartment, which is located on the 7th floor, indicates the joining to the structure of the son's consciousness and the external environment.

In the practice of resurrection there is one rather particular point that characterizes the attachment of the body to the structure, to the place where that body is located after biological death. The location where the body is placed is the place to which it is connected. The primary attachment area covers a radius of about two meters from the physical body. The total attachment area exists within about 50 meters from the grave, and further on there is already connection to the informational framework of the external world. Knowing about the attachment point and related aspects is important for the resurrection procedure, because the reverse transition from biological death in reality also means a transition through the attachment structure. And the person being resurrected, naturally, also has to be oriented towards leaving the attachment area. By the way, if we interpret the vision described by Emiliya Aleksandrovna from this standpoint, we can say that she saw the grave as a version of the attachment of the biological body to a specific fixed place.

Subsequent text in the statement by E.A. Rusanova is based on information she received from T.I. Kozlova (so the description of subsequent events can be obtained from both women).

From the text we see that after Emiliya Aleksandrovna came to me with the request to resurrect her son and shared this information with the son's ex-wife, T.I. Kozlova, T. I, Kozlova started seeing on the streets of Kaliningrad and Moscow people who looked like her ex-husband, A.E. Rusanov. Later, as she was traveling from Moscow to Kaliningrad on the Baltics on the train „Amber", she encountered the man, who had all the

439

characteristics of A.E. Rusanov, up close, directly in her train compartment.

When you read the description of this encounter provided by T.I. Kozlova, you may get the impression that she behaved too passively. But imagine that it is yourselves who are traveling by train; all of a sudden in the compartment you encounter a man who looks exactly like a relative whom you buried a few months before. And this man does not pay any attention to you. Do you think you would approach him and say: „Hi! What is it with you, don't you recognize me?" Or maybe you would freeze in amazement, unable to speak and never take a step because your legs would feel like jelly? Even though Tatyana Ivanovna does not describe her feelings during this encounter, one can imagine the whirlwind of sensations she was experiencing: surprise, confusion, embarrassment, and a suddenly appearing awareness of the real resurrection that had occurred against all odds. Against all odds because at the present time resurrection is still seen by many as a miracle, because the majority do not yet have a true understanding that resurrection is in fact a standard procedure and that soon resurrection will come to be perceived naturally, as a normal way of life.

But at this stage a man who suddenly sees in the train compartment next to himself a relative who was dead and buried, is incapable of reaching any conclusion, because he would not immediately accept the possible miracle, or is worried that something may be done wrong. So when reading the statement one needs to take into account the state of the person in these circumstances. This book specifically directs people to the understanding of true realities and makes it possible to figure out how one should behave under those circumstances.

Getting back to the story of Mrs. Rusanova, where she mentions that at *first T.I. Kozlova started encountering people who looked like A.E. Rusanov on the streets and then, during the trip from Moscow to Kaliningrad, she encountered the man who had all the characteristics of A.E. Rusanov, up close, directly in her train compartment.*

In connection to this story it is necessary to point out that those who have left, or in this case it would be better to say – those who are returning – are very good at perceiving the state of the people to whom they are returning, and under no circumstances would they subject those people to excess stress. So at first Rusanov A.E. started appearing at some distance away from his former wife, gradually leading her to accepting the possibility of his return, particularly since Kozlova T. I. already knew that the resurrection process had been started.

Therefore, when she writes that she saw people who looked like her former husband, in actual fact she was seeing A.E. Rusanov, who had already been resurrected.

It makes sense to clarify that the reason the resurrected behave so carefully and with such understanding is that those elements of resurrection were transmitted to their consciousness. And because they received the elements, they form a different psychological structure of their perception of reality. They, for example, consider, and their personal experiences confirm, that that life is eternal. They also develop a special attitude to the laws of the macrocosm. Many of those laws are absolutely correct for them, and they would never violate these laws.

They also know about the 50-meter attachment area, and after returning to the physical level for a while they stay beyond 50 meters from the people to whom they are returning.

After this first stage of contact, during which the person returning is perceived at the level of sensation, there is a transition to the second stage,

441

the stage of visualization, when the resurrected starts entering into closer contact with the living. We see that A.E. Rusanov appears already directly in the vicinity of his ex-wife, in the train compartment.

Note that at this stage the resurrected person develops a management technique, namely, management of the situation. This technical skill is given to the resurrected at the time of resurrection. As a result he is capable on his own to find and orchestrate situations which are necessary to establish contact with those who knew him and to whom he is returning.

Regarding the impression her son produced on his former wife in the train compartment, Emiliya Aleksandrovna writes as follows: „He had the likeness of appearance, manner, behavior, gestures and glance, but he appeared distant and lost. He was traveling with a man who sort of accompanied him, controlled him, but throughout the trip never called him by name."

Here we see in the actions of the resurrected person another element of the knowledge, namely, understanding of the state of the person who used to know him. Had he appeared alone, his ex-wife's concentration of attention on him could have been so intense that it would have made it difficult for her to gradually adapt, and could have interfered with the planned course of events.

Therefore an element is introduced in the situation to somewhat distract Kozlova's attention: the man, who accompanies the resurrected person. And it is not at all necessary for that second man to be a real person, in reality he could have been purely visual in nature, but I will leave these technical details aside for the purposes of this first book.

Earlier I mentioned the existence of the primary attachment within the radius of about two meters from the physical body. So, partial or significant concentration on the second man, when you view these events from the standpoint of the fine plane, corresponds to detachment from the primary zone, that is the area of the grave itself and the transition of this zone to the accompanying man. It is important to note that it does not have to be a man, it could be some object – for example, a car in which the resurrected person is traveling, or something else. The important part is the principle, the principle of detachment of the resurrected person from the primary zone.

Moving on. The fact that in the presence of Kozlova the companion never called Rusanov by name indicates that in that situation it could have led to sending Kozlova into shock, and as a result – to destruction of some of her cells. But as I already said, the resurrected person is finely tuned into the situation and feels the condition of the person in front of him, because he has been through the deeper stages of destruction and then restructuring of his consciousness. So, moving forward, he acts in a very circumspect manner.

There is a pivotal point in the statement by Emiliya Aleksandrovna. After the phrase we discussed above she writes: „T.I. Kozlova was surprised when my son, A.E. Rusanov....“ Rusanova talks not about a man who looked like her son; but she says „...when my son...“. Here we can see that after Kozlova told her about the encounter in the train compartment, Rusanova fully identified the resurrected person with her own son, who used to be dead and has now came back alive. I would like to add that in the future that was confirmed with certainty and, the above story was favorably resolved.

It is worth underscoring that spiritual identification is the main criterion indicating that the resurrection of the specific person had occurred.

The next phrase in the statement is: „Upon seeing some money (one thousand rubles of the new design), he clearly expressed that he was not familiar with this bank note design ".

When could we expect a similar reaction from an ordinary living man? In a situation in which at the time new bank note design was introduced, for example, while he traveled outside the country. Then he would have been surprised exactly in the same way coming across the new realities. At the time the new money was introduced A.E. Rusanov was located in the enclosed space of his grave. That space limited his consciousness as well, as it was close to his physical body. This shows that the consciousness of those who have gone, i.e. those who have gone through biological death, this consciousness is practically the same as the consciousness of those existing in the state normally referred to as life. That is why we observe similar reactions to analogous situations.

From this description one should not conclude that the described pattern of resurrection is a standard one. For the current time it is, actually, rather typical, due to the perception by modern society of the phenomenon of resurrection. In essence it reflects the actual laws of resurrection. In a situation like this everything depends to a great extent on the degree of preparedness of the living to the return of the family member or friend. It is possible for the entire process of resurrection to take little time. And in the near future, when at least part of society comes to understand that the process of resurrection is a normal standard procedure, resurrection will occur quickly, because of the readiness of society to accept this phenomenon.

The second chapter covers also the possibilities of practically instant resurrection, but for this the person who is performing the resurrection must have a very high level of spiritual development.

We review this situation again through the internal vision screen. We see how the resurrection occurs, the meeting with the ex-wife in the train compartment. We follow the process of resurrection of A.E. Rusanov. Grigori Petrovich created sort of an analogue to the planetary control system structure. He works through it. It is very convenient because the contact with the planetary computer is performed almost instantly. We see how through the consciousness he starts to form the framework of the body. This is a very important stage, and anyone who knows the technique would be capable of doing it. The man who performs the resurrection should first bring his brain and consciousness to the appropriate level of development. Only in this case can the consciousness of the deceased receive from the one performing the resurrection a sufficiently powerful impulse for the goal of return and accept it. After that it is necessary to help the consciousness of the resurrected person to stage the event of return to the circle of friends and relatives so as not to cause psychological trauma to them. And then he needs to catch up with the events that have moved on.

It looks like forming the body is not a serious issue at all. Information on it is always kept in the planetary computer and is never erased. The building materials are the atoms, which, in accordance with an activated program can form any organs. The most difficult part is the cells. Their structure is the most complicated..

Grigori Petrovich uses his consciousness to send an impulse to the man he is resurrecting to activate the program for regenerating organs and tissues.

The second impulse is sent to the soul. And it starts interacting with the consciousness.

Another impulse is sent to the relatives, so that their perception of information concerning death should not be so acute and over time it will

445

be forgotten like a dream.

First the outline of the shell appears, then the aura; structural assembly of all the organs is activated. The fissure in the ground appears. Consciousness appears on the surface and the soul starts filling the outline of the man with his mass of cells. When the outline is filled, the man stands up with his feet on the ground.

There is an odd feature there: his cells and aura seem sort of distended. Why? The soul was traveling on the levels, and it has not fully left there yet. Now everything is filled with information, and the cells assume their normal appearance.

The inscription on the grave fades. That's it, there was no death – there is just immortality.

But if those things happen, and it is recorded on video, there are books describing it – then why is this miracle not proclaimed on every corner? This is an interesting question, isn't it? The thing is that the informational field of the Earth very carefully monitors the reactions of people to information of that nature and sort of dampens it when people's consciousness is not ready to adequately perceive such events. So only those who have eyes to see and ears to hear can see it and know it. Which eyes and ears do I mean? You have to guess!

In any case, the ontological status of the man increases considerably. The implementation of the „philosophy of the common cause" is starting; as our great cosmic philosopher Nikolay Fedorov wrote over one hundred years ago. One of his main ideas becomes everyday practice. Of course it is not coming to pass exactly in the same manner as dreamt by the outstanding librarian of Rumyantsev Museum. But this is quite a normal thing: everyday life is both duller and richer than our fantasies.

Chapter 11

External forces were starting to have a stronger impact on my student Tamara. She had already been feeling unwell for a week with headaches that did not let up. Igor and I offered to help, but she was convinced that the headaches would pass soon, saying that the atmospheric pressure was to blame. Finally, she could take it no longer and asked us to examine her.

The three of us sat down in my office. Tamara was worried.

– Right now I have the feeling that someone is inside of me, constantly pushing me to start fights and get into arguments.

– Let's take a look together, – proposed Igor.

We turned on the inner vision screen. Tamara's aura was for some reason gray. When did she manage to change so? Nothing made sense. We tried to scan her, and saw someone else's silhouette behind her back. A demon was hiding there, an enormous one. It was immediately clear that this was not a rank and file brute, but one of the managers. It took its discovery calmly, baring its teeth and lifting Tamara by her neck with its claws, twisting her from side to side. Tamara was not doing well – here, in the physical plane. Tears were streaming from her eyes and she was choking.

– Let's have a talk, – proposed Igor.

– Let's, – agreed the demon, slackening its grip.

Tamara could now breathe, but she still felt poorly.

– You don't have a license to behave like that with her. You're violating the law, – said Igor, trying to bring the demon into the realm of jurisprudence.

– I am not,– objected the demon. – We have a license for her.

– Show me, – demanded Igor.

447

– I don't have it here. I left it downstairs, in the chancellery. Let's go down and I'll show it to you.

The demon was brash and cocky. It was clear that he was lying. He was trying to set a trap.

Igor took a step closer to him. But the demon immediately jumped back, lifting Tamara by her neck and whirling her around as if she were a rag doll.

Tamara was not well. She grabbed at her neck with her hands, gasping. Her face turned gray. What a terrible creature, trying to destroy a woman.

– What should we do? – asked Igor.

I kept silent. I was at a loss and feared that the demon would strangle her. Meanwhile, the demon, as if reading my thoughts, jumped further back and suddenly tore down the levels.

Naturally, we immediately transformed into St. George the Dragon Slayer, plunging after him in pursuit. But the nimble demon wove now to the right and now to the left with Tamara thrown over his shoulders like a sack of potatoes, bouncing around. The woman was completely senseless. She had lost her wits, couldn't understand anything – where was she being dragged and why?

Then we reached the lower levels, although we didn't think about this or guess at it. Just us against thousands. Well, we couldn't run away from them. They asked for it themselves, those mohaired creatures.

Igor tore out his sword and everything was just like in a fairy tale: one sweep of the sword created a street, while another sweep created an alley. The magical sword adapted itself to the task at hand. Where there were many evil spirits, it grew longer and in one fell swoop mowed down hundreds of the enemies. Where there were fewer evil spirits, it shortened so as not to tax the hand of the warrior. And the devils were also receiving endless kicks from my hooves. My height as compared to theirs was that of an elephant to a little mouse. Also, the ruby in my forehead was like a battle laser. If I just thought, just concentrated, hundreds of the other devils would vaporize. We mowed down three levels of them and it was just as though none of those evil spirits had ever existed. We also seized part of the fourth level and about half of the devil population living there.

It turned out to be a real massacre. The demon that had carried Tamara below threw her down and took to his heels. He understood, the parasite, that if he carried her any further down his levels, there would be none of them left.

Igor swept her up into the saddle, and we galloped up into the light of day.

We stepped out of space, and Tamara was lying on the sofa barely alive. Say what you will, but Igor and I saved our princess. It took her three days to recover.

But we were not allowed to rest that long. The next face-off started the next day.

After lunch at the Center's Moscow branch, the phone rang. It was a relative calling. He was almost in tears as he informed me that his car had been stolen. He had bought it recently and held his fine red Volkswagen dear. Kirill was hanging around nearby.

– Has something happened?

– My relative's car was stolen, – I confessed sincerely.

– Have you and Igor ever searched for a car?

– No.

– Who's stopping you from trying?

Kirill's proposal made sense to me. I called over Igor and the three of us sat down in the office and got to work. We were shown what happened

449

right away.

The car had been stolen by three young men. One of them was thin and had short hair. He was wearing a white t-shirt and blue sweatpants with white stripes down the sides. We tried to read his thoughts, but his brain was as smooth as a newborn's; he could really have given a fig. On his left elbow was a large scratch.

The other one was a little older, about 20. Heavyset. He was driving the car and was frightened.

The car had been stolen not long before. They stopped at a gas station. There was a telephone with metal buttons. Behind was a railroad line, with the Ucha River on the left and a church not far off on the right. This was Pushkino. The car thieves called someone with the nickname of Surok [woodchuck in Russian – Transl. note]. They spoke about how they would come when it got dark. So that he would be ready. Then they drove along a road parallel to the Yaroslavl Highway, in the direction of Sergiyev Posad. They stopped at a small store. My son's documents and money were lying in the glove compartment. They took the money and bought beer, vodka, and bananas. They drove along a parallel road by a traffic police post into incoming traffic. They drove on, passing towns of Talytsy, Rakhmanovo. Then they drove into the forest, quietly reinforcing themselves with beer and bananas. Waiting for it to get dark.

We could see what was transpiring very clearly, as if we were tearing down the highway along with them. From time to time we would stop our search and work on something else. We decided to stay at work and follow the car thieves for a little while. The victim called almost every hour to learn about the course of the investigation.

When it got dark, we started working again. The car thieves were on their way. Beyond the village of Golygino, right along the oncoming traf-

450

fic lane, they went around a corner in the direction of Abramtsevo. They tore on to Khotkovo. Garages. A great many. We read the sign at the entrance: State Concern Khimik. That was all. Nothing further was shown.

The person whom they called, Surok, wass waiting for them in a building next to the garages. He was standing by the window. It's not far off – about 50 meters. And everything was visible from here. There was an athletic field near the house and off to the right. A little to the left stood some sort of factory. Near the garages, at the entrance, was an abandoned or partially constructed plant. If we ended up going to the place we were then looking at, it wouldn't be hard to find our bearings.

The apartment where the car thieves were expected was on a higher floor, but the building was not very tall, probably about five stories.

Igor and I tried to look from both the street and the landing, but we couldn't see anything. Everything jammed up at the most interesting part.

Kirill proposed changing technology.

– Let's see if we can find anything out directly through the Earth's information field. You look and I will lead. I will escort you and cover you.

We had been so consumed by the chase that we had not even thought about a trap.

– Lead away.

In an instant we found ourselves in some sort of room of a light-gray color. A strange color, seemingly light, but mixed with some kind of dirt. In the middle of the room stood a pedestal in the form of a triangle. Its edges were cut off, so it was actually a hexagon. Higher up, on the foot, sat a console like a computer console.

Kirill was not with us in the room. He was guiding us from below through the inner vision screen.

– Hit the left key, – he said to Igor.

451

Igor extended his hand towards the console and clicked on the red keyboard.

Instantaneously, right before our very eyes, a screen appeared. It was very thin and transparent, like regular glass.

– Hit the key to the right and enter the password 'Migen.'

– What does 'Migen mean? – I asked lightheartedly, vaguely recalling some kind of unpleasant association with this name.

– It's my personal access code.

Igor clicked away at the keyboard and entered the password. Some numbers and a map of the location appeared on the screen right away.

We looked at the area. It really was the north-eastern part of the Moscow Region. I suddenly had the feeling that Kirill knew were the car was and that what was happening was not accidental. And, confirming my suspicions, the walls of the room began to vibrate as if they were having trouble maintaining the illusion of their existence. A moment later, they collapsed at the same time, like sheets of white-gray paper. The black boundlessness of space opened up before us. It was not empty. An enormous number of devils examined with surprise the intruders who had appeared from nowhere. Among them were really quite large demons. They gawked at us, sluggishly trying to understand what was going on. When they finally started to understand that two of their arch enemies had fallen into their hands, they immediately set out in our direction. The only thing we could do was fight them, but at that moment Kirill appeared next to us and shouted: – Everything is OK! This is Migen's plan! Stay where you are.

The devils stopped obediently and we started to retreat through some underground levels unknown to us.

When we left clairvoyant mode, Igor asked once again, – What is Migen?

– It's a masher, a seal in the chancellery.

– And perhaps it is the Ruler of Darkness? – my friend guessed unexpectedly.

Igor felt very unwell. He was still in a trance.

– His finger needs to be pricked so that he can come out of the trance, – fussed Kirill. A knife appeared in his hand from God knows where. He took Igor's finger and poked it with the point of the knife. At that last moment, Igor was able to jerk back his hand, weakening the pain.

– Is there any blood? – asked the little devil, worried.

– No, – answered Igor. He was still in a state of prostration.

– Let's prick him again.

– Maybe we don't really need to? – I ask, interrupting their conversation.

– No, you don't, – confirmed Igor. – It will pass.

– How was it that you were able to make white space in the darkness? – I wondered.

– Anything is possible, if you have knowledge, – said Kirill, disappointed with his failure to prick Igor's finger.

– Well, what can I say? Score one for you, – I said, acknowledging his cheap success.

Now I understood why the car disappeared. And it no longer held any interest for me.

* * *

Apparently, Lapshin had a good reason for hinting that the more heads the little dragon grows, the harder it is to get along with him later. For

453

some reason, my little dragon was raging, as if trying very hard to make me do something illegal. And this time too, as soon as Igor and I entered virtual space, we were invited to another face-off. The Dark Spirits had complained to the Creator about the unlawful acts Igor and I had committed. They reported that we had exceeded our powers, naturally leaving out anything about what they had done to provoke the situation.

The two heralds again announced a summons onto the battlefield. Someone wanted to reconsider the outcome of Armageddon, or maybe just get even with us. We transformed into the image of St. George the Dragon Slayer.

The arrangement was basically the same: three thrones, and alongside them, from whichever fairytale he was summoned, the actual Dragon Gorynych. A good-sized reptile, shifting from foot to foot with smoke puffing out of its mouth. And there was one more wonder – a naked maiden on a black horse. Her eyes were narrow, evil. Not a Russian maiden, but an Asian one. And her sword was not Russian either. It looked like a Polovtsian* one. Her spear was still in her hand.

The maiden was in a combative mood, and it was clear that she had no fondness for Igor and me. She beckoned us with her spear, and her eyes narrowed even more, even though this seemed impossible. And her horse took a step in our direction, but someone called to her from behind, stopping her. It appeared that the Ruler of Darkness Migen had not selected her as our opponent today. It would be more loathsome to fight Gorynych, of course, but we were there as soldiers. It was not for the money or the decorations that we were being asked to save the Earth. This is why we felt composure and clarity within.

The Lord was settling into his seat on a throne behind us. Apparent-

---

* A Turkic tribe that roamed in the Middle Ages – Transl. note.

ly, the levels that we laid waste to belonged to Gorynych and this Asian maiden.

– Are you prepared to undergo your second trial for your faith? – we were asked.

– We are, – said Igor, answering for us both.

– Know, – said the Lord, – that with your actions, you are helping people who come to me. You are helping your Earth. You are helping your family and loved ones rid themselves of that which persecutes them.

He made the sign of the cross over us.

– Go with me… Do not doubt anything… That which you are doing is the Truth.

We thanked Him and turned towards the battlefield. A legion was already standing in neat rows. We rode along the rows, looking into the eyes of each soldier. A battle is a battle, and before one it is never a bad idea to look into the faces of your dear fellow soldiers, who have gone forth to meet death with you more than once. We knew that the soldiers must have faith in us, not fear us. A soldier who today fears his commander may tomorrow fear his enemy.

We told them not to doubt our courage, because we were going to fight for our people, for our Earth, and for our Lord, who cannot be overpowered.

A circle burst into flames around the cross in the center of the battlefield. Whoever leaves it of his own will or is driven out by the enemy will lose strength, knowledge, and understanding. We rode around the legion one more time, giving each soldier a piece of Russian earth from our amulets. In exchange, each soldier gave us a small piece of land from his own native country. Now we had a common land and a common cause.

We took out a flask containing magical water. On it was inscribed, To

Victory! We gave the flask to each soldier to take three sips.

Then we were ready to take the field. Again, I was the horse and Igor was the rider. Gorynych had already started clawing up the ground in impatience. He was huge, bigger than us and, most likely, stronger. But, as Alexander Nevsky said: There is strength in the truth. And the truth was with us. And that is why we were not afraid of the loathsome Gorynych and went to face him calmly, courageously, and without any inner doubts.

We divided the circle in half. No sooner had we done this than Gorynych hurled a flame at us. What could modern-day flame throwers possibly have in comparison to this device? The stench of hydrogen sulfide enveloped us. Igor managed to take cover behind his shield, while I was protected by a magical horse blanket. But still it was hot, worse than in a sauna, and Igor still had to wield his sword. And here is what the fabled parasite was doing: he had not even entered the circle yet and was already putting all his might into smothering us with his odiferous hydrogen sulfide. It was nothing, though, we could hold up. It had been no easier with the Black Knight. Igor used the reins to tell me that we had to circle around the enemy from the side. I tore to the side, as fast as I could. Gorynych did not have a chance to turn his pates after us. They were knocking against each other, preventing him from carrying out his fire-breathing maneuvers.

Another two fighters appeared out of nowhere. A raven flew in from the side. Igor shot him down with a silver arrow at full gallop. A wolf was attempting to duck under my legs, but he wasn't having any luck. Igor snagged him with his spear easily. That was it, the end for the gray one. A voice sounded within us, The raven is eternal death. And the wolf is eternal death. You have now killed two eternal deaths.

Gorynych had finally untangled his crocodile heads and was preparing

456

to cause harm again with his flame-throwing squadron. Using his stirrups, Igor gave the command to fly right at him.

We raced closer, approaching him. Apparently he did not expect us to do anything so audacious. Great height is actually really not always that useful. It engenders arrogance in the head. And if you do not have just one head, but three, then this is more than just a problem, it is a diagnosis. Gorynych underestimated something about Igor and me. In the blink of an eye, his right head flew off his giraffe-like neck, followed by the middle head. To top that off, when I turned away from his bulk, moving around him sideways, Igor hacked with his sword at the beast's tail. In little more than a minute, the dragon had been made into an invalid.

But still, he managed to reach us at the last minute with his remaining jaws. He did not seize me with his dying teeth, but he did butt me in the backside with his head. We flew away from him head over heels, but at least we stayed on our territory, within the circle.

Stars were spinning in my head, nothing less than the entire Milky Way. Gorynych would have time to reach us – there was nothing we could do about that. But he had considerable problems of his own: missing heads, a missing tail. He wanted to take a step towards us, but he could not: now he was collapsing over onto his side, now his remaining head was tipping him forwards off balance. He was very badly maimed and not in good shape at all.

Igor suffered less. He was the first to stand up, and he started to help me up. The spinning in my head abated a little. I stood, reeling. And I still had to go into battle. Igor scrambled up on me. At that moment, he looked larger than Don Quixote after he was beaten with stones. We had no strength, but we had to fight. And then the words of Alexander Nevsky rang out within us: There is strength in the truth! He was right. We had no strength, but the truth was with us. Our truth was that we would finish off Gorynych. We gathered all our strength and approached. Galloping was no longer possible. But the fire-breather's stump was no better. Maybe even worse. I plodded up to his bulk, closer to his remaining head, so that Igor could reach it.

I felt my warrior tense up. He raised his sword and struck, but he was not able to chop off the beast's head and the wound closed up right away. He struck once more, dropping his sword. But he understood what had happened and gave a mental command for the sword to return to his hand. The sword was no ordinary one – it also understood commands. Igor struck again in martial rage, overcome with faith in the Lord and in the Russian Motherland.

Gorynych's last head fell off, but Igor could not keep himself in the saddle. He fell right under the head that he had chopped off himself. The head was at least the size of a shed. It pressed down on him with such force that he could not get out from under it. He lost all his senses under this weight. His twisting could not wrench him free.

I caught hold of his clothes with my teeth and pulled, digging in with my hooves. Somehow I managed to pull out my warrior.

Igor stood up shakily. Again he passed his sword over the bulk of the dragon, making a cross. Then, barely keeping hold of the saddle's pommel, he walked up to the three who were sitting on thrones in mute amazement, looking at their previously unconquerable Gorynych.

– Whosoever shall come to us with the sword shall die by the sword, – he said firmly, sternly looking at the three dark rulers. Then, squinting slightly at the naked beauty, he added,– Anyone, it seems, women too.

We turned and walked off to our side. The Lord said, – Come with me into my Kingdom.

And he disappeared. But where was it, the Kingdom?

We looked: thousands and thousands of people were walking somewhere. We were no longer a horse and his warrior, but instead looked like everyone else. The shirts we were wearing were linen and were tied around the waist with rope. We entered the columns of people and followed them, slowly because we had no strength.

Suddenly five elders appeared by the road. Each one held an apple in his right hand and in his left hand.

– Take them, they said. – Build up your strength.

We looked at the apples, but there was something strange about them. They were spinning like tops.

– No, we don't need your apples.

– Take them, – entreated the elders. – The Lord betrayed you. He did not give you the apple of eternal youth.

– Begone! – bade Igor. – Otherwise, you will answer for your words.

They disappeared. New seductions were standing along the road. Women with apples. They were speaking against the Lord, trying to seduce with their charms.

A sword materialized in Igor's hand, and they disappeared right away. Five children arose in their place. They held apple halves in their hands.

– Take this! – they beseeched. – You will gain eternal life. The Lord won't give anything like this to you.

– Go away! – ordered Igor. – Our children would never speak like that.

We managed to reach the gates, which were large and iron-sided. The walls were high, white. Beyond them stood an alabaster city. Other elders waited by the entrance.

The gates opened onto a cobbled pathway leading to a garden. The Lord himself was waiting for us, smiling. A vessel holding water stood next to Him.

We kneeled before Him. He picked up a dipper and sprinkled water over us. He sprinkled once, our strength returned; a second time, our wounds healed; a third time, and all the evil spirits from the dragon's blood slipped off our bodies and crawled out of our souls.

He washed us with water and gave us three apples from His garden.

– Throw one down on the earth so that there will be a harvest, – he bade. – Give the second to the people, so that they have enough strength to last until My Advent. Divide the third up among yourselves, your families, and friends.

He blessed us.

We exited through the gates and did as the Lord said. We threw one apple onto the ground. We gave another to the blessed people. The third we divided among ourselves, our families, and friends, many of whom were with the soldiers in the legion.

We returned to the battlefield. Picking up the cross, we focused all our will on it and moved Gorynych's corpse into the Bardo channel of the lower levels. That was it. We had cleaned up our territory. Some information remained – traces of presence of Dark Spirits. We picked up a white ray and made a white cloud. We cleaned their space.

Holy elders appeared.

– You are on the right path, do not doubt it, – they said. – For the victory which you have brought, you will be endowed with the energy of the Absolute. The Lord thanks you for not doubting him and not listening to His blasphemers. A new path to knowledge has been opened for you. Take from it deeply, and not just from the surface. A chariot lies between the third and fourth levels. It needs to be turned upright. The Lord is with you!

– As we are with him, – Igor and I answered in unison.

We descended into Bardo. Between the third and fourth levels stood a huge man holding a trident. It was the new God Androgin. He was looking, waiting.

Next to him an enormous chariot lay on its side. It was much bigger than us.

Since the Lord ordered us to do this, our strength must be known to him. Igor and I set about our task together, setting the chariot right without any real difficulty. It must have been the apples. We drove in the bushings.

Suddenly three fiery horses appeared next to us. They hitched themselves up to the chariot. The God climbed up into it. He was smiling.

– You are on the true path, a path that is seen by few. – The voice was thunderous, resonant. – Help people. Fear nothing, even the persecution you will face on Earth. You must pass through everything, endure everything. Separate the light from the dark. You have been given the right to deliver judgment. No one can block your path, but along the way many will dare to obstruct your way and impede your progress. I will say it again: Do not doubt yourselves. Your path has been predetermined by He whom no one can impede.

He is so large that we can only see up to his waist. But the ring on his hand is unmistakable. It is the Creator Himself – the Father of the Gods.

How can it be that archetypal figures suddenly become direct participants in current events and, indeed, in a most active way influence not only what is happening with me and my family, but also the possibilities of both physical and spiritual personal development?

Vitaly Yurevich and Tatyana Serafimovna Tikhoplav, scientists from St. Petersburg, have presented most interesting material in their book Pivotal Turn, which to some extent clarifies what happened:

461

Today specialists from the Institute of Quantum Genetics are trying to decode the mysterious text of DNA molecules. Their discoveries point more and more to the fact that in the beginning there was the Word. Scientists believe that DNA is a text just like a book, but that it can be read starting from any letter because there is no break between words. Reading this text starting with every subsequent letter produces more and more new texts. What's more, the text can be read backwards, if the row is flat. If the chain of text is unfolded in three-dimensional space, as in a cube, then the text can be read in all directions. This text is not stationary. It is constantly moving, changing, because our chromosomes breathe and sway, giving rise to an enormous number of texts.

Work with linguists and mathematicians at Moscow State University has shown that the structure of human speech and texts from books is mathematically close to the structure of DNA sequencing, i.e. these are actually texts in languages that are as yet unknown to us. Cells actually do speak with one another as we do with each other. The genetic apparatus knows infinitely many languages.

The program that is recorded in DNA could not have appeared as a result of Darwin's evolution. Recording such an enormous amount of information requires time, time far in excess of the time the Universe has existed.

The renowned microbiologist Michael Denton has confirmed this: Neither of the two fundamental axioms of Darwin's macroevolutionary theory has been validated by one single empirical discovery or scientific advance since 1859. As we now know, when Charles Darwin said that he broke out into a cold sweat when he was examining the structure of elements in a living organism in his later years: such organisms could not have formed on their own. They had to have had a Supreme Creator.

On the same topic Charles Thaxton wrote: "Do we have evidence that life owes its origins to intelligence? Yes! This evidence is the analogy between the sequence of nucleotides in a DNA chain and the sequence of letters in a book.... There is a structural equivalence between DNA code and written language. The analogy between human languages (which are all without exception products of intellect) and DNA may serve as a basis for the conclusion that DNA is also a result of intellectual activity."

It is already clear that the wave genomes of the animal and plant worlds are governed by the same universal mechanism – Speech, fragments of which researchers have learned how to simulate. Many years of intensive research have shown convincing proof that the development of languages and human speech follows the same rules that genetics does! DNA texts, human written speech, and oral speech carry out identical management and regulatory functions, but on different scales and within different spheres of application. DNA texts function genetically on the cellular and histological level, while human speech is used for communication.

It would appear that Cosmic intelligence has created some copies of itself and is working to develop them. At the first stage, they cannot be used in complicated programs. The main task of such organisms, facing survival as self-sufficient and self-developed organisms, is to grasp the moral laws of a social community. The program becomes more sophisticated at the next levels: the inevitable - under conditions of earthly evolution - battle must now take into account not only the personal progression of the individual, but also his spiritual alignment with the concept of society, or, more importantly, with a higher ideal captured in the image of the Creator.

And this is when the confrontation between Kashchey the Immortal and the Dragon Gorynych, both within, in one's consciousness, and without, in social life, takes place. During this entirely real fight, a procedure takes place that cleanses the spirit of the negative past and checks the level of its qualities and development.

This same Dragon Gorynych represents a part of Earth's historical past, the epoch of the dinosaurs. The spinal cord in human beings is still called a reptilian complex. And this is not accidental. But, for example, in dinosaurs the thought process was lodged in the spinal cord, at the level of the sacrum. This means that in life they had, if it can be put this way, a rearward reaction. Imagine how much could happen as a signal travelled to the neck, to the head, and back again just to cause a reaction to an event. It's enough to make you crazy. Now this is not possible with human beings because they have two brains – one in the spinal cord and one in the head. If, of course, the latter works. So when it comes time to move from the brain at the level of the sacrum to the brain that is on the neck, something like a high school graduation exam takes place. Your further advancement towards the distinctly defined ideal for humankind depends on the results of this exam.

* * *

After all these events, our abilities to heal increased exponentially. We felt that with just a little bit more, we would be able not only to cure incurable diseases, but also resurrect people. In fact, we already knew how to do this; we just had to try it out in practice. But we would need the consent of relatives, the consent of the soul of the person to be resurrected, and also an analysis of the lives that the deceased had lived up until then. After

464

all, people are different. It would be nice to help primarily good people, those who had helped someone themselves.

Something strange was going on with Kirill. He was the first to get to work and the last to leave. He was working so hard that it seemed as though he could handle everyone's work on his own. He was railing against Lapshin and taking advantage of any chance he got to tell us that he had definitely decided to go with us. But how did he see this path? And how did Igor and I see it? I do not think that we saw the same thing. Can it really be that millions of years have not delivered him from vanity, have not given him wisdom? Sometimes he would burst out with:

– You know that I'm hanging on a ledge right now. Things are hard for me. You have to help me.

– You mean that you owe someone money?

– You don't understand. I'm the very very last in the line.

– Oh, so that's how it is! – exclaimed Igor. – Not just the last, but the very last squared.

– But this was my only chance to have a son! – said Kirill in desperation. – I was prepared to annihilate the entire Earth for him. If I do not have a son, then I will never be reincarnated again.

– So you were prepared to annihilate everything for your son? And billions of other lives are what, nothing? – I tried to ascertain, curious. – And millions of other children? Only you and your little son!

– Man is such scum! – The boy Kirill hissed evilly, and his dark eyes for a moment shone with the abyss. There was nothing in them – no light, no life, no Earth.

Everything was clear to him, but he was clinging to his last hope. His last hope squared.

– OK. I'm going to see Lapshin in Theodosia. I'll sniff out what's

465

going on there and let you know.

Igor and I shrugged.

– Go wherever you want. You are as free as a bird.

– I'll leave you my mark, – said Kirill, and a round piece of paper with figures drawn on it appeared in his hand. You can use it at any time to connect telepathically with me.

He shoved it into my folder containing notes that was lying on the table.

That evening, while Igor and I were traveling home on the commuter train, I remembered this piece of paper.

– Should we take a look at what he shoved in there?

Igor turned on the inner vision screen and scanned the paper.

– It's the stamp of the Ruler of Darkness Migen. – We received our answer right away. – He can use it to keep a constant watch on what you are doing.

OK. We ripped up the paper and threw it out the window. A good boy, Kirill… Loves children. True, not all of them in a row, but only his own, who did not yet exist.

Kirill actually did leave for Theodosia the next day. Like he said, for intelligence gathering. Just Malchish Kibalchish* [the Boy Nipper Pipper], not demons of darkness.

Well, what of it? It was somehow easier to breathe without him. We decided to take a look at the levels. But even on the first level we started to have a sense of uneasiness, a feeling of vague alarm. Twelve doors. Behind them are zodiacal energies that help heal, restore, and resurrect. The Creator's stamp on one of the doors was broken. There was an intruder.

* The young hero of a Soviet war tale who dies at the hands
of the enemy, rather than reveal a military secret.

466

We quickly collected a cross from the eighth level and took it with us through the door. The energy in the room was drawn up into the cross. Now through it the Lord himself could see what was happening here.

In a corner, an enormous demon was trying to fade into the darkness. He was frightened: he knew that nothing good could come of our meeting. He happened to be from one of the levels that Goryncyh ruled over. A vacancy opened up, and he decided to curry favor. He was displaying – how to put it? – initiative. Well, well...

– Why did you come here? – asked Igor.

As a former police official, he was able to pose questions diplomatically. It was just a few words, but the intonation, the look... Even a demon cannot withstand this, especially if he is being cornered by a cross.

– The Ruler of Darkness ordered me to break in and take this energy, – admitted the demon frankly.

– Why didn't you take it?

– It kept slipping away from me. I spent a whole hour chasing after it.

– How did you get in here? After all, the passage through the Bardo channel is secured by the Creator's seal.

– We have secret approaches, – said the demon. I imagined how pleased the Lord would be to hear such a confession.

– And who is Lapshin? – I suggested the question and Igor sternly repeated it.

– The Ruler of Darkness uses him for identifying future adversaries. He knew that you would come. Under the terms of his agreement with the Creator, he has the right to make the first move. He wanted to make effective use of this.

– So why didn't he use it?

– That Lapshin.... – The demon almost choked with outrage. – He got too big for his britches. He thought only about himself and wanted to use the knowledge he had discovered for his own personal power. He should have exposed you and either lured you over to his side or told our people in the government about you.

– You have people in the government? Who? – demanded Igor, with a threatening intonation in his voice.

The demon wavered, then sputtered out a tongue twister: – One speaks, the other discusses, the third has money, and the fourth knows all.

– Names, give me names!

– I don't know. I am the highest demon over the lowest. Those above me intimidate me, while I abuse the ones below. Who is going to tell me about something like that?

– How can I find them? – pressed Igor. The prisoner wavered. His frightful pig-like snout furrowed. But the Lord's cross pressured him into telling the truth.

– You know them all. Three have dark hair with a bald spot in the front. They all look alike. Very brisk in their ways.

– And the fourth?

– He is not bald and exchanges a few words with everyone.

– And the grande dame who was with your ruler at the last battle? Who is she?

– The goddess of the lust, – said the demon. – She is harmless when a man fails to take notice of her. Indifference defeats her. But when she gets attention, she can fight for a day or two. It's the same as battling yourself.

The voice of the Lord thundered from the cross: – You will see everything, but you will not be able to say anything. Go back to the kingdom that you created for yourselves.

We stood to the side, and the demon dashed by us.

468

– Those doors which were sealed you may now open, – said the Lord. – This will be your school. Send your disciples here. The saints will teach them how to heal themselves and others. Only people sent by you may come here for knowledge. You may walk around all the remaining levels on this side, but did not bring anyone else. My blessings upon you!

We thanked the Lord, carried the cross back to its place, and left the levels.

* * *

The next Friday evening we invited to the Center our best students, those whose inner vision screens worked well. We told them that from now on we would be holding an unusual master class at our Center that would be taught by saints.

The students looked at us with surprise, even though they were used to the unusual here. They calmly slipped on their patches and turned on their internal vision screens.

Everyone was ready. We asked them to hold hands so that they would not get lost in the boundless space of another world. They looked around, thinking that the whole setup seemed strange. They were used to working individually or in smalls groups, but now there were many of us. We were together, leading people to a school that the Lord had given us permission to run. It was the moment of truth: Would the others see the school that Igor and I saw? And would they be able to enter it if we were not next to them?

But everything went better than we expected. We showed our students the path and when we led them to the school, the saints were already waiting for us. The classroom doors stood open and each student was taken to

469

the place where his or her health problems could be resolved.

– Be polite and grateful, – we instructed those who had, on our recommendation, received the right to ascend to a new level of their development. – Bear in mind that you will be given knowledge by holy people.

After classes, both the children and the adults spoke effusively with one another about their training on their own bodies. They were shown which illnesses they had and were taught how to treat them.

Most importantly, they would now be able to access the school at any time, whenever they had the need. They could do this anywhere: at home, at work, during a trip.

In this school our students for the first time learned exactly what role collective consciousness, collective soul, and collective energy play in life on Earth. That these concepts are not fabrications flying from the minds of esoteric idealists, but actual reality. By the way, the Communist Party of the Soviet Union prided itself on its collective mind. Apparently, its bosses were no strangers to mysticism.

Here I would like to cite one more excerpt from Grigori Petrovich Grabovoi's book "The Resurrection of People and Eternal Life – Our New Reality," which can in the most direct manner provide a commentary on what happened with our students. Indeed, elevating one's level of consciousness is the correct way to change oneself and the surrounding world.

One current position holds that the outside world does not depend on us, that it exists on its own, so to speak, objectively, and that all a person can do is observe this world and study its laws so that they can be used for the good of people.

In fact, we should think about why it happened that people have such an impression. A person sees that the sun rises every morning and sets every evening, that the seasons change regularly, in the same sequence, that the North Star can always be found in the same place in the sky, and that an object dropped from a hand will always fall downwards, like Newton's famous apple. All these phenomena are constantly occurring one after the other, and man forms an impression that these events are taking place independent of his existence, that they are objective events that are not subject to his will. In other words, that he is dealing with an objective world that exists independently of him. But this is precisely man's great error.

To determine what is actually going on, we must introduce the concept of a collective consciousness. Collective consciousness is the combined consciousness of all people. Later we will see that the consciousness of other beings, for example animals, and all living things for that matter, should also be included in the collective consciousness.

A stable set of beliefs exists in the collective consciousness. These beliefs are stable because they are in the middle. In other words, they are the result of the averaging out of all people.

Let's look at a specific example so that we can better see what it is we are talking about. Imagine that we are flipping a coin. Can we say with any certainty if it will come up heads or tails? If it is a standard coin, then we cannot say. But what if we flip the coin, let's say, seven times? It's the same. It may come up heads several times or it may come up tails all seven times. Even if we set up a ratio of how many times heads comes up to how many times tales comes up, we still cannot determine what this figure would be in the examples above without using clairvoyance. We cannot say, for example, what number this figure will equal after seven flips.

However, if we flip the coin several thousand times, then we can say in advance that the ratio of heads to tails will tend towards one. If we flip the coin several million times, this number will be virtually equal to one. So it is possible to predict a result when the coin is flipped many, many times. This is no accident. The fact is that with a large number of trials or cases, what is known as a statistical regularity emerges. (This refers to a well-known law of large numbers – A.P.).

Thus, several individual trials will not uncover any regularity and the result will appear accidental. But if we look at a very large number of events, then statistical regularities emerge.

Many such regularities surround us. For example, look closely at a computer's keyboard. You can see that the letters on the keyboard are not in alphabetical order. They are laid out in some sort unique order, apparently following some kind of rule. But which one?

The letters that are used most frequently are in the center of the keyboard, while the ones that are used less frequently are on the sides. This makes sense because it is easier to use the index fingers than the little fingers.

How can we know which letters are the most frequently used? One way would be to give a computer a command to read many books and determine which letters occur frequently, which ones appear less often, and which ones are rarely seen at all. A computer can calculate the probability of each letter's appearance in the text. The letters with the highest probability of appearing in the text are positioned in the center of the keyboard.

Consider this. If we want to know the probability that some letter, let's say A, will appear in a word randomly selected from the text, we will not be able to find an answer to this question. But if we take many books containing many words and, accordingly, letters, then we will have statistical regularity and we will be able to determine the probability of its appearance in the text.

This type of information can be used by printing presses to put to-gether type cases. Not all the letters of the alphabet need to be cast in the same amounts, but instead letters can be prepared in the amounts proportional to the probability of their appearance in the text.

This same concept is used to compile frequency dictionaries. After reading many books, particularly classics, a computer can put together a list of the most commonly used words. These kinds of dictionaries are particularly useful for studying a foreign language. For example, 3,000 of the most frequently used words in the English language make up 90 percent of the text of a work of fiction. By contrast, Webster's Dictionary contains several hundred thousand words. Thus, we can see how using statistical regularity can simplify the study of another language. With just 3,000 of the most commonly occurring words, you can already read and speak another language.

But let's return to our main topic. Each person has his own set of beliefs, beliefs on everything, and they can differ greatly from the beliefs of another person. But if we take all people – and this is a very great number – then all these beliefs are averaged out. As a result, the collective consciousness has a stable set of beliefs about different things. And it is this collective set of beliefs that is understood by people to be objective reality. An illusion is created specifically by the stability of this resulting set of beliefs, even though this stability is simply the result of averaging out a large number of objects, in this case the beliefs that exist in the consciousness of people.

For example, when I conduct a diagnostic exam of a person who has come to me for help, I see that the condition of his body is constantly in flux, more often than not within very large bounds. But if I send this person for an x-ray, the screen will show a stable picture. The catch here is that the equipment gives readings connected to the belief set of the collective consciousness about the given situation.

And now we are ready to formulate a very important principle:

OUR CONSCIOUSNESS ACCEPTS AS REALITY THAT WHICH EXISTS IN OUR CONSCIOUNESS.

When you are thinking, that about which you are thinking is as real to your consciousness as that which is taking place around you and as that which, for example, you see with your own eyes, through regular vision.

This principle is fundamental because when you combine what you think with events in external, supposedly objective, reality, when you combine these things at the level of action, you can affect the materialization of objects, you can bring to life.

It is as though there are two realities: a reality within consciousness is one and a reality outside of consciousness is the other, the one that is perceived of as stable.

That said, it must be understood that all objects in the surrounding world – let's say a table, a chair, a car – all these objects, every particle of them, every element of the world, is built upon the collective conscious-ness of living people. And therefore, if even just one part of consciousness is changed, the world starts to change. And so, incidentally, it is necessary to retransform without destroying, but by creating through creative know-ledge. So, when we look at the surrounding world, what we are actually looking at is not actual stability, but the most convenient space for living beings and objects, obtained as a result of averaging. To be more precise, we understand the collective reality in the sense of space-time. And there-fore, our Earth, for example, or our physical bodies, are simply the result of the unification of the consciousness of all people, or, more precisely, of all creations in general, people and living creatures alike.

474

If we know this principle, then we can say that resurrection is simply the right technological addition to the structure of collective relationships.

So, to repeat. Everything that surrounds us – the Earth, the Sun, stars, space, the entire world – all this has in reality been created on the structure of consciousness, including the consciousness of the Creator. Therefore, when we know what the spirit is, what consciousness is, we can resurrect, we can create space, we can build a world, and we can generally perform any creative actions.

Practically, it is possible to change reality because reality was created at the appropriate time through the decision-making process of the consciousness of every individual and every object of information.

This means that into order to resurrect, in order to have immortality, in order for each person to have a happy life, each person has to adopt this point of view. Each person has to arrive at a decision about this path. And the more people that decide to select such a path, the path of an eternal and happy life, the faster reality will start to undergo a transformation in this direction.

So, Yevtushenko's formulation about the alder catkin that "When we change, the world changes" is correct. This is a thoroughly exhaustive commentary on our experiences. Everything exists in this world – the Creator, the Holy Spirit, and Christ – because everything exists in our consciousness. Just like we ourselves do. In their consciousness! Everything within everything…. As above, so below…. There's not really anything new about these ideas. It's simply that our level of perception of them is qualitatively different. In ancient times, the world view of the masses was magical. Priests represented science and guarded its secrets. Why has a rational trend prevailed? Why has the Aristotelian and Cartesian world view

475

triumphed over 2,000 years? Did the supreme bearers of teachings err in betraying universal aims for their own selfish motives? Or was this wrinkle in the development of science – this move towards mechanical thinking, towards atheism – objectively necessary for the development of nous.

Indeed, despite the influence of so-called materialism and rationality, faith in non-traditional knowledge has lingered in people. It has lingered in the popular mind in sorcerers and witches, in the enlightened layers of astrology, in the search for the philosopher's stone, in the elixir of immortality. In the serious scientific studies of Jakob Böhme, Emanuel Swedenborg, Friedrich Mesmer, and other inquisitive minds. The belief was reflected in epos and literature. Even though Russian literature is comparatively young, it contains many works dedicated to attempts at understanding the supernatural. I'm not talking about Gogol or Odoyevsky and their fantastic tales, but about other authors, perhaps less well-known, but having a scientific bent. Pisemsky's thick "Masons," Mitrofan Ladyzhensky's "Mystical Trilogy," Sluchevsky's "Letters from Beyond," Bryusov's "Fiery Angel," and the historical and mystical novels of Vsevolod Solovyov and Mikhail Volkonsky – it's not possible to count them all. But all the same, collective belief leaned towards mechanical reality. Christ was increasingly supplanted by thoughts that "if you don't lie, you won't sell," and "an honest day's work won't get you a house made of stone." And almost everyone wanted to live in a house of stone. Not in a small monastery, but in satisfaction and prosperity.

Duplicity and double standards exist at all levels of society. In Volkonsky's Two Magicians, one sorcerer reproaches the other: "Instead of using the knowledge revealed to you for good and truth, for the benefit of other people, for treating them with charity, you started to reap benefits for yourself, to think only of yourself... And your power started

476

weakening." But these words are also about humankind en masse, in the collective consciousness. Otherwise, humankind would not have bowed down before the golden calf and other gods and idols of the Israel of the Old Testament.

"He that has ears to hear, let him hear." Are the populations of Russia and other countries prepared to embrace a new situation in the world, much less the fact of its creation? Let's recall how intensely the Soviet government advocated for a healthy way of life, primarily in the areas of physical education, instruction in basic medical skills, harmonious family relationships, and rules for "public facilities." There were dozens of scientific and academic institutes and armies of instructors at companies, health resorts, vacation hotels, and sometimes even residential buildings. They tried to encompass the movements of young and old. But how much of an effect did this have? People en masse preferred to live the old way. Articles about heroes who had overcome their ailments and achieved phenomenal results, people like Valentin Dikul, Shavarsh Karapetyan* and many others, were splattered across the pages of newspapers. Ordinary people would read these articles with amazement and envy ("if only I could do that"), but would not pursue this desire. It was the same with public life: issues about autonomy, working in unions, etc., etc. Pretty much everyone understands that "the only people worthy of life and liberty are those who go to fight for them every day." But in real life, they wait with open mouths for manna to fall, either from God or the Kremlin. Try to puzzle this out on your own, and maybe one day you will be able to reenergize a person who is near and dear to you.

I had already spotted two people – Mama and Boris Andreyevich

---

* Dikul is a circus performer who made a miraculous recovery from a broken back. Karapetyan is a finswimmer who saved 20 people from drowning after their trolleybus drove into a reservoir.

Mozhayev. I met them at their place on the third level. We were not allowed to approach one another or embrace. We spoke at a distance so that their bodies of that place would not be harmed by direct contact. Mama was not saying much, but Boris Andreyevich had something to complain about.

– We are rarely allowed to look at what is there, on earth. And sometimes we refuse the chance to take a look. My soul aches at what I see.

He was wearing a short gray raincoat. He knew that, having died in our world, he had not really died at all, but had returned as it were through the looking glass – to the other end of a figure eight, the symbol of infinity. In this place, their collective consciousness also forms all the conditions for life – work, cars, houses. For us this is an illusion. For them it is reality. But they know that they will still have to return to the earth to complete the incarnation program. And Mozhayev knew that if my plan worked, he would be the first to undergo incarnation with his memory intact, that is, with the experience of all his incarnations.

He could not understand why I had become such a big shot in the noumenal world and why I could speak freely on these topics. But there was no way he could not believe my words, especially since the saint in charge of their level right nearby.

– I know about my grandsons. If you see Milda, tell her that that I remember how we went on vacation together in '56. It was a lot of fun. Autumn, family. There were an iron twin bed and a stove in our room. Together we coated that stove with clay.

– It was autumn. We went for a walk in the park. Puddles. Flared pants. I swept the ground with them. We dreamed about children, made plans for the future – study, work. I remember my couch. This was already in the later years, in Moscow. I had a favorite book, in a red binding. I'm telling you this so that she'll believe you. Otherwise she'll think you were a dream.

And then he angrily went off again about general things.

– You have a real mess there, folks. Everyone is deceiving one another.

Later I was preparing to call his widow, Milda Emilyevna. But how can you tell someone about something like this? She would think that it was a dream, and that would be in the best case. I decided to wait a little, until the book came out. In the overall context, it would be easier to understand, both for Milda Emilyevna and for all the others.

While I was speaking with Boris Andreyevich, Mama remembered something about us, from our distant past, and Igor, who was able to read her mind, later asked me:

– What, you were so poor that you didn't have sleds?

– We couldn't have been any poorer, – I confirmed. – Mama worked as a typist at the factory "40 Years of October". She worked on a typewriter. Her salary was 40 rubles, and that was before the monetary reforms of '61. With three children on her hands. Remember, she raised us on her own. She went to bed at night after washing clothes and preparing food. Then, in the morning, at about 5:00am, she was back in the kitchen. To feed us and send us off to school.

– So you didn't have a sled? – Igor harped on. – Did you have a washbowl?

– We did. It was old, nickel-plated. I found it somewhere in the dumpster. I threaded a shoelace through a hole and dragged it behind me. I rode it down hills. I would get in it and fly down the hill like crazy.

– Hmph, – clucked Igor. An Academician and sledding in a washbowl.

– It was a magnificent device! I flew down the hills faster than anybody. I recalled the past with delight.

– With a shoelace?

479

– Exactly, with a shoelace. There was a hole in the washbowl. I threaded a rope through it and dragged it behind me. It rattled as I walked down the street. Brilliant!

– I see, I see, – acknowledged Igor.

– You know, it was so great! There was no way those kids on the sleds could overtake me.

– I see, – Igor acknowledged again.

– It was better to go sledding in washbowls than on sleds, – I went on, insistent on demonstrating the advantages of my childhood means of transport.

– Yes, yes…

– What else did Mama show you?

– Patched clothes.

– Yes, Mama patched everything. All my clothes were patches upon patches.

– She showed me sugar and oil or butter? You loved these.

– Sugar and sunflower oil? – I clarified.

– No. Bread and butter with sugar sprinkled on top.

– Right. Sugar with butter. But if it was sunflower oil, then I used salt.

– Bread soaked in butter, just like water, the sugar dissolving and melting away. And she showed me some kind of book, very worn out… She said it was the only one to read, that there were no others…

– I still have it, I've kept it.

– She showed me her housecoat. It was old. She had no other.

– We were very poor, – I reminded Igor. – She earned 40 rubles a month with three children!

– You lived in a room. Was everyone in one room?

– Yes. We used the couch as a partition.

480

– She said she wouldn't agree to take another room. She was given a large room, but it was heated by a stove, which had to be fed. When, she said, will I get the time to do that?

– Exactly. That's how it was.

– She was given another room, a much larger one. But the ceilings were not good. She said, I hadn't taken it.

– She lay down to sleep at night. And what she did? How did she have the time? And then to have to feed the stove? Of course she would not have had the time.

– She had a basket or a string bag where she kept needles, thread…

– Yes, she did.

– Like a hamper. She said, I had kept everything there.

– Then they bought me a violin, but I never did learn how to play it. They tied a pillow underneath my chin… I ran my bow over the strings again and again, but I just couldn't get the hang of it. My heart wasn't in it. But I did love to read books.

– This is what can take place at the level of the soul. Everything is in reality. She is aware of everything and sees everything. I was just reading everything off of her. She remembers, she knows everything. She definitely sees everything. This is spiritual vision. On the other hand, they seem to see everything with their eyes. This means that whatever they imagine, they see with their eyes. They perceive everything differently. Their eyes have significance. They see with their souls and with their eyes. You still see visual images, but the eyes have significance. She tried to talk you into becoming a director, but you kept your silence…. You were silent, silent, silent.

– You can see my side too. What kind of responsibility would that have been? And I was still little.

– What do you mean? You can do it, your mother reproached you.

– I could have. But first one publishing company grew, then another. It takes a long time to drag one publishing house and then another to the top. And when you reach the top, someone can give you a kick... And everything goes tumbling backwards, and very quickly too.

– Yes. Mozhayev was carrying on a conversation about some film. It wasn't clear... Boris Andreyevich resembled the hero of the film, resembled Fyodor from the film. He had the same character – you could grate away at him, but nothing could keep him down... At first he was not accepted into the Communist Party. Then they wanted to expel him. Then the people who persecuted him started inviting him to different celebrations, angling to become his friends. He said: I never paid any attention to any party whatsoever. I was invited, expelled... It really had no bearing on me at all.

– He was a very wise man. And independent. He didn't get into hand-to-hand fights with those authoritative writers over trifles. He kept his distance: hello, goodbye, yes, yes, no, no – and that was it. He never let them see what was in his soul and kept himself out of their secretarial rat race, where the person you join is the one you attack, – I explained to Igor.

– Why was he saying all this? Does this mean that they see physical bodies like we see living people? – asked Igor.

I didn't say anything. I was thinking about collective consciousness.

Chapter 12

Now when we entered another space, we immediately found ourselves in the place where we wanted to be. It is especially useful to look down from the apex of the triangular energomagnetic structure, which soars over the Earth's North Pole. The lower levels are also visible from here. This time, they were still empty after the recent massacre that Igor and I unleashed when we were saving Tamara. On the lower platform, near the fiery seething of the Earth's core, stood three thrones. Two of them were empty. The Ruler of Darkness had, apparently, found his scapegoats. And he was right. Someone had to answer for the mess we had created. Androgin appeared. We kneeled down before him. He ordered us to stand.

– What was started must be finished, – he said. – There is a pouch behind Migen's throne. It holds your Russian land. They stole it a long time ago, but they don't know what to do with it. We have to go get it. Are you afraid to go there?

And the God pointed to the place to which we would have to descend.

– Your legion is already waiting, along with the lion and the eagle. The Lord himself will watch over your negotiations. The law requires them to give you the land. But if they attack – and there are many of them there – it will be difficult for you. Do you understand?

Igor sighed and waved his arm as if he were chopping away with a sword.

– If you're scared of devils, then don't go to hell.

– You're right about that. – Androgin roared with thunderous laughter. The familiar ring sparkled on his hand when he brought it to his mouth.

Androgin vanished and in his place our troops, the lion, and the eagle appeared all at once. We embraced our soldiers, bidding each other fare-well just in case. And down we went.

The evil spirits went crazy. Migen looked at us ferociously. The mute demon, the one we had caught out in the levels, was mumbling something, pointing at us with his hand, or maybe his paw, as if he were the only one who was sharp-sighted enough to notice us. And behind the thrones – Oh my goodness! – were innumerable devils. They were scrambling over each other, baring their teeth, ready to attack. But Migen did not give the command. He was making his own complicated calculations: about this very moment between the past and the future, about the Creator and our role in the polarity of Good and Evil.

– Why have you come here? – he asked.

From everything it is clear that it is difficult for him to speak with us, taxing. Like it might be for a lord to speak with a serf or a criminal with a prosecutor.

Igor silently set down the cross, which he had prudently taken from the eighth level before our campaign.

– Why did you drag the cross with you? – frowned Migen.

– The Lord himself will be a witness in case one of the devils violates the law.

– Are you aware of the kind of power that I have? – The ferocity of the Ruler of Darkness started to emerge. – A wave of my hand and nothing will remain of you.

– Sure, sure. You're so terrifying that you're even scared of yourself, confirmed Igor.

We exchanged glances. The devils, choking with rage, were trotting about on their pig-like hooves, ready to throw themselves at us. And that naked woman, the goddess of lust. Also dreaming, apparently, of close contact, of a fight. Well, what can you say! As the saying goes, what the heart bids, the soul desires.

– Our faith is strong. As far as our susceptibility to fear is concerned, you can figure that out for yourself, no doubt. So why don't you just nicely hand over that which we earned in honest battle – our Russian land.

– Are you going to fight?

– On the battlefield, in the Kingdom of Heaven. That's what the law stipulates. So that the Lord can see everything.

– What's your Lord to me? – he asked spitefully, mockingly. – As Pontius Pilate said, "What is the truth?"

Igor, an old hand at being a soldier, barked out all the statutes so that the evil-doer would not doubt our faith or our Lord.

– Our Lord is our faith, our Motherland, our people. He has never deserted us and we will never desert Him, never leave Him.

The woman behind us started leaping about purposively. We could see her reflection in the eyes of the Ruler of Darkness. Suddenly, hissing snakes took the place of the hair on her head. They were trying to make us turn around with their racket. But we did not. The mute demon had warned us in time, and we could see her through the pupils of the Ruler of Darkness.

She took one step, then another, and started to turn to stone. Now her eyes were filled with terror. It was probably the first time that such fundamental setbacks were taking place in her vile body.

The Ruler of Darkness was astonished, but still did not lose his hope of outwitting us.

– Why are you rooted to the ground? he said to Igor. Strike her! She was the first who wanted to attack you!

– We have no business with her, – answered Igor. – We came to speak

485

with you.

After his words, the goddess of lust disintegrated into pieces, as if she had never existed.

– We earned the right to this land, – snarled Migen. – We defeated your knight during the last Armageddon.

– During the last one, yes, – admitted Igor. – But not now.

– Fine, – agreed the Ruler of Darkness unexpectedly. I have it in a pouch here. But there are three pouches. Who will make the selection? The horse with its hoof or you with your hand? But be careful you don't lose everything.

Three bags, each tied with a knot. Igor wavered, trying to sense which one contained his native land. One pouch extended itself out to him – it held birch trees, our rivers, wide-open expanses. The soul could sense these. The other ones held a sense of malice, of darkness.

– Give me that one, – said Igor, taking the middle pouch without any fear.

– Who's stopping you? – hissed Migen.

– Not you, – answered Igor cockily, turning me around. We returned to our side with our legion, the eagle, and the lion.

The Lord himself met us upon our exit from the Bardo channel. The saints were with him. He made the sign of the cross over us, taking the pouch into his hand.

– This land came at a high price, – said the Lord.

It was clear how agitated and worried He was. All the saints were rejoicing behind Him.

– This is not just land, it is My strength! If you set out on a dangerous path again, I will give you and your legion a handful of it to take with you. – He blessed the legion. He blessed us once again and let us go.

486

He had tears in his eyes. It was hard for him to cope with his feelings. He had been waiting a long, long time for this joyous moment.

* * *

Everyone was talking about the loss of the Kursk, Russia's best submarine cruiser, in the Barents Sea. Igor and I decided to see what had actually happened there.

We turned on our inner vision screens. Everything was clearly visible from the North Pole. We found the location of the accident. We started looking at events in the order of which they occurred. Our information was not matching what officials were saying. But were they really to be believed? For politicians, the truth lies wherever it can bring benefit.

Here is what we saw several days after the accident...

08.16.2000 08:30 We saw a vessel lying on the sea bottom. There was a dent in the middle part. The nose was torn open.

The cause of the accident was a collision with an American submarine. It was standing motionless. The Kursk approached it. It was right next to the American submarine. Visibility was very poor. There was a lot of silt in the water because of the strong current. The Kursk came to rest alongside the American submarine, coming out into the line of fire. It opened its torpedo hatches. The Americans understood that they had found themselves in the wrong place at the wrong time. There was nowhere to retreat. The American vessel for some reason moved forward, probably because it wanted to dive under our ship and get out of the line of fire, but it struck the submarine cruiser in the side. The officer navigating our cruiser was thrown backwards. His hand caught on something on the instrument panel. The Kursk lurched downwards, nose first. It shoved out

487

of the way the American ship, which struck the body of the Kursk with its tail, damaging its propeller. The Kursk went down quickly, nose first, striking the seabed. There was some kind of explosion. With a piercing sound, the Americans retreated to neutral waters 10-12 kilometers away. During the vessel's retreat, more damage was done to the propeller and its parts. The propeller was grinding against something, unable to withstand the stress. Something had gone wrong with their boat as well. It settled on the seabed. The crew numbered almost 70 people. There were wounded and, possibly, fatalities.

08.17.2000 21:10 A rescue vessel tried to dock with the hatch on the nose. There were two people inside it. They did not feel well – they were tired and their blood pressure was rising. They numbly kept trying to do the same thing over and over, attempting to dock with the hatch under poor visibility conditions and in a turbulent sea. They would keep hitting the cruiser and getting carried off to the side. Nothing worked for them.

08.19.2000 8:10 We were in the boat, in the compartments. Some of the sailors were still alive. The rescuers were not able to enter the vessel and open the jammed hatch. They had no skills. The situation was terrible. Commanders take on the responsibility for training rescuers in specific emergency situations and they believe in a rosy future: what if the rescue actually succeeds? We can't say that they were idiots, but there was so-mething inept about the way they were conducting themselves.

The temperature was dropping. Half of those still alive were in comas.

Special equipment should have been ordered for the damaged hatch from factories in Severodvinsk. The people inside were half-dead.

Our equipment was not able to handle this problem. Officials were most likely aware of this, but could not make up their minds about what to do.

They feared that the reactor had not been shut down!

They feared pulling the submarine out of the seabed!

They feared towing it to shore!

They feared opening the hatch: What if there was radiation there!

They feared there would be some sort of blast from within!

They feared everything!

Where were the divers? Why weren't they being used? If we didn't have any, we could have asked other countries. Only sad questions. And the only responses were the inscrutable, cold portraits on television of admirals and politicians, offended by the information hysteria.

08.19.2000 17:30 We were next to the ship. We went down lower. The module had attached. The hatch was open. There, below, were people who were still alive. They were lying in the 8th and 9th compartments. It looked as though there were four rescuers. They descended into the ship. Two were standing by the doors. They could not open them. Beyond the hatch was an unsubmerged compartment. People were alive there, albeit in a very bad state. Their blood pressure was too high. The rescuers had been there for a long time, but they were not able to open the door. They had some sort of tool with a pipe.

The inner vision screen gave an analysis:

The danger involved in opening the hatch was really quite great. If the powerful pressure were to shoot out (that very same loud blast that they feared), then the rescue module would be torn off its landing place and water would rush into the ship. Then the rescuers would perish.

The British had a submarine. They were sailing from afar with 100 percent certainty. For some reason they had both divers and equipment.

How much time they lost. Now they would try to convince everyone that nothing could have been done.

08.20.2000 08:20 Our module was trying to approach the stern. The weather was good. They had already entered the submarine. They did not open the hatch into the compartment. The greatest efforts were directed at inspection. There was no life in the nose. The consciousnesses of 10 to 12 people were fading in the stern.

Our people did not want to do anything more than evaluate the situation, observe, and intercept espionage activities. They had taken up the position of observers.

The British rescuers made it unequivocally clear to our leaders working on the situation that the latter had deliberately sunk the submarine and its crew. The picture of the investigation was also changing. The British and Norwegians were giving a complete picture of the events. They asked, "Are you planning on waiting a month to dive down there?" They said that they were coming face to face with Russian irresponsibility. "You have many people, and you do not value them," they reproached.

Now the divers were working below. They were moving to the left and to the right. They were inspecting the casing. Within a half hour to an hour a picture of the accident would be ready.

An analysis of the situation of those who were conditionally alive. They had no desire to live. Unbearable pressure. Suffocation.

17:15 The divers descended four at a time. The front end was submerged. The middle section as well, but the rear section was not entirely. Water was trickling in and filling up the submarine very slowly. A fight for life was taking place on the submarine – they were doing everything possible.

19:40 Nothing was happening. There was water in the taper pipe, but no bodies. Our people had already been there.

The impact that the six-ton rescue vehicle had made upon docking increased the flow through the plugs and gags (??) that the sailors had put in during the first hours after the accident. With every hour, more and more water was pouring into the ship. Where it had not been before, it was now.

Prognosis phase.

The chance of saving people was none. The situation was worsening with every minute. Water was pouring in faster than before.

The people's blood was hardly moving. It was as if it was congealing. But it was still warm. There was a chance to save them, but again there was the time factor. Everything was done so that the rescuers would not have enough of it. The blood vessels in many of the peoples' heads burst. Everything looked like hot cereal. That was the price of the seven hours it took to lower the rescuers to the Kursk.

There were no complaints about the Norwegians. They were beyond professional. They repaired the damage. The module was able to dock. The danger was the excessive pressure inside. But the Norwegians were ready and their equipment ran smoothly.

* * *

We saw these events when we docked with a specific information thread leaving the Earth's information field. This thread stretched from the sailors and officers who were perishing on the Kursk. They were still tied to their physical bodies, even though from the materialistic point of view there were dead. This fact is of extreme importance. It meant that we were seeing through their consciousness. They themselves were not yet aware that they were dead. Therefore, following them we were able to get a slightly distorted impression of events. They thought that they were alive. And consequently we perceived them as alive. But in reality, this did not

491

correspond with what was happening. I know that my words will seem improbable, but am I the only one who thinks that what I have just written about is possible? We will not turn to foreign authorities on the subject, like Dr. Raymond Moody, who described life after death. It happens frequently that we completely ignore our own, more powerful prophets only because they live next to us, right close by.

I turn again to Grigori Grabovoi's book. After all, this is a person who does not just speak, but can actually do what he is talking about.

In a state of high consciousness, a person may be capable of performing actions that his everyday, wakeful consciousness would consider improbable, impossible, and fantastical. Like, for example, communicating with the dead. One can learn how to see the dead and communicate with them. And one can help them return here. Because the problem is that only some of them are able to return to our world under their own efforts.
It should also be noted that those whom we call deceased have departed only from the point of view of everyday, wakeful consciousness.

Therefore, however strange it may be for the relatives and close friends of the sailors on the Kursk to hear this, I want to say the following: Those whom you believed to be deceased have not died. They have actually moved into another world. And this world is no less real than ours.

There's one more lesson to be learned from the Kursk catastrophe. It has been learned by many, including military officials, politicians, and scholars. Not by everyone, naturally. We are rapidly moving away from the time of the USSR, when the concepts of "think first of your Motherland, and then of yourself" and "today the most important things are not your personal matters, but the results of the workday" reigned. Of course, we have to think about our Motherland, but not in the sense of service to the state, meaning the Empire of Caesar, but in the sense of showing concern about the people, about each human soul. We must restore the kingdom of the soul in every human being.

What a dramatic difference between the fates of the Komsomol*, which sank over 10 years ago, and the Kursk! Now the loss of a nuclear-powered ship rouses all of society. And in the case of the Kursk, society forced the government to assume a more human face and to identify the casualties out loud and by name. To show concern for relatives and, for once, to accept foreign aid. It would appear that this trend towards spirituality is taking place not only in Russia, since memorial services for the Kursk crew were held in other countries as well.

The era of the reign of violence on the planet is coming to a close. In the coming years, humankind will rapidly become more and more spiritual.

* * *

The 13th Moscow International Book Fair gathered hundreds of participants, including almost 70 foreign publishing houses. We prepared a huge sign announcing that this was the 70th anniversary of "Khudlit" and hung it on the side wall of the exhibition booth. As in previous years, our office was not that large, only 19 meters. But this was three meters more than the previous year. At the fair in 1996, our booth was only 6 meters. These additional meters, which had come to us with great difficulty,

*A Soviet submarine that sank in the Norwegian Sea in 1967.

493

were only ours and well-deserved. No one had extended a hand to our government enterprise, even though functionaries had spoken about our belonging to a united government team. The State Publishing Committee, having once written into my contract a paragraph about required government assistance for the publishing house, was not in a condition to meet its obligations. The new leaders of the Ministry on Publishing, although not lacking funds, removed "Khudlit" with demonstrative consistency from its list of projects already approved by the Federal Book Publishing Commission for financial support.

So our additional meters for the exhibition booth were proof of our slow but steady return to the Olympus of publishing. There cannot be an Olympus without a Pegasus! Otherwise, what kind of Olympus would it be?

And there were more books in our booth. We were very proud of many of them, for example the Golden Collection series. This truly represented the pinnacle of the printing art: the bindings were made from genuine leather, the main text was on Verge paper, and the exclusive design was produced by the best artists. The books were recognized by the Federal Book Publishing Commission as the best books of the year. This project carried us through a very hard time after the government default in August 1998.

But our sign attracted not only well-wishers, of which "Khudlit" has traditionally had many. There were also those who were for some reason very irritated by the publishing house's tenacious unwillingness to die and not be resurrected. The first premonition of the impending storm was Irina Yakovlevna Kainarskaya's refusal to discuss the topic that she had initiated about the impending consolidation of the publishing house.

– Forget everything I said, – she told me. – There's been a change in the wind. Maybe you will be merged with "Sovremennik" and possibly

494

moved to a different building. I take back everything I said. It's all up to Grigoryev. Go see him.

The second signal of trouble came right on the heels of the first. The newspaper "Kultura" [meaning "Culture"] (No. 38) published an article by its correspondent Grandovaya entitled "The 13th International Book Fair." This review devoted special space to our publishing house. And I would even say that it displayed a particular bias. This perpetually cheerful lady suddenly felt dejected:

"But I became unspeakably sad standing near the booth of "Khudlit"," which is celebrating its 70th anniversary this year and was once the mother of all Soviet publishing houses.

"According to one of the editors who has worked here for many years, publishing reforms hold nothing good for "Khudlit" because the same director will stay in place!

"That very same old Arkady Petrov, who contrived to 'invest' the modest government funds allocated to the publishing house in issuing keepsake books in leather bindings. These folios, which were thankfully not handwritten, have still not been sold. Meanwhile, the publishing house does not have enough funds to finish releasing literature, mainly classics, that was started as far back as the years of stagnation. Nobody even thinks about contemporary literature when the author does not want to publish at his own expense.

"The deputy minister of publishing in charge of publishing reforms probably knows all about this. Vladimir Viktorovich probably knows how to make "Khudlit" become our pride once again. Who would know, if not Vladimir Viktorovich, the renowned publisher and one of the founders of the famed publishing house "Vagrius"? Now there's someone whose business is steadily growing every year!

495

"In her opening comments to the 13th Moscow International Book Fair, Valentina Ivanovna Matvienko, who found herself next to the "cute donkey" at the stand of "Vagrius", broke into a smile when she noted that in its eight-year history, "Vagrius" has succeeded not only in forming its own circle of authors, but also in creating its own aesthetics marked by refinement of form and thought."

The reproach about the modest government funds that I contrived to "invest" in issuing keepsake books in leather bindings was particularly remarkable. If they had only given one kopeck towards these books! And it is unlikely that there is any basis to the idea that Vladimir Viktorovich Grigoryev knows what to do. At any rate, in a year and a half he has not gotten around to sharing his experience with the director of "Khudlit"." What's more, he has never even met with him once or expressed the desire to do so.

This representative of the second oldest profession lied, clumsily hiding behind the back of an anonymous editor who "has been working at "Khudlit" for many years." And how enthusiastic she was in the compliments she paid to the head of "Vagrius"," who also happens to be the deputy minister of publishing! A smart one, that, able to keep her ears pricked up no worse than the little donkey on the "Vagrius" logo. It is entirely possible that for her words she will soon be given a permanent position with those who service his stable.

Of course, I could protest that it has been a long time since Grandovaya's own *"Kultura"* looked as respectable as it once did. In any case, it is clearly behind *SPID-Info* and *"Moskovsky Komsomolets"** in

* Spid-info is a monthly about celebrities and their lives; "Moskovsky Komsomolet"s
is a daily paper covering general news with a sensationalist slant.

terms of both quality and circulation. But we would do better to limit ourselves to the conclusion that the very same "editor who had worked at "Khudlit" for many years" came to. He said: "I never thought that a journalist from *"Kultura"* would go as far as to use her own newspaper to publicly wipe a donkey's ass. Even if this anti-cultural act was not the only fee that she received for this, I am still very sorry for her."

Me too, Ms. Grandovaya. But after all, every person decides for himself where and with what to wipe. Like every other person on the Earth, you have the right to choose. It is unlikely that you would advise someone to impinge upon your choice. You made it, and the consequences are on you.

* * *

Kirill arrived. The "spy" had returned from Theodosiya. He had a cake in one hand and a bag containing expensive cognac in the other. He was radiant. He said that Lapshin had asked him to say hello. In these exact words: "You will all be washed away by water, but I will live a thousand years."

Kirill pronounced these words and smiled. Then, just in case, so that we didn't misunderstand, he added:

– But you know in connection with which events.

We sat down at the table.

– Tell us.

– I had very little contact with him there. We met twice. I spent most of my time sitting on Mount Mitridat and thinking. There's absolutely no future with Lapshin. He built up all the circles there with children – there was no channel. I have made a firm decision to work with you.

– Why are you so confident that the Center will take you? – I asked.

497

Kirill's face paled. His smile slipped from his face, which again became taut around his cheekbones.

– But we already agreed that when I returned… You promised me that you would think about it and decide.

– That's exactly what we've done. When we extended a hand to you, what did you put in it? Migen's seal. See how badly that looks?

– You're making a mistake, – Kirill said with great effort. Then, thinking a little, he added, – A fatal one.

– Where's the mistake? – Now Igor was starting to show an interest.

– You need me.

– Why?

– You know why.

I– f we knew, we wouldn't be asking…

– I'm like a cloud. – Kirill started to play the fool in his customary way. – I cannot be taken, probed, and locked up somewhere, but I am needed by everyone.

– Why are you needed? – Igor was pointlessly trying to break his habit of beating around the bush.

– You still think I've come from them, – said Kirill, pointing his hand downwards.

– Where are you from then, such a good person with the seal of the Ruler of Darkness?

– From the Holy Spirit.

This bold statement really made us lose our tempers.

– Well! – exclaimed Igor and I in unison, as if we were in the theater, turning to face one another.

– We saw the Holy Spirit this morning and He did not tell us anything good about you, – I dropped carelessly.

498

– It's true. The Holy Spirit said nothing about His new son Kirill, – confirmed Igor in a serious manner.

– You are making a fatal mistake, – said Kirill, again trying to scare us. – First of all, you do not know the way. Second of all, I can destroy the Earth.

Yes, the new school was educating interesting children. He was standing resolutely, trying to scare us with threats of destroying the Earth. We did not play games like that in our childhood years. The times were certainly changing. But there were probably boys like this, we just kept a different company.

– Do you have the red button with you? – I inquired.

Kirill seemed ill at ease for some reason. He drawled out uncertainly:

– No.

There was a battle being waged within him. He did not know how to make up his mind.

– It has become unbearable on Earth because of you, – he complained. And then, out of nowhere, – I love you all. I will work, I will serve you.

I got up from the table.

– That's it Kirill. We extended our hand to you, and what did you place in it? If you move out any further on your ledge, you will fall...

I left the room. In time. Dear Olga Ivanovna Koyokina had arrived. She had already been waiting for half an hour. Out of consideration, she had not wanted to interrupt our private conversation with the demon.

I took her by the hand and led her to a different room. We spoke about the future program of cooperation with the Scientific Research Institute on Traditional Healing Methods.

Kirill stuck his head in through the door twice while we were speaking. Apparently, he had worn down his tongue on Igor's rock-like rigidity and was coming to complain. There it was, the fatal reputation of a good person! It was time to change his image.

Koyokina could not withstand such an insolent hint that it was someone else's turn.

– People are probably waiting for you, – she said delicately, giving up her right to conversation.

– They can wait, – I reassured her.

And we went over the research program again, point by point.

We finally finished. I said goodbye and went out into the hallway. Our secretary Svetlana Ivanovna had prepared tea for me. Everyone else had already had theirs while we were talking. I was the last. I went to the Center director's office. On the table stood a teapot and a little bowl with cookies.

Kirill followed right behind me as if nothing had ever happened. He took his cup out of the cupboard. It was a unique cup, with a special inscription. He sat down across from me, not looking at all uncomfortable. He poured himself some tea and got right to the point:

– You know that there will be a trial after you die and that you will be questioned about my sufferings? And I am suffering greatly right now.– The expression on his face matched the tone of the monologue he had pronounced.

– What do we have to do with this? – I asked about the upcoming judicial proceedings.

– I broke off my ties with them there, – Kirill said, again pointing emphatically downwards. – And you won't take me here.

– Why? – I tried to determine yet again through the crumbs of the cookie I was nibbling.

The boy stabbed his gaze into me meaningfully, not in the way of a child. He was turning his goblet with his fingers. On the rim of the goblet was the significant inscription: "The Lord. The Master."

– Do you know what the name Kirill means? – he asked suddenly.

– What?

He jabbed his finger at the inscription on the goblet.

– You don't say! – I exclaimed, marveling at his subtle way of stating his claims.

– And what does the name Arkady mean? – I inquired in turn.

– Arch, arcade, – explained Kirill, displaying his esoteric literacy.

– Correct! – I confirmed. – You had an arch across seven spaces. You did not spot it. See, look.

I took a piece of paper and started drawing.

– We were introduced to Lapshin in the fall of 1996, right?

– Yes, – confirmed Kirill.

– A strange number. Two nines and one six. The code of my fate also contained two nines and two sixes. The date of my birth is 08.26.1946 [in Russian this date would be written 26.08.1946 – Transl. note], again two sixes and two nines. Let's take, as prescribed, every second number: 6.8.9.6. You yourself know that an eight is the significant sign of infinity and immortality, if, or course, it is slightly slanted. You already had two sixes – one from Lapshin and another from one very serious comrade. You needed a third.

– I told him, – roared Kirill. – He wanted to outwit everyone. Both Migen and the Lord! He wanted to become an independent Archon!

– Here, of course, you are right, – I said, sympathizing with Kirill. – And then there was that money that he took from me for a film about himself and never returned. Igor and I checked specially – the money was exactly equivalent to thirty pieces of silver at the current rate. Don't you see what an ingenious plot it was? Two thousand years ago during the secret Lord's Supper, Satan entered Judah as the latter was taking a drink of the wine in his goblet and made a substitution. He forced this physical body to the Sanhedrin to betray Jesus for 30 silver pieces. Right?

– Right, – confirmed Kirill unwillingly.

– Since the Creator gave you the first move under the terms of your previous victory in Armageddon, you also received the sacrificial lamb and the missing sixes. Note, two in the code of one person. Lapshin made a mistake in counting the second and third. He did not know that two sixes were in one person. This could not have even occurred to him. That is why he took stock of me and did not believe that this was the link that he was missing.

– The darned goat, – roared Kirill, but this oath was clearly not meant for me.

– Yes, exactly, – I agreed. – Remember what it says in the Bible: "Dark forces serve the Saints, since they have been blinded by the Holy Spirit."

– Then what? – demanded Kirill, clearly curious about the intrigue.

– I even have these numbers in my office. They should be completely clear to you: 2+2+2=6. The dragon in the protective quadrant could also grow up to six heads. This was not a plain old dragon, but one in crowns. So, what is still unclear to you here?

Kirill was silent, thinking things through.

– Why are there two sixes in one person? – he asked suddenly.

– I'm sorry, but I can't say anything about that yet, – I apologized. Your guys there are clever and quick on the draw. I'll tell you what I can now and save the rest for sometime later.

Kirill did not argue. And what would be the point? He already knew my nature.

– So, to return to the silver pieces. Lapshin took them and did not return them. On the one hand, they were like a ransom. I used this money to pay my ransom. For that six, which had already been counted towards you. On the other hand, these coins were payment to him for treason.

– Whom did he betray? – This boy was businesslike and focused. It was clear from everything that he would not forget anything or forgive anyone.

– Migen! – I exclaimed, shocking him with my answer. – Pardon the expression, but he pissed away your entire Communist Party. Now my two sixes have been upended and turned into nines. And the Arch-arcade has passed you by. Others now walk along it, do you understand?

– Yes, – confirmed Kirill gloomily.

– Now you must address me not by my name, but by my surname. What is my surname?

– Petrov, – pronounced the demon.

– And the meaning?

– From Peter. Stone.

– Yes, – I confirmed. – The stumbling stone, if the first opportunity of the archway is not taken. So, sorry. You've come up against a rock, master.

Kirill paled. He wanted to cry.

– Do you want me to get down on my knees?

He was prepared to collapse onto the floor, but Igor saved him from this embarrassing act by entering the room.

– Are you having some tea? – he asked, taking a seat.

– No, we're playing at democracy. Kirill is proposing to get in line with all the others and follow them.

– That's it, that's it, that's it! I'm sick of this, – protested Igor. – I am going to the restroom and not coming back. This is what your play has

503

come to.

But a minute later, changing his mind, he turned to Kirill:

– Let's do the following, if you can't wait to get in line. Let's look at the options.

– Let's, – said Kirill, pleased at least at the chance of some sort of dialogue.

– So, – said Igor. – I am a shepherd and you are a lamb. I am about to approach the edge of an abyss and jump…

– Go ahead, – agreed Kirill.

– Who will be responsible?

Kirill shrugged his shoulders, as if to say, figure it out for yourself.

– Fine, – agreed Igor. – Now you are the shepherd and I am the lamb. I'm about to get lost. Who is responsible?

– What does this have to do with me? – Kirill was again trying to avoid responsibility.

– You see, you never think anything has to do with you, you are always innocent. You don't want to be a sheep or a shepherd. There's one more option. You can be a black sheep. Your soul is fainthearted and hideously spoiled.

– I cannot return. – Kirill was again whining about his own problems. – I am the very, very last in the line. I can never be resurrected again without a son.

– He's going on about the very, very last again. Perhaps I lack experience in otherworldly intrigues, like one of Suvorov's soldiers in the emperor's court. Here's how I see it: if you really are a young man with an all-Russian passport, then it is a little early for you to be thinking about offspring. If you are a five-and-a-half-million year old demon, why didn't you get yourself some direct descendents, faithful students, or anyone else who could have given you historical immortality? Why don't you just live like a person, like everyone lives, proposed Igor.

The demon was silent. His eyes showed despair. The very, very last in a line. That meant that there would be no one else.

– I'm going back to Lapshin. We will come to Moscow and crush you, he said, suddenly switching to open threats. We have learned how to work with global entities of the elements.

– I'm not scared, – I responded.

– Me neither, – acknowledged Igor.

– We do not betray our friends. Nor do we fear our enemies, – I explained to the horned boy who was five-and-a-half-million years old. – And certainly not because someone is bidding us to be devoted and brave. This is just our internal nature. It cannot be altered. Is that clear?

– I have perished! – he screamed.

– Oh would you cut it out! Study, work, live like everyone else. But if you are afraid of living, go hide in a dark corner and cover yourself with a rag. Wait for the time of changes.

I left. I couldn't look at him anymore. It was repugnant.

* * *

Here is why I am thankful to Kirill, that Demon – Tempter: He gave me departure or "reference" points for understanding (relatively, of course) all the events that were happening with me. Humankind on Earth is a foundling hospital, a nursery school for raising 144,000 new Creators of new Universes...

As it is written in the Bible, the wind blows wherever it pleases. The expression Zeitgeist emerged several hundred years ago. It is an entirely mystical category of existence that does not lend itself to rational explanation. "Such was the Zeitgeist: the most mysterious and most elusive, yet still real, force in history," lamented Fyodor Stepun, one of the luminaries of Russian society abroad, in his memoirs "What Was and What Might Have Been."

As a witness, Stepun is observant and tolerant, in other words, he was never judgmental and always tried to hold himself above the situation. "According to my observations, in the late 19th and especially early 20th centuries every single Russian family, including even the imperial family, had its own relative who was more or less radical, its own household revolutionary. In conservative noble families, these revolutionaries were usually ordinary liberals, in families from the liberal intelligentsia, they were socialists, and in working families after 1905*, they were sometimes Bolsheviks. We cannot say that all these secret revolutionaries were people of ideas and sacrifice. A very large percentage of them was composed of talented underdogs, ambitious idlers, self-deceiving babblers, and visionary womanizers (at that time, a left-leaning phrase had a great effect on Russian women) carried to the left by radical winds."

The history of Russia over the last three centuries is especially rich in mysticism. "Especially" because this fact is present in a whole array of documents. At the same time, it had been described in detail and explained by sensible historians. But there are too many riddles for a sane, ordinary mind. Why, in the Warsaw fashion, did the gallant editor, poet, and translator Ivan Kalyayev become a bomber and a murderer? And what about the elegant, well-bred, and highly educated Dmitry Pisarev is only known to his descendents as a nihilist, a rejectionist of moral and aesthetic principles ("Boots are more elevated than Shakespeare"), who advised

* Russia experienced widespread unrest in 1905, resulting in the creation of a constitutional monarchy.

people to behave "as they wished, in a manner profitable and convenient to them"? Why did the family of the happy Simbirsk official Ulyanov raise both the regicide Aleksander and the cannibal Vladimir*? And the female revolutionaries: Sofiya Perovskaya, Vera Figner, Mariya Spiridonova – who drove these happy baronesses into the world of Dostoyevsky?

Absolutely everyone is a victim of Zeitgeist. There was a reason why Evgeny Trubetskoy called the Russian revolution national and of a kind that "hitherto has not taken place in the world. Everyone participated in this revolution, everyone made it... all social forces in the country in general." Another great Russian philosopher, Georgy Fedotov, wrote about this in his article "Revolution is Coming," where he listed and explained the guilt of each class of Russian society in the catastrophe.

This Zeitgeist is constantly and continually blowing. In one direction or the other. Has it been long since we sang along with the song of the genius Pakhmutova** "Our homeland is revolution..."? Scholars have not been able to come up with a rational explanation of this historical influence. Gustav Shpet, the Russian philosopher whose life ended in Stalin's Gulag, tried to arrive at an understanding of the concept of "spirit." One of his colleagues called him the "Dorian Grey of Russian philosophy." But even a mystical sobriquet like this did not help Shpet understand the essence of this phenomenon. In "Introduction to Ethnic Psychology," Shpet analyzes six descriptions of the concept of "spirit." Unfortunately, his theoretical studies do not add anything special to common thinking on the subject.

Modern science has been trying to destroy the mystical halo surrounding Zeitgeist. It is familiar with the "hundredth monkey effect."

* Lenin's original surname was Ulyanov and Aleksander was his older brother.
** Aleksandra Nikolayevna Pakhmutova (b. 1929) is a renowned Soviet/Russian composer.

507

Here is what happened: at a preserve on a small Japanese island, a young female monkey came up with the idea of washing potatoes before eating them. Shortly thereafter, her comrades in the preserve started following her example – first two or three, and then more and more. When the number of fastidious monkeys approached one hundred, observers noticed that at another preserve on a neighboring island, monkeys had started washing potatoes and en masse besides. Let's say that on the first island mimicry was involved, but none of the monkeys traveled to the neighboring island to share their best practices!

The wind blows wherever it pleases. Ideas are carried on air.

But under which laws and along which air (historical) currents are they carried?

I came away from all these reflections with the conviction that everything has its time. We cannot give monkeys the nuclear launch button, but it is high time that they learned how to eat clean potatoes. The entire history of mankind is a school. It is education in the laws of creation. Not only physical and material laws, but also moral and spiritual ones. However, there are many very talented but slovenly and headstrong students behind the desk of this school. Meanwhile, the exam is taken not only by the people, but the nation (The Bible clearly states about Israel that the Old Testament is the story of how God tried to inject wisdom into the unwise people that he loved). Every person takes this exam, every individual on his own. Believers have known about this for a long time – will a person be "saved" or not. But the situation is much more serious.

Our Orthodox tradition offers believers a dilemma: a righteous life or a sinful life. In the end, heaven or hell. The problem is actually more complicated. The old arrangement worked for our not terribly literate babushkas. As a generation, we are at a different level of knowledge. And the demand from us is different, all the more so since the possibilities before us are qualitatively different than they used to be...

It is another matter that the ideals remain the same. The spirit blows where it chooses and with whom it chooses, but it carries with it the eternal principles of Good and Evil. And the question standing before a person is: Which will you choose?

Meanwhile, we receive hints and warnings from the first years of life. Take at least those very same folk tales and fairy tales. Vladimir Odoyevsky (nicknamed the Russian Faust) has a well-known children's tale called "Johnny Frost," which is about how two sisters – Rukodelnitsa [literally, "needlewoman" – Transl. note] and Lenivitsa [literally, "idler" – Transl. note] – who descend into the Kingdom of Frost and find out what they have earned for their labors. The tale is naïve and didactic, but that is just the point. The most common and the most hackneyed truths are also the most timeless and enduring truths. And they are the ones that are placed in our heads during childhood. What will you choose? What can you give a person close to you? Or do you think you can only take?

On this depends whether you are an individual in God's image or not. An individuality is a creator who is trying to create something for people or give them something. How successful you are at this is a matter of time and the speed at which you master the rungs of Jacob's ladder. Individuals build their own Jacob's ladder and ascend it towards their ideal (or Ideal – words, words, words...). A being that does not create this ladder is not an individuality, because an individuality is a creator. Our demon, that teenager Kirill, is not an individual. My tongue has trouble even pronouncing him a person. So let's call him a restless little imp.

* * *

509

More and more people were coming to the Center. This was surprising because we had not advertised anywhere. The few articles that journalists had written about us were never published: editors found it impossible to believe that something like this could be possible. Even the article by the Academician Ivliyev "Aesculapians from the Nooshpere" was rejected by several publications at once. I was not surprised by this reaction. Three years ago, I myself would not have believed that people who did not have even an elementary medical education could be cured from serious afflictions.

But you cannot ignore the ones who have been cured.

Dasha Gorokhova, deaf since childhood, now attends lectures at the institute. Nastya Kvakova – who was nearly blind from a brain tumor and who had stomach and duodenal ulcers – now dreams of getting married and working at our Center. She has already typed up my articles on the computer. Who could now remember that no so long ago she could not see and did not want to live? The doctors remain silent or say: Anything can happen!

Things do happen, of course, from time to time. But for some reason, not with them. But if all this happens almost every day in one place, then how can that be explained?

Here is a recent case. A woman received excess radiation at work. Her organs had been to all intents and purposes destroyed. She had cancer and her kidneys had stopped functioning. To avoid this unbearable pain, her consciousness had turned off her nervous system. She had not months or weeks to live, but days.

This woman's husband came to us because not one facility under the Ministry of Health wanted to even try to do something in this hopeless situation. He came as if guided by the hand of Providence. My good friend

510

Dmitry Gavrilovich Sokolov, Academician of the Medical Technology Academy, happened to stop by at the same time. He is an assistant to the renowned Mikhail Ivanovich Fomin, the author of "Integrated Medicine."

Listening to our client's story about what happened to his wife, Sokolov suddenly took a colored diagram out of his briefcase and started telling us about it.

– These here are aggressive radicals, – he started to explain. – These are the ones that drive cells and molecules of the organism first to disease and then to degeneration.

– Is there any way to neutralize them? I asked.

– Yes, a saturation of electrons must be created in the body. Electrons are extremely fast particles and the electron wind that they form can wipe out accumulated aggressive radicals very quickly. Medicine usually uses antioxidant preparations in such cases, but they enter the blood through the digestive system when the main negative events are taking place in tissue cells. So if you can create an electron wind in this woman's body, you really will have a chance of saving her.

Dmitry Gavrilovich was already familiar with some of the miraculous healings that we had accomplished, so he was entirely serious when he offered us his diagram.

We turned on our inner visions screens. We entered the dying woman's biofield through the photograph of her that her husband had brought, and we started scanning her organism.

The aggressive radicals – radioactive particles – were very clearly visible. It was like her entire body was engulfed in flames. Solid red: her body was burning, burning in the direct sense of the word – radiation was setting it on fire. We brought the electron particles up on the screen: it looked exactly like Sokolov's diagram. We launched the process of electron wind in real time. And a miracle: like benign protectors, the electrons attacked the billions of radioactive enemies burning the body and started destroying them, establishing new internal connections, neutralizing and cleaning them like a vacuum cleaner made of cells.

Two weeks later, this woman's husband told us that she was feeling so much better that she was able to read books and was longing to get up from her bed. We forbade this. She needed to preserve her strength because the repair of her tissues and organs destroyed by radiation still lay ahead. In this battle, each grain of strength was worth its weight in gold. But she still got up a week later. Her happy husband brought us tons of cakes, setting them one on top of the other to make a tower.

In addition to our work here, however, we also had work to do there. When we were in Theodosiya, Lapshin told me that Mamay once hid in the Crimea one of the most important sacral attributes – the Golden Steed. Prince Vyacheslav had a statue of the Earth Mother and he was promised the staff of power. The third symbol he needed to be able to acquire absolute power on Earth was that very same Golden Steed. Why were they all so drawn to gold? Would a real horse have been worse? The Golden Steed once belonged to St. George the Dragon Slayer, but then became the possession of the Golden Horde. St. George had a strange relationship and complex scores to settle with the Volga khans. So Igor and I started looking for the steed to help us get a jump on Lapshin. And, strange as it may seem, we found it, just not where we thought it would be. The steed was hidden in one of the caves not far from the Crimean town of Sudak.

In order to move the horse through the interspace tunnel, we had to first dematerialize it in the information structure. We moved it to the levels where the mighty time-worn warrior, known to different peoples by different names, had sat motionless on the steps of the staircase for several

512

centuries already. We stood the steed next to him and, using the techniques that we had recently been trained in, we gave the steed the impulse it needed to assume its regular form.

The Golden Steed started to grow quickly before our eyes. St. George watched this miracle with amazement. The steed had on a harness, a saddle, a saddle blanket with small bells, and a red saddle. St. George stood with difficulty, approached his friend whom he had not seen for hundreds of years, took him by the rein with one hand, ran his hand over his mane with the other, and suddenly nestled his gray head into the steed's neck. A teardrop ran down the wrinkled cheek of the old soldier. And the steed, as if understanding his feelings, also tried to press his body to his master.

Not wanting to interrupt their meeting, we quietly vanished from St. George the Dragon Slayer's staircase.

Then in the same manner we collected from Lapshin's statue – the same woman for whom he had organized shamanistic ceremonies – its informational essence and raised it to the upper platform. There there was a mountain where a platform had been built for this statue, once stolen by evil spirits. We returned her to her rightful place. The sun was shining behind her back, piercing her through and through, and from the forehead of the Earth Mother figure, where she wore a headband with a stone, a ray shot out and fell below, onto our planet. Now the object that remained with Lapshin had no informational essence, and he was not able manipulate it to serve his interests.

There was one more object – the staff of power. Lapshin had only been promised it. But where was the one who made the promise?

We found it several days later under the throne of the Ruler of Darkness and collected it along with the banner of St. Andrew the "First-Called" Apostle, which was also lying around nearby, along with a very ancient book covered with a thick layer of dust. The letters of the title did not shine clearly through the dust, but we did not try to read them. We were not the owners of this book, and it was not up to us to flip through its pages. No one dared to interfere with us. We dragged the enormous staff through the levels to the upper platform with difficulty. A place had already been prepared for it to the left of the Earth Mother. And it started working right away. We anchored the banner next to the staff and it unfurled, revealing the inscription "For Faith in Christ." We also placed the book right there – a spot had been prepared for it.

This was not a physical level, but a spiritual level. But what would take place in the world would happen here first. If today St. Andrew's banner started fluttering proudly on the spiritual level that meant that good fortune would soon come to the state with this flag.

Everything was now in its place and the rays joined: the flag, the staff, and Earth Mother. A bit lower on the steps sat St. George the Dragon Slayer – who bore a strong resemblance to Ilya Muromets* of the epic poems – looking at his steed. The steed was also looking at him. They were pleased with one another.

* * *

Thus ends the first part of my story. In the future, if I am permitted, I will tell more. It is up to the reader to decide if this book is a revelation or if it is an amusing fairy tale.

In the famous play of the Calderon, the shy prince, upon learning that "life is a dream," becomes a courageous soldier and a wise ruler. I hope that my readers, upon learning about the relativity of life in this world, will

* Literally Elijah of Murom, a legendary powerful warrior who was also thought to be a real person.

start to look at is as a stage in eternal life, as an exam that requires wisdom, courage, and greatness of spirit to pass. But these are not buzzwords.

Humankind en masse still believes that is was created for happiness, like a bird was created for flying. It is much more captivated by civilization than it is by culture. Many commonly believe that civilization and culture are to all intents and purposes one and the same. For example, that television is an achievement of civilization and a tool of culture.

Meanwhile, the difference between the two is fundamental. Civilization was built on the supremacy of scientific and technical elements, while culture was built on philosophical and aesthetic elements. Culture is human-based and civilization is machine-based. Culture is idealistic, while civilization is utilitarian. Culture has a unique and national character, while civilization is cosmopolitan and anonymous. Culture is grounded in beliefs and traditions: it tends towards conservatism. Civilization is ageless and impatient for something new, something technically or economically perfect. Culture represents the work of individuals, whereas civilization represents mankind's collective efforts. The ideal of culture is the assimilation of the most diverse aspects of the human soul. The ideal of civilization is total power. The dominant factor in culture is duty. Finally, the dominant factor of civilization is the satisfaction of needs.

Why have I been so tiresome about explaining this difference, which the best of humankind have understood and felt so well? Because the dialectic of the relationship between culture and civilization – the barometer of society's spirituality – is far from simple. Lack of spirituality is fatal for the human race. It leads it away from the lofty tasks and goals of divine order to the lower levels of objective reality.

Enough has been said about the meaning of collective consciousness, its establishment, and changes to it. But is the collective spirituality of a

515

specific nation, people, or all humankind possible? I don't know. It would appear, however, that individual spirituality is a sin, the recognition of a sin, and the aspiration to atone for this sin. Each person must build his own Jacob's ladder and must climb up it. And each will be rewarded according to his just deserts.

So, dear reader, do not get carried away and start thinking that a new era is beginning and that all you will have to do is reap its blessings. The era is indeed new, but the demand from you is the same. Only through the labor of your soul and through your contribution to the new collective consciousness will you gain access to it. I wish you success in this honorable endeavor.

Book started on 06.06.2000. Finished on 09.09.2000.

Contents

Arcady
Petrov

CREATION OF THE UNIVERSE

SAVE YOURSELF

Cover Design: A. Tomilin

For further information on the contents of this book contact:

SVET centre, Hamburg, Germany, www.svet-centre.eu

Jelezky publishing, Hamburg 2011

CPSIA information can be obtained at www.ICGtesting.com
Printed in the USA
LVOW010513021212

309686LV00003B/342/P